This volume is the first to look in detail at the important relationship, initially studied in 1871 by Bowditch, between the strength of the heart beat and the interval between beats. Although this topic has been somewhat neglected, it is now recognised that it provides a key to unlock the mysteries of excitation–contraction coupling and has important implications in advancing our understanding of the functioning of the heart. The book draws together the work and experience of leading international research workers in this field. Collectively, the contributors illuminate the underlying mechanisms involved, their expression in both isolated muscle and the intact heart, and speculate on further avenues of research which will help to reconcile some of the remaining controversies.

The volume will be of interest to cardiologists, physiologists and all those concerned with the function of the heart.

THE INTERVAL–FORCE RELATIONSHIP OF THE HEART: BOWDITCH REVISITED

THE INTERVAL–FORCE RELATIONSHIP OF THE HEART: BOWDITCH REVISITED

Edited by

MARK I. M. NOBLE
Weston Professor of Cardiovascular Medicine
Charing Cross and Westminister Medical School
University of London

and

W. A. SEED
Professor of Medicine
Charing Cross and Westminister Medical School
University of London

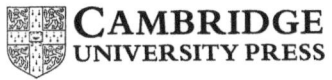 CAMBRIDGE
UNIVERSITY PRESS

CAMBRIDGE UNIVERSITY PRESS
Cambridge, New York, Melbourne, Madrid, Cape Town,
Singapore, São Paulo, Delhi, Tokyo, Mexico City

Cambridge University Press
The Edinburgh Building, Cambridge CB2 8RU, UK

Published in the United States of America by Cambridge University Press, New York

www.cambridge.org
Information on this title: www.cambridge.org/9780521116985

First published 1992
First paperback edition 2011

A catalogue record for this publication is available from the British Library

Library of Congress Cataloguing in Publication data
The Interval–Force relationship of the heart: Bowditch revisited /
edited by Mark I. M. Noble and W. A. Seed.
    p.   cm.
Includes index.
ISBN 0 521 40022 8 hardback
1. Heart–Contraction. 1. Noble, Mark I. M.   II. Seed, W.A.
[DNLM: 1. Blood Pressure. 2. Myocardial Contraction—physiology.
3. Systole. WG 280 I619]
QP113.I58 1992
612.1'71–dc20
DNLM/DLC
for Library of Congress 91–47867 CIP

ISBN 978-0-521-40022-0 Hardback
ISBN 978-0-521-11698-5 Paperback

Contents

**Part 4: The expression of interval–force phenomena in cardiac
   muscle**

Contributors

D. G. Allen
Department of Physiology F-13, University of Sydney, NSW 2006, Australia

P. Arlock
Department of Zoophysiology, University of Lund, 221 85 Lund, Sweden

M. Boyett
Department of Physiology, Worsley Medical and Dental Building, The University, Leeds LS2 9JT, UK

D. Burkhoff
Cardiology Division, The Johns Hopkins Hospital, Carnegie 568, 600 N Wolfe St, Baltimore, MD 21205, USA

I. C. Cooper
Department of Cardiology, St Thomas' Hospital, London SE1, UK

W. Deppert
Philosophisches Seminar der Christian-Albrechts-Universität, 2300 Kiel, Germany

J. E. Frampton
Department of Physiology, Worsley Medical and Dental Building, The University, Leeds LS2 9JT, UK

S. M. Harrison
Department of Physiology, Worsley Medical and Dental Building, The University, Leeds LS2 9JT, UK

S. M. Hardman
Department of Medicine, Charing Cross and Westminister Medical School, Fulham Palace Road, London W6 8RF, UK

W. C. Hunter
Departments of Medicine and Biomedical Engineering, The Johns Hopkins Medical Hospital, Baltimore, MD 21205, USA

M. Jóhannsson
Department of Pharmacology, University of Iceland, PO Box 8216, 128 Reykjavik, Iceland

T. Kenner
Physiologisches Institut der Karl-Franzens-Universität Graz, Harrachgasse 21, A 8010 Graz, Austria

M. S. Kirby
Department of Physiology, Worsley Medical and Dental Building, The University, Leeds LS2 9JT, UK

M. J. Lab
Department of Physiology, Charing Cross and Westminister Medical School, Fulham Palace Road, London W6 8RF, UK

G. A. Langer
Cardiovascular Research Laboratories, UCLA School of Medicine, 10833 Le Conte Avenue, Los Angeles, CA 90024-1760, USA

A. J. Levi
Department of Physiology, Worsley Medical and Dental Building, The University, Leeds LS2 9JT, UK

B. Lewartowski
Department of Clinical Physiology, Medical Centre of Postgraduate Education, Marymoncka 99, 01-813 Warsaw, Poland

R. K. Lie
Centre for Medical Ethics, University of Oslo, Norway

B. Lohff
Institut für beschichte der Medizin der Christian-Albrechts-Universität, 2300 Kiel, Germany

E. McCall
Department of Physiology, Worsley Medical and Dental Building, The University, Leeds LS2 9JT, UK

D. R. Milner
Department of Physiology, Worsley Medical and Dental Building, The University, Leeds LS2 9JT, UK

S. E. J. N. Mörner
Department of Pharmacology, University of Lund, 221 85 Lund, Sweden

M. I. M. Noble
Academic Unit of Cardiovascular Medicine, Charing Cross and Westminster Medical School, Horseferry Road, London SW1P 2AR, UK

C. H. Orchard
Department of Physiology, Worsley Medical and Dental Building, The University, Leeds LS2 9JT, UK

K. Pfeiffer
Physiologisches Institut der Karl-Franzens-Universität Graz, Harrachgasse 21, A8010 Graz, Austria

U. Ravens
Universitätsklinikum Essen, Pharmakologisches Institut, Hufelandstrasse 55, 4300 Essen, Germany

J. Schaefer
International Institute for Theoretical Cardiology, Am Orbtal 1, 6482 Bad Orb, Germany

W. A. Seed
Department of Medicine, Charing Cross and Westminster Medical School, Fulham Palace Road, London W6 8RF, UK

C. I. Spencer
Departments of Physiology and Medicine, Charing Cross and Westminster Medical School, Fulham Palace Road, London W6 8RF, UK

H. ter Keurs
Department of Medical Physiology, The University of Calgary, Health Sciences Centre, 3330 Hospital Drive NW, Calgary, Alberta T2N 4N1, Canada

B. Wohlfart
Department of Clinical Physiology, University of Lund, 221 85 Lund, Sweden

David Yue
Department of Biomedical Engineering, The Johns Hopkins University School of Medicine, 720 Rutland Avenue, Baltimore, MD 21205, USA

Introduction

The purpose of the present book is to bring together current ideas of the interval–force relationship, as propounded by some of the main contributors to current research on the subject, and to review the evolution of our knowledge of the subject since the publication of Bowditch's original paper in 1871.

Unlike the other important intrinsic controlling system of heart muscle – the length–tension relation – the force–interval relationship has been relatively neglected. Professor Jochen Schaefer (who first fired our own interest in the subject) and his collaborators consider the historic reasons for this neglect in the first chapter of the book, which includes their translation of Bowditch's paper. Their discussion is of considerable interest from a general point of view, since it illustrates how the fate of scientific contributions may depend on factors other than their intrinsic value. Later sections of the book address the basic cellular mechanisms which underlie interval–force processes, the ways in which these processes manifest themselves in the mechanical behaviour of cardiac muscle, and their relevance to the function of the intact heart. To our knowledge, systematic reviews of these topics have not been brought together before. Our other justification is the recent upsurge of interest in interval–force events.

A number of ambiguities in terminology need comment. The first concerns the main topic itself, which is variously referred to as the force–frequency, force–interval, interval–strength, or interval–force relationship. We have not attempted uniformity in this book, though we prefer the latter term because it identifies the independent and dependent variables appropriately (compare length–tension), and embraces events related to single as well as repetitive stimuli. Two other ambiguities which arise are related first to the use of the term 'force', and secondly to the precise meaning of the term 'staircase' or 'Treppe'.

Dimensions of 'force'

Force is measured in dimensions of mass times acceleration (e.g. 1 kg m s^{-2} = 1 newton). When force is expressed per unit of cross-sectional area of muscle (N m^2), it is termed a stress. The term *tension* is widely used, usually in a non-specific way to indicate either force or stress. Pressure is also force per unit area, but this time exerted within the cavity of the ventricle rather than across the cross-sections of the muscle. The rate of rise of force, stress or pressure obviously divides these variables by time. In our opinion, the inconsistency with which these terms are used in force–interval descriptions only affects the quantitative magnitude of the variable being used. When they are used comparatively as a function of interval or frequency, the same relationships will emerge. Again, therefore, we have not attempted to impose uniformity. The situation which differs fundamentally from these circumstances is that of cardiac ejection. The confusion that arises from including ejection variables has plagued the study of interval–force relationships in the intact heart. Thus in considering the effects of interval or frequency, we must exclude effects on variables such as stroke volume if we wish to confine ourselves to the intrinsic mechanisms within muscle that Bowditch described. In this book such exclusion has generally been followed, but since the clinical relevance of interval–force processes is a legitimate interest, their possible influence on ejection variables in the intact heart is discussed at the end of the book.

'Staircase' or 'Treppe'

There are three ways in which these terms are used, schematically represented in Fig. 1:

1. Following a prolonged period of rest, stimulation of the muscle causes a progressive increase of force to a plateau (Fig. 1(*a*)).
2. Following a period of low frequency stimulation, stimulation of the muscle at a higher frequency results (after an initial decrease in force) in a similar pattern of increase to that shown in 1(*a*) (Fig. 1(*b*)).
3. During steady-state stimulation, the final plateau of force may progressively rise with increasing steady-state frequency (Fig. 1(*c*)).

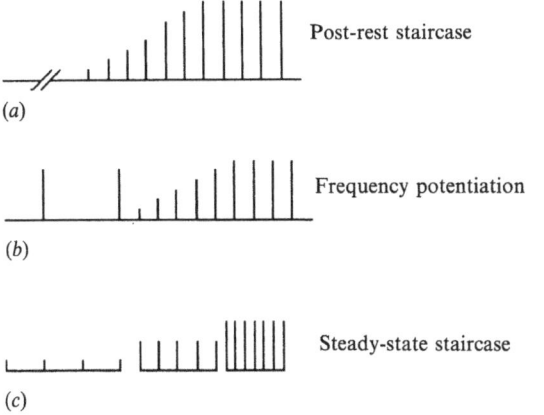

(a)

(b)

(c)

Fig. 1. Schematic representation of 'staircase' or 'Treppe'.

The first two examples involve the same underlying mechanism and, in our opinion, could simply be termed 'Treppe'. However, the reader should be prepared to meet other terminologies. Of particular note is that of Koch-Weser and Blinks (1963), who described a 'positive inotropic effect of activation (PIEA)'. The reason for coining this term was to separate it from the initial drop in force (Fig. 1(b)) which they termed the 'negative inotropic effect of activation (NIEA)'. The latter term has lost its *raison d'être* because this is now recognized to be incomplete mechanical restitution (see chapter by Jóhannsson). For this reason, PIEA has also dropped out of fashion, although it remains a reasonable term. One could argue that the term 'frequency potentiation' is the most appropriate. This mechanism is also responsible for the strong beat that follows a return to the low frequency. The third application of the term 'staircase' (Fig. 1(c)) has a different meaning because the final steady state force depends on the balance between the effects of incomplete mechanical restitution and frequency potentiation. Thus, as long as the latter dominates, force does increase more or less stepwise, but if incomplete mechanical restitution dominates there may be a decrease in force, as occurs in rat ventricular muscle. This has led to the very misleading terms 'negative staircase' our 'negative Treppe'. Our preferred terminology for this effect is 'steady state interval–force relationship'.

Bowditch described nearly all these phenomena and also post-extra-systolic potentiation, an important interval–force relationship that has escaped terminological ambiguity more than the others. However, we should point out that there is no necessity for the premature beat which imparts potentiation to the ones which follow to be an extrasystole in the clinical sense of that word, i.e. a beat originating from an abnormal site in the heart. Thus the phenomenon might more accurately be called 'post-premature-beat potentiation'.

The sub-cellular sites involved in force–interval phenomena

In Fig. 2 we present a remarkable record of steady state interval–force responses in a single cell. This confirms the assumption that we have all made that force–interval phenomena do reside in the myocytes themselves. However, the frog is not typical of the species usually studied because it has little internal store of activator. This is a subject to be discussed in considerable detail in this book, and a subject of considerable controversy as to its subcellular site.

The experiment illustrated in Fig. 2 is of some interest in showing that the steady-state interval–force phenomenon need not depend on any of the postulated internal mechanisms of calcium handling that dominate the thinking of our co-authors and ourselves. Thus we should emphasise that our book is really confined to the consideration of properties of mammalian myocardium. Even with this limitation, the material available for discussion is excessive, and the selection for presentation to a certain

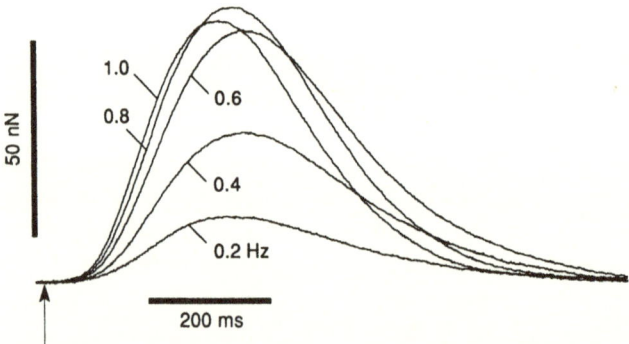

Fig. 2. The isometric contraction of a single frog ventricular heart cell was measured using an ultrasensitive force probe. The cell was field-stimulated, initially at a rate of 0.2 Hz. The stimulus rate was then increased in a cumulative, stepwise fashion to 1.0 Hz. The tenth twitch obtained at each new stimulus rate is shown. The increase in stimulus rate resulted in an increased initial rate of rise and a decreased time to peak of contraction. At the highest stimulus rates, the rate of relaxation also increased. The arrow indicates the onset of the stimulus pulse. (From Tung, L. (1987). By copyright permission of the Biophysical Society.)

extent arbitrary. We therefore apologise to the many scientists whose excellent approaches to this subject are not covered, while expressing our great thanks to our contributors for the effort they have put into their contributions. One name in particular is missing – that of Kiichi Sagawa. We have in our files a typically cheerful and optimistic letter from him about the chapter he intended to contribute with Dan Burkhoff. In the event, his death intervened. His contributions to cardiac mechanics need little chronicling, and many chapters of this book attest his more recent work on interval–force processes. In common with many of the contributors to this book, we shall miss his friendship and enthusiasm deeply.

M. I. M. Noble

W. A. Seed

References

Koch-Weser, J. & Blinks, J. R. (1963). The influence of the interval between beats on myocardial contractility. *Pharmacological Reviews*, **15**, 601–52.

Tung, L. (1987). Force–frequency relation in single frog ventricular heart cells. *Biophysical Journal*, **51**, 111a.

Part 1

On the peculiarities of excitability which the fibres of cardiac muscle show[1,2]

H. P. BOWDITCH

From the Physiological Institute at Leipzig, introduced by the scientific member C. Ludwig (With 22 wood engravings)

The excised frog heart can be filled with fluids of various compositions and the cavity changes can be examined by a manometer to determine the number and the range of its beats. This preparation therefore seemed to me to be very suitable for the study of the conditions under which the excitation processes of the heart fatigue and recover. During the execution of this project, it very soon became evident that this purpose could only be realised if the peculiarities of fatiguing and recovering cardiac muscle could be known to a more precise extent. To the solution of this limited task, for which I had the kindhearted support of Professor C. Ludwig, I first had to direct my attention.

The preparation which I needed for my experiments, I procured by putting a glass cannula in the cavity of the ventricle, advancing it from the auricle of the excised heart and tying it approximately at the border of the upper third of the wall of the ventricle. In this way, the muscle fibres of the lower two-thirds of the chamber, which I shall call in short, 'The Apex of the Heart', could be severed from its living connection with the auricle (and from the ring of the ventricle bordering the atrio-ventricular groove) and thereby, as known, could be deprived of the control of endogenous cardiac stimuli. It was necessary to fill the cavity of the apex of the ventricle (via the cannula) with fluid and to connect it to a manometer. The extent of its contractions could be measured in the same way as is done in the intact heart, by movement of the amount of fluid in the manometer. In using the great advantages which this sensitive way of determining the twitches allows, one should not forget that there are also shortcomings and that it is not free from special difficulties.

---

[1] Originally published in 1871 in German as: 'Über die Eigenthümlichkeiten der Reizbarkeit, welche die Muskelfasern des Herzens zeigen'.

[2] A historical note about the work follows on pp. 31–39.

Its first flaw is that nothing else is known to us about the relation between the linear shortening of the muscle and the volume of the ejected fluid. We could assume that volume is related to the linear muscle dimension cubed, so that the curve of the ejected volumes plotted versus the increasing shortening of the muscle fibres (abscissa) is concave toward the abscissa.

At this stage of our insight we are forced to measure twitches of the apex of the ventricle (which we want to compare with each other) with exactly the same filling of its cavity. Only with this precondition does the height of the manometer displacement accurately register the size of the twitch.

The manometer introduces another blemish, in that, with progressing twitches and the consequent increase of fluid in the manometer arm, the weight which has to be lifted by the heart is changed (see Fig. I). Therefore,

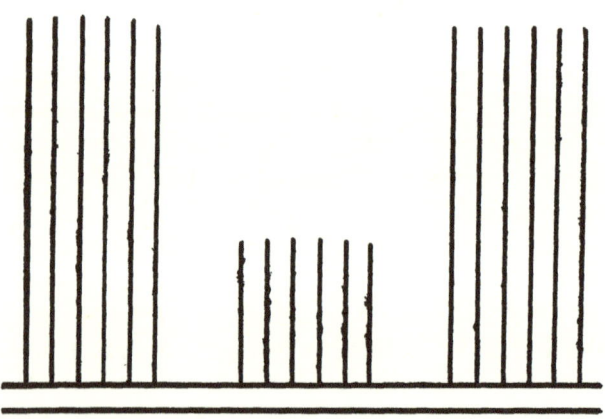

Fig. I.   Water-   Mercury-   Water-Manometer

all series of experiments for which the constancy of the weight is a necessity have to be excluded. The influence of the weight on the recorded amplitude of the cardiac twitches becomes evident if the same preparation (in spite of the fact that it had been brought to the same degree of filling and had been stimulated in precisely the same way) would eject quite unequal volumes when the specific weight of the fluid, with which the manometer had been filled, was changed.

In the recordings illustrated in Fig. I, the excursion of the water-manometer ($=17$ mm) is more than twice that in the mercury-manometer ($=7$ mm). The increase in pressure, which in the latter case is produced by the mercury column (which is lifted above the position of equilibrium), is more than ten times as high as the one present in the water manometer ($= 2 \times 7 \times 13.6$). In spite of the foregoing considerations, I still gave preference to the mercury-manometer. I did so because it is easier to handle and because in the subsequent series of experiments, the interrelationship of the lifting height to the carried weight did not matter.

It was necessary to expose the apex of the heart to easily graded stimuli which could be delivered at arbitrary but regular intervals. To this end, an apparatus served me which was built according to the model which had been put together and successfully used by K. Kronecker, consisting of

1. The recording manometer which was writing the variable positions of its mercury column with light liquid ink (solution of aniline blue) on the
2. paper of a rotating drum. To facilitate the observation and to save paper, the cog of the clockwork was stopped after each half revolution, so that the drum itself was standing still during the twitch, but moved on for approximately 2 mm after completion of the twitch.
3. A small bottle as proposed by Mariotte which kept the filling of the apex of the heart constant during the duration of the experiment. In the tube which connected the cavity of the bottle with that of the cardiac apex,
4. a stopcock of glass was inserted, which could be closed during the twitch and opened again afterwards with the help of an electromagnet.
5. Electrodes which could not be polarised and which
6. conducted only the opening pulse (shock) to the ventricle using a sliding apparatus.
7. A cogwheel on a clockwork which would interrupt the electrical current which went through the primary spiral of the inductor at regular but arbitrarily changeable intervals.
8. A relay to make the main current independent of the contacts of the clockwork.

Because the items which are mentioned under the first six numerals (except the electric magnetic stopcock), have been described in these transactions before, I can confine myself to the apparatus depicted in Figures II, III and IV and a short explanation.

The known frog manometer (Fig. II) carried at its free end, a perforated glass cap in order to guide the light floater made of a fine straw: at the upper end of the latter, a very fine glass spring (b) was lacquered on, filled with an aniline-solution which inscribed the reading of the manometer

Fig. II. III. IV.

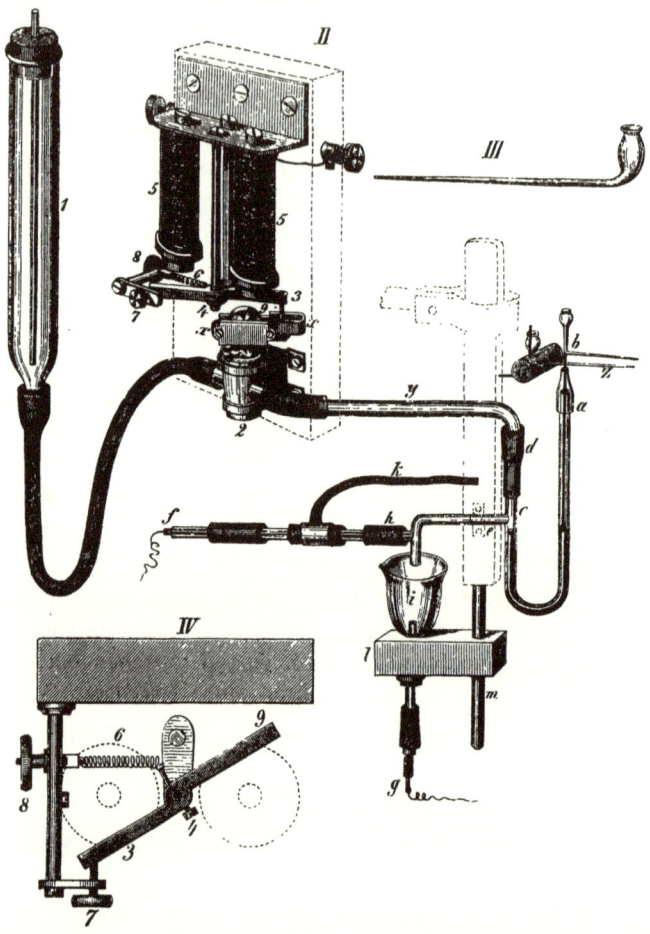

on the smooth paper of the drum. Fig. III shows the spring at its natural
size. The second shaft of the manometer opens at (c) and (d). The opening
(c) leads into the rectangularly bent tube (e), on the descending shaft to
which a rubber tube connected the ventricular cannula. The electrodes
which led the induction-current to the heart ended in the apparatus at (f)
and (g); these consisted (according to the directions given by du Bios) of
glass tubes in which a zinc amalgam rod was put, which was surrounded
by a solution of sulphate acid zinc oxide. At their cardiac ends, the tubes
were closed by a stopper made of cotton which had been submerged into
$\frac{1}{2}$% NaCl solution. At their other end, a tube of flexible rubber connected
them to the zinc rod. The electrode (f) was in connection with the fluid
contents of the heart apex by the tubule (h) which had been connected

to the descending shaft of the rectangular tube. The electrode (g) led to the bell shaped glass (i); the latter was filled during the experiment with serum to such an extent that it reached to the upper rim of the small glass bell (i); thereby, it was possible to keep the height of the serum always the same, because every drop that had been filtered through the cardiac wall had to run through the spout.

The electrode (f) was kept in its position by the wire (k): the small glass bell (i) rested on the perforated prism made of cork (l), which could be moved on the rod (m). The apparatus which controlled the degree of filling consisted in the beginning, of a small Mariotte bottle (1), which would be brought to the desired height by a holding device (not depicted in the drawing). The lower part of the bottle was connected with the glasscock (2) by the tube of flexible rubber. The stopcock could be opened and closed by means of a small spiral spring and an electromagnet. The time in which the one or the other occurred, had been chosen in such a manner that the pressure bottle was shut off from the ventricle when the latter was contracting. However, there was an open communication between both of them when the ventricle was limp. The necessary guidance for the cone of the stopcock was achieved by the armature (3) which is shown in Fig. II from the side and in Fig. IV in plan view. The rodshaped armature (3) rotated in the horizontal plane around the vertical axis (4). If the magnetism in the iron cores (5, 5) was developed, the rod lay parallel to the line which connected the centre of the bases of both iron cores. If however, the magnetism disappeared in the latter, the rod (3) was pulled by the spiral spring (6) (Fig. IV) into the position which it shows in this figure. The excursion which the rod could reach by the pull of the spring, was limited by the screw (7), which was located in a small crossbeam on a brass column on which the screw (8) was located (Fig. IV): this served to increase the tension of the spiral spring. The movement which the armature (3) exerted was transferred by means of a small pivot (9) to the clamp (x), which embraced the cone of the stopcock (2). The pivot (9) had (within the clamp (x)) some room to move, as can be seen in Fig. II. Beyond the stopcock, there was a small tube (y), which led (after a rectangular bend) to the opening of the second manometer tube. To mark the position of equilibrium of the mercury-column in the manometer, there was a glass spring (z) which was fixed by a cork at the rack to which the manometer was fixed. Since the spring which was floating on the mercury had been brought to the height of mercury equilibrium before fixation on the ventricle, and because it was kept in this position during the total rotation of the drum, it was possible to find (at any optional section of the cardiac curve) the height by which the curve had risen above the position of the mercury equilibrium.

The wheel, which is referred to as a contact breaker and which is listed under number (7) in the table of my instruments, was driven by clockwork supplied with a centrifugal pendulum. The contact breaker should open and close the electrical current at regularly recurring intervals in such a way that one could choose optionally between the intervals of 1, 2, 3, 4, 5, 10, 15, 20, 30 and 60 seconds. Furthermore, if one desired, the current could be opened immediately after its closure, or closed during a longer interval of time. The contact breaker, which achieved this, was constructed and executed by the watchmaker B. Zachariae in Leipzig; it consisted of a wheel being driven by clockwork on the rim of which were cut multiple rows of teeth. There was an adjustable angular lever, one of whose arms was leading to the cog-wheel, whilst the other was in contact with a knob of platinum (Figs. V and VI). The exact description of the apparatus may begin with the angular level. Both of its arms (a) and (b) which were inclined at a sharp angle (Fig. VI in plan view) were revolving around a vertical axis. The arm (a) was pointing to the cog-wheel (A) at the rim of which it could drag. The arm (b) was connected to a spiral spring which pressed it against the small button (c), provided that the arm (b) was not kept fixed by a higher force. Because one of the terminals of the battery ended in the small button (c) and the other one in the lever-arm (b), the flow of the current depended on their mutual contact. At times when a tooth of the wheel (A) pushed the arm (a) in front of itself (and in consequence also pulled arm (b) behind), the current was interrupted. If arm (a) slid down from the progressing tooth, the spiral spring drove back arm (b) in the opposite direction to the stop at the small button (c).

The ability to change the time interval between two consecutive current flows was achieved as follows: The circumference of the wheel (A) rotates four rows of teeth (of 60, 30, 20, and 15 pieces each) once a minute. In addition, 12 small pins are located on the upper plane of the wheel (A). At the moment at which arm (a) was opposite the pins or rows of teeth, the flow of the current recurred after 1, 2, 3, 4, or 5 seconds. To prolong the interval beyond this period, one removed 6, 8, 9, 10 or 11 pins, by which intervals of 12,[3], 15, 20, 30 and 60 seconds were made possible. The rows of teeth could also be set against arm (a) at will, by locating the contact pieces on slider (B), which could be elevated by the

---

[3] Apparently a misprint or miscalculation has occurred here, because removing 6 pins would give an interval of 10, not 12 seconds.

Fig. V. VI.

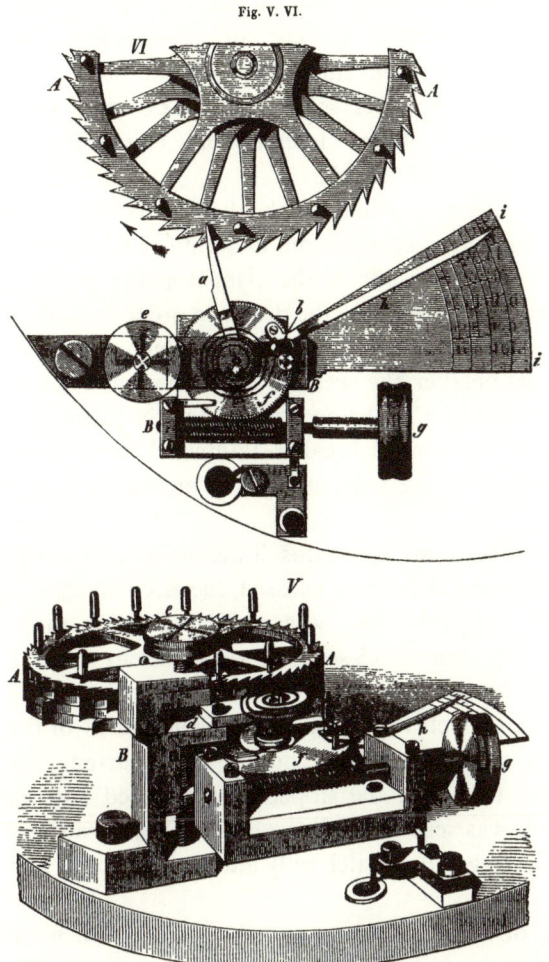

screw (e) and the guiding plate (d). The fulfilment of the second requirement (optional distribution of the total time for an interval between the flow and the interruption of the current), was realised because the arm (a) could be held by the tooth which was grabbing it for different periods of time. If this happened, the arm (when it had glided down) was momentarily taken up again by the succeeding tooth, the duration of the flow of current dropping to a minimum. In the other case (where the grabbed tooth was released instantaneously), the duration of the interruption was minimised. To achieve this, the device which was enabling contact with the slider (B) was set on the disc (f), itself geared with its toothing rim into the screw (g). Screw (g) could change the direction by which arm (a) pointed to the circumference of the wheel (A). Because the duration of current flow, or the interruption of the current, depended on the position of the disc (f), it was very convenient to mark the position of the arm (a) by a pointer (h) on the clockface (i–i); these positions were equivalent to a certain duration of flow interruption. This could be achieved at any time very easily and reliably.

The electrical current for which this contact breaker had been constructed produced the stimulating induction current and, in addition, magnetised two pairs of iron cores, namely the one at the glass-stopcock and the other one at the blade of the device rotating the drum. In order to achieve this, a strong current of high amperage was necessary which could not conduct through the contact breaker; the need for a relay became evident. By this, the main current could be kept flowing whereas the current of the relay was interrupted by the contact breaker. I adjusted the latter in such a way that the duration of the contact breaker amounted to 0.5 seconds.

According to the positioning of my apparatus, if the main current was flowing, the blade of the rotating drum was released, the electromagnetic stopcock opened and an induction beat was produced, being made ineffective by attenuation. The time of 0.5 seconds was sufficient to bring the contents of the heart to the pressure of the filling bottle, and to make the drum perform a rotation which would lead to a displacement of the paper by approximately 1 to 2 mm. If after this the main current was interrupted, the blade was held fast, the stopcock was closed and an interrupting induction beat was sent through the heart. This, because of its long latent stimulation, triggered a twitch only after the stopcock had been closed.

For the understanding of the experiments and the full assessment of the apparatus, a few more remarks should serve. The application of the ink facilitated the experiment extraordinarily. Its use was more accurate than that of smoke as its easily flowing solution wrote on smooth English paper. The sliding pen which was in use had been made according to the description of A. Fick (1869). The specifications on the strength of stimulation in the following paper accordingly do not describe the distances of the coils, but the size of the induction intensity; the maximum strength that could be reached was estimated to be 1000.

The stimuli which were conducted to the apex of the heart shorted to the wall of the ventricle; accordingly the stimuli must also have stimulated the muscle and not only the nerves. Because the electrode, reaching into the glass bell filled with serum, was vertical, special caution was needed to avoid the accumulation of small air bubbles under the stopper made of cotton. I do not think it unnecessary to point out that I was aware of this source of error. I start the description of my experiments with the chapter:

1. that deals with the **relation between the numbers of stimuli and the number of cardiac twitches**.

If the apex of the heart is stimulated at regular intervals by equal induction pulses, it either contracts after each stimulus or the number of the twitches is larger or smaller than the number of the stimuli. These three different kinds of response will be called: the regular, the supernumerary, and the discontinuous pulse or beat sequence.

The supernumerary sequence of beats occurred in my experiments rarely, and only then if the ventricle had not been ligated deep enough. Since this seems to be a fault of my experiments, I shall not take it into consideration further. This, of course, does not mean that the supernumerary sequence of beats is not worthy of special consideration. On the contrary, I consider that the relationships between this phenomenon and those which we are dealing with in this paper are very close. If the ventricle is tied deep enough, discontinuous and regular pulses can be produced at will by mere changes in the strength or sequence of the induction pulses.

First, I shall speak about the dependence of the sequence of pulses on the strength of the induction shock. If the strength of the induction shocks is gradually increased from low values, quite soon a point is reached at which the stimulation induces a twitch. If one maintains this strength and allows the induction pulses to follow at regular intervals, not every one of them will lead to a contraction. Thus, the number of stimuli exceed the number of pulses significantly. If, however, the strength of the induction shocks is increased further and further, the number of contractions also grows, without however equalling that of the stimuli. Little by little, one is reaching a value at which the sequence of pulses is becoming regular, i.e. that each stimulus is followed by a twitch. Occasionally, however, it happens that, in spite of a great intensity of the induction currents, no regular sequence of pulses can be obtained. When this occurred, the relation between the number of contractions and the number of stimuli approached unity. In order to document these communications, I shall give some examples: see over.

The discontinuous sequence of pulses may be transformed into a regular one, by increasing the interval between two stimuli of unchanged strength (but also by the fact that with unchanging strength of the stimulus, the

Intervals between two stimuli = 6 seconds.

strength of the stimuli	100	105	110	120	130	140		
number of twitches/ number of stimuli =	0.0	0.07	0.10	0.20	0.66	1.00		

Intervals between two stimuli = 4 seconds

strength of the stimuli	100	110	90	80	90	110	130	150
number of twitches/ number of stimuli =	0.04	1.0	0.17	0.30	0.88	0.77	0.82	1.0

Intervals between two stimuli = 6 seconds

strength of the stimuli	200	207	215	222	230	237		
number of twitches/ number of stimuli =	0.0	0.7	0.14	0.24	0.59	0.87		

interval between two of them is increased). In the examples below, the intervals were changed in an ascending and descending order.

Strength of the stimulus = 140

Interval in seconds		4	6	4				
number of contractions/ number of stimuli =		0.58	1.00	0.57				

strength of the stimulus = 150

interval in seconds	5	10	5	4	3	4	5	10
number of contractions/ number of stimuli =	0.74	0.97	0.87	0.71	0.73	0.80	0.95	1.0

Instead of searching for a given intensity of the induction current which at a particular interval would generate the regular sequence of pulses, one can also proceed vice versa, i.e. one can ascertain the threshold current at which (for varying intervals) the pulses are just still regular. In the execution of these experiments, one expects that with increasing length of the interval, the intensity of the stimulus could appreciably decrease before the regular sequence of pulses became a discontinuous one. This only happened in a very limited fashion. One may therefore conclude that large differences of the interval may be compensated for, by small changes of stimulus strength. A few examples may serve as an illustration. For the understanding of these examples, one has to note that, with the mentioned intensities of the induction current which are listed after the rubric 'strength of stimulation', the pulse sequence becomes regular when the induction pulses occur at the given intervals.

interval (in seconds)	10	3	4	4	3
strength of stimulation	42	43	41	45	46

and at another heart apex:

interval (in seconds)	3	4	3	5
strength of stimulation	80	74	74	68

Should one not feel urged by these and similar series of experiments to regard the above mentioned assumption as a well-founded fact, one should nevertheless be careful not to see a refutation in its imperfect confirmation. In the properties of the heart itself lie the reasons which make it difficult, yes even impossible, to furnish the proof.

The heart-muscle itself has the remarkable peculiarity that its sensitivity to stimulus strength changes as the result of the twitches which it has executed. Thus, after a longer series of contractions, a weaker stimulus than before this series suffices to trigger a regular sequence of pulses.

One's attention to the influence which the preceding twitches exert, is drawn if one uses the same stimulus with the same interval multiple times successively. Under these circumstances, the quotient of the number of twitches over the number of stimuli grows in size gradually. It may equal unity, so that a stimulus, the intensity of which did not suffice originally to induce a regular sequence of pulses, gradually becomes sufficient. For instance, I shall refer to the following observations: If the apex of a heart was stimulated by an induction shock of intensity 52 at intervals of 6 seconds, 100-times successively, the apex of the heart contracted in consequence of the first to the tenth stimulus twice, of the 11th to the 20th stimulus twice, of the 21st to the 30th stimulus twice, of the 31st to the 40th 6 times, of the 41st to the 50th stimulus 7 times, of the 51st to the 60th stimulus 6 times, of the 61st to the 70th stimulus 5 times, of the 71st to the 80th stimulus 9 times, of the 81st to the 90th stimulus 10 times, of the 91st to the 100th stimulus 10 times. Thus, the ratio of the twitches to the stimuli had increased from 0.2 to 1.0 with some variations.

In another case, in which the intensity of the strength of stimulation amounted to 52 also, and the interval to 6 seconds, the ratio grew during 40 stimuli for each 10 of them from 0.2 to 0.4, to 0.8 and finally reached 1.0. The growing sensitivity which the heart apex gains after many successively executed twitches is substantiated by the observation that the intensity of the induction current which is necessary to induce a regular sequence of pulses may decrease, in the course of a longer series of experiments. As an example, the following may serve:

Interval 5 seconds

strength of stimulation	200	300	200	150	100	110	115
number of twitches/ number of stimuli	0.0	1.0	1.0	1.0	0.27	0.8	0.9

If, thereafter, the same heart apex was stimulated at intervals of 10 seconds, the strength of stimulation was related to the ratio between the number of stimuli and the number of twitches as illustrated by the following numerical series. In the upper line I have listed the strengths of stimulation and, in the second, the respective proportional numbers:

115	90	110	115	105	100	90	80	70	65
0.0	0.6	1.0	1.0	1.0	1.0	1.0	1.0	1.0	0.7

70	68	66	60	55	50	46	42	38	42	40	42
1.0	1.0	1.0	1.0	1.0	1.0	1.0	1.0	0.0	0.9	0.2	0.7

Observations such as these speak quite expressively for the fact that the sensitivity of the apex of the heart is increased by the executed twitches, because the same strength of stimulation alternately leads to either a discontinuous or to a regular sequence of pulses, depending on the preceding response. In the discontinuous sequence of pulses, the twitches (without following a special rule), may either appear or fail to appear; I think it necessary to point out this behaviour and to illustrate it by the reproduction of some recordings, see Figs VII and VIII.

After having looked at these figures, one will see how difficult it is to describe their contents by word precisely; to use a quotient can merely be a stopgap. Its application is solely excusable because it was only thereby possible to come closer to the understanding of some very peculiar facts.

Fig. VII.

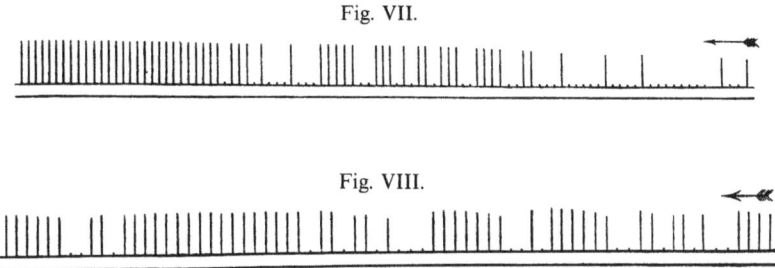

Fig. VIII.

Every dot on the baseline marks an induction shock

If one envisages the heights to which the twitching apex of the heart is able to drive the mercury, it is immediately evident that the extent of the twitch does not show any dependence on the mode of its recurrence.

In both series of experiments, the twitch may be equal or unequal, and if the latter occurs, the twitch can be greater or smaller in the discontinuous series than in the regular one. From this behaviour one can infer that the stimulus which induces a discontinuous series is sufficient to elicit the maximum twitch of which cardiac muscle is capable. However, since this cannot be done all the time, we are forced to give this phenomenon, in contrast to the stimulus which can achieve it, a special name. I shall call the stimulus which always induces a twitch as often as it occurs, the *unfailing* stimulus, whereas the one which can induce the maximal twitch only occasionally may be called the *adequate* stimulus.

That the adequate stimulus is not an unfailing one cannot be due to a fatigue of the muscle mass. Such exhaustion would not explain why the twitch, if it occurs in a discontinuous series, is not smaller than in the regular one. Even less could it be reconciled with the assumption that the frequent repetition of the same stimulus (in the same interval) could change an initially adequate into an unfailing stimulus.

If the heart muscle reacts to natural stimuli in a similar way, we would have found a new reason for the intermittent pulse especially found in those hearts whose inhibitory nerves are out of action. If, at the moment, I hesitate to apply the phenomena which the apex of the heart are showing to the intact heart, it is because of the ligature which has been put around the musculature to ensure the fixation of the cannula. Why should the ligation of the ventricle not act similarly to the one in the atrium? And if this would be the case, an inhibitory stimulus would be present which is lacking in the intact heart. This hypothesis receives some confirmation by an observation which I made incidentally but did not follow (unfortunately). It is that the strength of the stimulus which will induce a regular

sequence of pulses has to increase considerably if one adds a new ligature
to the existing one; this sometimes has to be done if the first tie around
the cannula was not tight enough.

Sometimes the introduction of fresh serum into the cavity of the apex
of the heart is effective in the opposite way to the ligature. Quite often
one can lower the strength of the stimulus considerably after such a
change, without losing its character of being unfailing.

2. **On the extent of the cardiac twitch.** For the size which the twitch
can reach, the time which passes between it and a preceding contraction
is of such importance, that above all it is necessary to consider its effect.
Here, it is always presupposed that the cavity of the cardiac apex is filled
with fresh reddish serum of rabbit blood, and that the stimulus which is
effective at regular intervals, is not only maximal but that its strength is
unfailing.

If before the beginning of a series of consecutive, equally intensive,
stimuli with intervals of approximately 4 to 6 seconds, the apex of the
heart had been in perfect rest over several minutes, a series of twitches is
induced as depicted in Figs IX and X. The records come from two
different hearts; IX worked with a mercury-manometer, X with a water-
manometer.

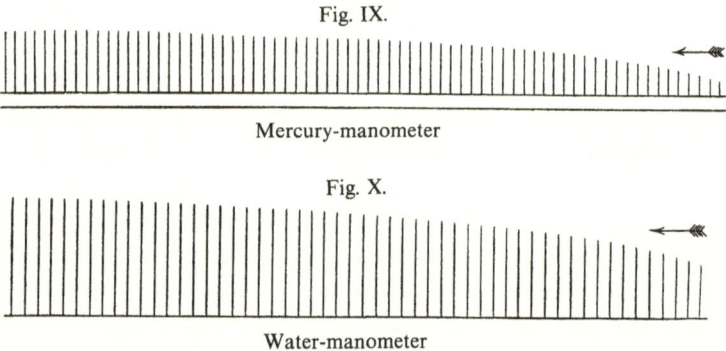

Fig. IX.

Mercury-manometer

Fig. X.

Water-manometer

The first twitch, elicited after a minute-long pause, is the smallest, and
each following one increases in size in such a way that with the rising
number of twitches, the amount of increase gets smaller and smaller until
it completely vanishes. The subsequent twitches have the same size. I call
such a sequence of twitches a *Treppe* (*staircase*). The steps of different
Treppen obtained in the same heart show various deviations with respect
to their minimal and maximal sizes, as well as to their connecting links.
Therefore, the next task was to look at the reasons for these variations

and especially the dependence on strength, direction and interval of the stimulating induction current.

It is evident that the shape which the *Treppe* takes is absolutely independent of the direction and strength of the induction current. This was expected from the very beginning, because the stimuli applied were maximal. I nevertheless have convinced myself by the most thoroughly executed experiments, that the extent of the first, the increment of the next and the size of the maximal twitch were not influenced by the aforementioned properties of the stimulus.

If one lets at least five minutes pass between two consecutive series of experiments, all twitches are small or completely equal, or only deviating within the limits of error of the measurement. This, in spite of the fact that the direction of the currents is sometimes ascending, sometimes descending, and of different intensities.

In order to obtain a number of comparable observations, I rested the apex of the heart for 5 minutes and then stimulated it by two stimuli, of which the second followed the first by an interval of some seconds. Thereafter the apex of the heart was rested again for another 5 minutes, and again a pair of stimuli was given with a similar interval and so forth. Whereas the pauses and the intervals between the stimuli stayed the same, the intensity of the current was manifoldly changed. Twelve pairs of twitches were obtained which are listed in the following table (see over).

To appreciate the exactness with which these numbers depict the independence of the growth of the twitches from the properties of the stimulus, one has to realise that the twitch height (because of the known properties of the manometer) could only be recorded at half the real amplitude. Since the numbers reflect the full value of the height, the error of measurement is doubled. Because upstrokes with values of 0.1 mm recorded by ink on the paper, undoubtedly fall in the range of error, differences of less than ± 0.2 mm between a pair of observations cannot be taken as significant. Thus the agreement between the differences which consecutive pairs of twitches show is very great indeed. However, the upper four pairs are equal among themselves but show a 0.4 mm difference from the four last ones, which also are equal among themselves. This may indicate that with the passage of time the muscle mass of the apex of the heart could experience marked changes in its characteristics. If this is accepted and observations are only compared when they were obtained with intervals which are not too far apart, the conclusiveness of the results does not leave much to be desired. All experiments which I performed according to this plan have yielded the same result.

Treppe Number	Twitch Number	Height of manometer column lifted (mm)	Strength of induction shock	Difference in manometer heights (mm)	Direction of induction current
I	1	11.0	90	1.4	Rising
	2	12.4	90		
II	1	11.0	90	1.4	,,
	2	12.4	100		
III	1	11.0	90	1.4	,,
	2	12.4	90		
IV	1	11.0	90	1.4	,,
	2	12.4	120		
V	1	10.4	90	1.8	,,
	2	12.2	120		
VI	1	10.2	90	1.2	,,
	2	11.4	130		
VII	1	11.0	90	1.4	,,
	2	12.4	90		
VIII	1	11.0	78	1.6	,,
	2	12.6	78		
IX	1	11.0	90	1.8	,,
	2	12.8	90		
X	1	11.0	90	1.8	,,
	2	12.8	150		
XI	1	11.0	90	1.8	,,
	2	12.8	90		
XII	1	11.0	90	1.8	Falling
	2	12.8	90		

We have seen that the size of the smallest twitch and the increase between two consecutive twitches at the same interval are independent of the strength and the direction of the stimuli. The same proof is left for the maximum of the twitches. However, this has already been confirmed during the extensive series of observations (which have been performed on the adequate and unfailing stimulus), mentioned on page 14 in this manuscript.

However, the effects are quite different if the interval which separates two consecutive beats is changed. Because the stimuli can be regarded as useless without twitches, it would be more correct to speak of an interval between twitches instead of between stimuli. The latter expression can therefore only be justified as long as one speaks of unfailing stimuli. In order to portray the dependence of twitch amplitude on the interval between the stimuli, one can proceed in different fashions.

a. After a pause of two to five minutes, one lets two consecutive twitches follow each other. The interval which separates one pair of twitches from another should be made variable following a certain rule. For instance, the interval can last 4 seconds between the first pair, 6 seconds between the second and so forth, up to a minute, and then one decreases the interval again in a descending fashion to 4 seconds. An experiment which is performed in such a manner shows that the first contractions of all pairs are almost if not completely equally large. The second twitches of the pair however, are unequally large; and in general larger than the first twitches. The amount by which they exceed the height of the first twitch is related to the length of the interval between the twitches that belong to one pair. The picture to which such a series of observations leads is in the following figure (XI).

Fig. XI

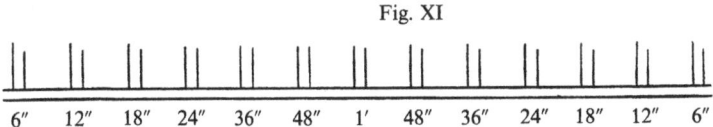

| 6″ | 12″ | 18″ | 24″ | 36″ | 48″ | 1′ | 48″ | 36″ | 24″ | 18″ | 12″ | 6″ |

b. As with the increase between two consecutive beats, so also the highest step the *Treppe* can obtain is determined by the interval of the stimuli. This assertion can easily be proven in the following way; one sends unfailing stimuli with a given interval to the apex of the heart until the height of the twitches no longer increases. This is done for a series of different intervals. It is desirable to change the duration of the interval according to a certain rule in an ascending and a descending fashion. As examples of this kind, I want to emphasize two which have been obtained with different apexes of heart. In the upper row of numbers, the intervals are listed in seconds, in the lower row, the maxima of the height of the twitches. Below each interval the greatest height is listed which could be obtained by its application (see over).

From these rows it can be seen, that the greatest height which the apex of the heart (which had been filled with pure serum) can generate is apparent with an interval between 4 to 5 seconds. If the interval is prolonged the height will decrease continuously, until it (according to the individuality of the heart) reaches a minimum at a pause of five minutes; it does not fall further after a longer period of rest. Nonetheless, the extent

						I.						
seconds	60	30	15	10	5	4	3	2	4	5	15	60
mm	12.0	14.0	16.0	17.0	18.0	18.0	16.4	14.4	15.2	15.2	14.4	10.0

			II.		
seconds	5	60	30	20	5
mm	24.4	10.6	15.4	17.6	23.2

of the twitches does decline if the interval is shortened from four to two seconds. I rarely went to shorter intervals because the twitches either merge to a tetanus or do not become more frequent. The behaviour of cardiac muscle towards quickly successive stimuli needs a special study, which considers changing excitability depending on the season of the year.

With knowledge of the inherent properties, it is not difficult to predict if a twitch of the apex of the heart will be greater or smaller than a preceding or later one, if the succession of the stimuli is known. Only comparison of two twitches which are not separated by a larger number of contractions is legitimate, because under this condition new influences come to bear.

The interdependence between twitch height, number and sequence is not completely described by the expression which is derived from the *Treppe*. This is not quite self-evident because the apex of the heart, as every other muscle, loses working capacity in the course of the performed work. A greater number of unfailing stimuli causes the contractions to decrease gradually until they finally disappear. On the way in which this fatiguing occurs, I can say the following: if one plots the heights of contractions following the descriptions of H. Kronecker, one sees that the line is either straight or descending to the abscissa by a convexity which is directed towards the abscissa. In skeletal leg muscle, the curve of fatigue would have pointed its concavity towards the abscissa, so that the decrease in the extent of the twitches during fatigue would have been the contrary picture to its ascending character in the *Treppe*. About the reason for the apparent extent of fatigue of cardiac muscle decreasing with the growing number of contractions, I dare not speculate because of a lack of experiments. The interval of the stimuli exerts a visible influence on the steepness with which the curve of fatigue declines. Also on this aspect I have to refrain from an extensive explanation and can only restrict myself to the presentation of two of my pertinent observations (Figs XII and XIII).

Fig. XII.

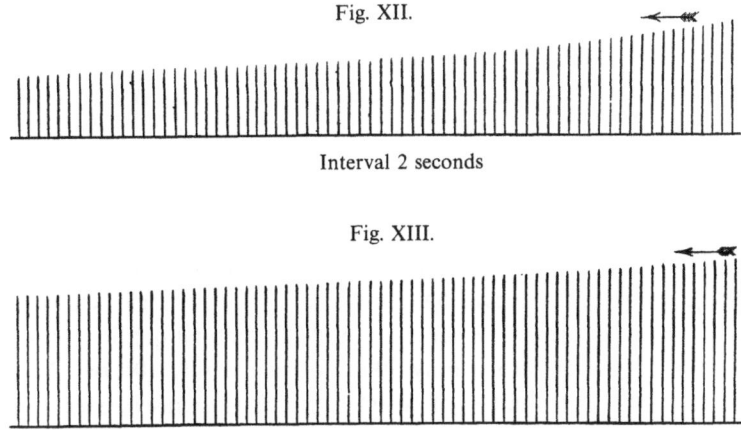

Interval 2 seconds

Fig. XIII.

Interval 4 seconds

If in consequence of fatigue, the twitches of the apex of the heart finally get too small to lift the mercury visibly, one can make a comparison with fatiguing skeletal muscle by replacing the serum with which the ventricle has been working up until now by new serum. The working capacity which the heart thereby gains is not insignificant, but it is far less than was present originally. If the apex of the heart is fatigued for the second time by the executed twitches it can recover again following a new change of the serum, but the efficiency attainable will be smaller than that produced by the first change in serum. If one continues in this way with the fatiguing and the exchange of the serum, a point will finally be reached at which the addition of new serum is completely ineffective. The following wood engraving may serve as an example for this, in many aspects, remarkable behaviour. In order to understand this, it is necessary to observe that instead of the recorded twitches only the decline of the line of fatiguing has been drawn, and the abscissa across which it runs has been shortened. Its length has been taken as proportional to the number of twitches which have been performed from the maximum to their disappearance.

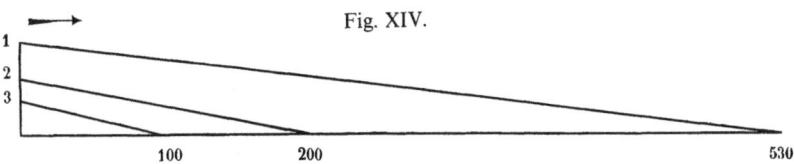

Fig. XIV.

The uppermost of the three lines depicts the decline of the fatiguing of the fresh apex of the heart; the length of the abscissa corresponds to 530 twitches; the second line shows the fatiguing after the first change in serum; the length of the abscissa represents 200 twitches; the third line finally shows the fatiguing after the second change in serum; the length of the abscissa corresponds to 100 twitches. By comparison of the lines of fatiguing, it is evident that, with each new recovery, not only the maximum of the twitch gets smaller, but that the steepness of its decline increases.

In addition to the insights which can be gained from skeletal muscle, the apex of the heart offers a new one, which relates to the importance which the qualities of the serum have in regard to the muscle which is fatigued to various degrees. The same amount of identical quality serum made possible at first 500, then only 200 and finally only 100 twitches. Thus, less than half the number of twitches which the muscle executed after the first recovery either changed the serum as much as the ones which the fresh apex of the heart had performed or, if this is not the case, the serum has to be richer in recuperating substances if it has to restore a fatigued instead of a fresh muscle. Also on this important alternative further experiments have to decide.

Apart from the endurance and the size of twitch, fatigued muscle does not differ from fresh; namely, the inherent stepwise increase of the height of the twitches and the dependence of the latter on the stimulus interval are retained.

The excitability of the heart becomes quite different if its cavity is filled with other fluids instead of with pure serum, or if poison is added to the serum. Because the new phenomena explain the hitherto mentioned observations, their description will follow immediately.

A. A solution of 0.5 g NaCl and 4.0 g gum arabic in 100 parts of water

I tried this fluid to save some of the serum. The most striking deviation by the heart that was filled with this gum was shown by its behaviour after a longer period of rest. If after this period of rest the regular sequence of stimuli was reintroduced, the stepwise increase of successive twitches would be missing. The same apex of the heart was alternately filled with serum, with gum solution and again with serum. Fig. XV shows the result of an experiment.

In other experiments, a maximum was reached after only one or two twitches. Such aberrant *Treppen* occurred more often after very long than after short pauses. Normally with lengthing of the resting period, the first

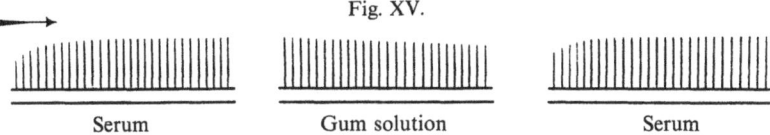

Fig. XV.

| Serum | Gum solution | Serum |

of the twitches to be triggered decreased, but with gum solution, the first of the triggered twitches increased according to the duration of the resting period, and this to a not insignificant degree, if one allowed the aforementioned time to extend to 10 minutes. Consequently, the apex of the heart behaves like any other cross-striated muscle, but it seems only qualitatively, since the recovery was much more powerful than in skeletal muscle, which I have seen perform work in the experiments of my friend Kronecker. The capacity of work performance which had been gained during the resting period did not decline as rapidly as in ordinary skeletal muscle. In the following figure (XVI), the heights of the twitches are

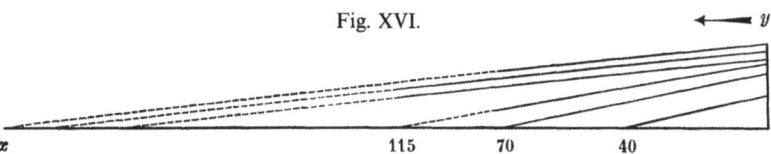

Fig. XVI.

depicted on the y axis while the lengths on the x axis are proportional to the numbers of executed twitches. Each of the 6 lines corresponds to a series of contractions which started 7 to 10 minutes after the conclusion of the preceding ones. The drawn part of this line has been constructed according to the number of actually performed beats, whereas the dotted part has been drawn under the premise that the decline in the height of the twitches would continue in a linear fashion. The numbers below the abscissa indicate the beat number corresponding to that point.

In other aspects, everything which has been observed concerning the adequate and unfailing stimulus is also completely valid in gum solution.

B. Solution of muscarine in rabbit serum

This poison which has become famous through the investigations of Schmiedeberg was added to the serum of rabbit blood which filled the cavity of the apex of the heart. The preparation was exposed to a series of stimuli before the poisoning. It hereby was evident (Fig. XVII), that during the stepwise increase of the twitches, the minimal and maximal

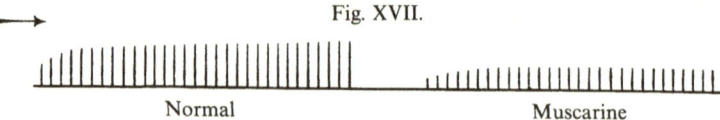

Fig. XVII.

Normal   Muscarine

twitch, and also the increase from one beat to the next became distinctly smaller during the poisoning.

From this it follows that with stimuli of equal intervals, the maximum of the twitch is always greater in the unpoisoned heart than in the one that had received muscarine. With intervals shorter than 4 seconds, the height of the twitch increases further with decreasing interval, so that the greatest beat appeared when the stimuli occurred every two seconds. Because with this short interval the twitches increase very significantly, the possibility cannot be excluded that the maximum of the twitch which a poisoned heart may reach after a 1 second interval is larger than the one that would be reached under the same circumstances in the unpoisoned heart. These effects become evident if at least 10 minutes have passed. If the poisoned heart is forced to perform numerous twitches, then the effect of the muscarine disappears gradually in the course of 1–2 hours; if this has happened, the apex of the heart can be poisoned again by a new dose of muscarine.

Because the possibility is conceivable that the muscarine is lowering the elastic coefficient of the cardiac wall, and since if this happened the smaller extent of the twitch of the apex of the heart may have been due to a lessened elastic tension of the wall, I increased the latter by filling the resting heart with a higher pressure than usual. This increase in pressure, however, did prove to be quite ineffective as to the extent of the twitch; the latter one stayed unchanged, and additionally was not altered if the resting heart was under 30 or 100 mm water column. With the exception of the aforementioned, the muscarine poisoned apex of the heart behaved in all aspects like the unpoisoned.

C. Solution of atropine in rabbit serum

Atropine was employed here as an antidote to muscarine. In Fig. XVIII, series of twitches were obtained in three different states: (a) has been produced by the unpoisoned heart, (b) by the one that was poisoned by muscarine, (c) by atropine.

With atropine, the stepwise increase of the twitches could be abolished, whereas with muscarine it was prominent to a greater degree.

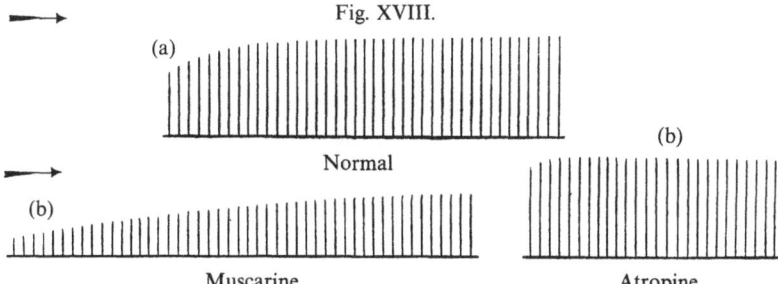

Fig. XVIII.

The absolute heights of the twitches during poisoning with atropine are greater than in the unpoisoned state. How large the difference can be, is shown in the following records, of which (a) was obtained before, and (b) after the poisoning with atropine (Fig. XIX).

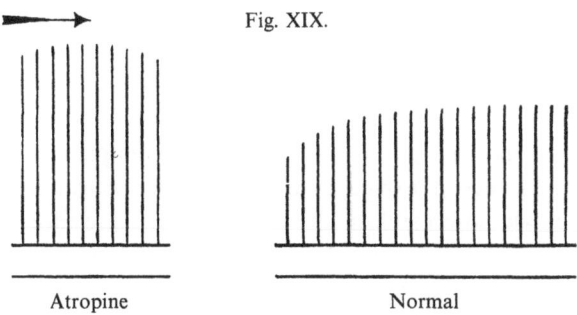

Fig. XIX.

The dosages of atropine which are necessary to achieve these effects have to be called large (0.6 mg) in comparison to those which one has to use, according to Schmiedeberg, in the intact heart. In all other respects the atropine-poisoned heart behaved like the unpoisoned one.

D. *Solution of Delphinin in rabbit serum*[4]

[4] Bowditch reported at length on the arrhythmogenic properties of this alkaloid, and on its effects in raising the electrical threshold for stimulation and eliminating the *Treppe*. In view of its limited interest this material, together with two figures has been excluded. The cardiac actions of delphinin can be found in: Bowman, W. C. & Rand, M. J. (1980). *Textbook of Pharmacology*, Blackwell Scientific Publications, Oxford. Second edition, p. 2254. The deleted text and figures are contained in the original translation (see footnote p. 31).

E. Changes of temperature

In earlier experiments, especially of those of Cyon (1866) it is known that with increasing temperature, the extent and working capacity of ventricular systole in the intact heart decreases. Whether this is due to a change in the natural endogenous cardiac stimuli, or the excitability of the muscular substance is unknown. From a study of the apex behaviour of the heart under the application of a constant and maximal stimulus, the opportunity arose to try and prevent the usual decrease of the twitch caused by atropine.

With increased temperature, the twitches decreased in height in spite of the maximal stimuli. The rule according to which this occurs resembles the one which is underlying the increase in the extent of the twitches with the staircase. A line which is connecting the upper points of the consecutive twitches results in a slightly bent curve which turns its concavity towards the abscissa, see Fig. XXII.

Fig. XXII

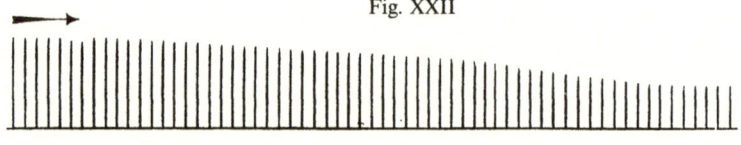

Application of atropine had no positive effect. During temperature increase, the heart that had been poisoned by atropine behaved exactly like the unpoisoned one. Measurements in the warmed heart are more difficult as the serum loses its recuperating property. In a series of experiments in which one started with a low temperature, increased the temperature and returned to the original one, the result is that the twitch with the renewed cooling of the apex of the heart, does not return to the same height which it showed before the warming. The twitch reaches its former height only if the old serum has been replaced by fresh.

F. Ligature of the atrium

From the experiments of Coats (1869) it is already evident that electrical stimulation of the ventricle during excitation of the vagus leads to smaller twitches.

With my improved equipment it seemed of interest to me to study if, by means of the regularly recurring electrical stimulus in a heart whose inhibitory nerves were excited, the phenomenon which we called *Treppe* could be induced. I suppressed the inherent twitches of the heart by a ligature around the atrium and stimulated the ventricles at regular intervals. *Treppe* could be produced which was similar in appearance to that in the muscarine-poisoned heart. In one case for example, it required 54 beats, at 2 second intervals, to increase from an initial twitch of 2 mm to the maximum of 17 mm. I could not follow this promising experiment any further because of lack of time.

To what extent are the results described above suitable to advance our thinking about the processes in the inside of muscle fibres and especially in those of the heart?[5]

1. The interdependence of the size of a cardiac twitch on the number of the preceding contractions, and on the interval between it and the preceding twitch, (the phenomenon of fatigue by work and its recovery by rest) is similar to findings in other muscles, if the heart is either filled with sodium-chloride gum solution or has been poisoned with atropine. This could be explained by the supposition that in the surviving muscle, there is a certain store of a substance from which, in the time between two twitches, a limited amount is transformed into such a state that on the introduction of a stimulus a twitch is produced, and that substance is used for work. Both the rate at which this alteration of the mass proceeds and the maximum force produced by this alteration, depends upon the stored amount of that transmutable substance, for not only does the extent of the twitches decline compared to previous twitches, but also, at longer intervals the original height of the twitch can no longer be obtained.

Such presuppositions do not suffice, however, to explain the characteristics which the ventricle shows when filled either with serum intoxicated with muscarine, or under vagal stimulation. But this very explanation is incompatible with the observation that, up to a certain limit, the size of the twitch declines with the duration of the interval. Since the heart muscle gains in its twitch capacity during a period of rest, one has to postulate for the observations during stimulation of the vagus nerve, poisoning with atropine, etc, that during the pause where there is no twitch (in contrast to the circumstances which increase the extent of contraction), factors develop which try to decrease the size of twitch. These later influences might be best compared with the influence of friction, because by their appearance, the occurrence of the twitch is not impeded, but only its

[5] In what follows (the 'Discussion'), we present as precise a translation as possible. Where ambiguities arise about which preparation is being referred to, they cannot be resolved from the original text.

excursion will be diminished. Hence, we could say each twitch would result from two directly opposing influences, an accelerating and an attenuating one.

Further information about this reduction in twitch height can be obained from regularly repeated stimulations. In an executed twitch, the attenuating circumstances will partly be destroyed, and in the recovery period be restored, so that the fatiguing and the recuperating influences are valid for the attenuating, as well as the accelerating influence, the difference being that the recovery of the first progresses more slowly than the latter; in consequence of this, the extent of the twitch increases with declining stimulation intervals. The strength with which the influence of the attenuation is brought to bear increases considerably under the conditions that are made probable, if not definite, by the support of a stimulation of a nerve; should this stimulation (similar to the one which leads to an increase of the excursion) be a triggered movement? If the conditions which produce an attenuation have developed to a great extent during a long period of rest, it can only be countermanded by a series of twitches to the size with which they are otherwise effective, at a given interval. This is a complete analogy to the time that the ordinary muscle needs to recover. If the cardiac muscle, due to continuously increasing number of twitches, is progressing towards death, the accelerating and decelerating influences will disappear to the same extent and the size of the twitches can be influenced in the same direction.

Because the development of the attenuating conditions in heart muscle can only be observed under certain circumstances, it remains doubtful on one hand, if the normal heart can develop them. Not all cross-striated muscles show them under certain conditions. Evidence for attenuation has been shown from the phenomena observed by Wendt (1859)[6] which have been described as secondary modification.

2. The induction current of the smallest strength which can evoke a cardiac twitch, does not cause the weakest of all twitches, and twitch height does not reach an unsurpassable maximum if the intensity of the stimulating current is increased. In our experiments, the induction current either induced a twitch or not; and if it did so, it provoked the most extensive twitch which that induction current could produce. The reason why the apex of the heart contracts to a different extent lies in the variable properties of the muscle fibre itself.

---

[6] This is a reference to a point which was (and is!) controversial, namely the influence of experimental conditions on the scale of force–interval effects.

3. If an induction current exceeds a so-called maximal limit, it will provoke a twitch in ordinary cross-striated muscle as often as it is applied; in the heart, however, this is only possible when the current is increased considerably beyond that needed to produce a twitch. One could say that, by the differences between the intensities of the adequate to the unfailing stimulus, the heart possesses some kind of a replacement property, which is that it can increase, within certain limits of the strength of current, from the minimal to the maximal extent of its twitch. By proposing such an analogy one has to beware of the fact that factors affecting the reliability of an induction current in producing a twitch are not simple. The present observations make it clear that a stimulus of only adequate strength, and at long intervals (seconds) was sometimes effective and sometimes not, but no external cause for these differences could be seen.

Therefore, we were left with the assumption that the excitability of the heart does not represent a state of equilibrium, but that it is a swiftly changing event, since the degrees of excitability towards the weaker stimuli can appear and disappear like waves, which rise and fall in an irregular sequence over the constant level of the unfailing stimulus. This variable sensitivity was in contrast to the reproducible effects produced by the unfailing stimulus. In these circumstances, the intensity of the induction current did not have to be increased, even when twitch height had decreased either due to poisoning with muscarine, or fatigue. The only change which occurred fairly frequently was when the unfailing stimulus was near the lower strengths of current, and the heart had performed a larger number of beats of equal intervals. With a longer period of rest, the sensitivity declined which was attenuated by a series of twitches. From these observations, the following consideration was proposed:

stimulation of the vagus, ligature of the atrium and poisoning with muscarine provoke in the intact heart, two series of phenomena: (i) a loss of contractions and (ii) a decrease of the size of those which can be generated. Can both of these have the same cause? The loss of the twitches can be explained in two different ways; either by the fact that the sensitivity of the muscle fibre to the stimulus is getting smaller, so that a stimulus which was previously unfailing becomes only adequate, or by the fact that the stimulus itself is losing strength. Since during poisoning with muscarine the induction current did not have to be increased in order to stay unfailing, it would appear that the second of the mentioned possibilities is more plausible. Notwithstanding this, we have to allow that the induction current as a stimulus has many properties, which are dissimilar to natural cardiac stimuli, and furthermore, that in my experiments it was not possible to grade the stimuli finely enough.

4. Since the normal apex of the heart does not contract spontaneously, it is justified to assume that endogenous cardiac stimuli originate in the atrium or in the atrio-ventricular groove. In the delphinin-intoxicated heart, however, the apex of the heart shows inherent twitches, which seem to be similar to normal heart beats in terms of their energy and time course, and the more or less regular sequence. Therefore, it would appear that the apex of the heart, by incorporation of a trace quantity of delphinin, can be transformed into a 'normal heart'. Whether indeed, the endogenous stimuli which excite the delphinin-intoxicated apex of the heart are identical, or not, to those which originate from the atrium, cannot be decided. However, it is again evident that cardiac muscle is essentially different from the usual cross-striated muscle in so far that the cross-striated muscle will develop a long-lasting tetanus if poisoned by delphinin (Weyland, 1870), but will not show any kind of endogenously caused twitches.

References

Coats (1869). These transactions.

Cyon (1866). These transactions.

Fick, A. (1968). Investigations from the phys. laboratory of the Technical School of Zurich, Vienna 1869, p. 38.

Wendt (1859). *Reichardt und Du Bois-Reymonds Archiv* 1859; 537 and 1861; 781.

Weyland (1870), In Eckhard's contribution Vol. V, pp. 51 and 68.

Historical note on the translation of H. P. Bowditch's paper 'Über die Eigenthümlichkeiten der Reizbarkeit, welche die Muskelfasern des Herzens zeigen' (On the peculiarities of excitability which the fibres of cardiac muscle show)[1]

Berichte der Königlich-Sächsischen Gesellschaft der Wissenschaften, Mathematisch-physische Classe, 1871, 23, 652–689

J. SCHAEFER, W. DEPPERT, R. K. LIE, B. LOHFF AND M. I. M. NOBLE

For some discoveries in science, it seems to take decades before their importance is recognised, and before they gain the acknowledgement denied to them at the time of first publication. The 'staircase' phenomenon which was described in Bowditch's paper of 1871 belongs in this category. While other important observations in the publication immediately earned a wide recognition, the importance of the 'Treppe-Phänomen', though mentioned, was not recognised for a long time. It was Hadju & Szent-Györgi (1952) who pointed out that 'whatever is the ultimate cause, the staircase must be the direct impression of the functional state of the actomyosin system, which is governed mainly by the temperature and ions'. It was probably because of Hadju & Szent-Györgi's

---

[1] The original translation was accomplished under the auspices of the International Institute for Theoretical Cardiology, and presented to members of the British Society for Cardiovascular Research at an Interval–Force Symposium in 1988. That was a literal translation which of necessity retained the somewhat obscure style of the original (high) German. In the present book, we have tried to reduce this basic text to a more understandable modern English form. This has included some shortening and paraphrasing of the original, and occasional judgements about Bowditch's meaning in the presence of some uncertainty. This may inadvertently have changed his meaning in some instances, but we think that the new version will nevertheless be more useful. The interested reader is referred to the original translation, accompanied by the original German version, which is available from Professor Schaefer at the IIfTC.

publication that Bowditch's description of the relationship between
stimulus interval and force development became recognised as relevant
to modern cardiovascular research. Fishman & Richards (1964) stated
that 'the staircase effect . . . received little investigative attention for over
half a century, but suddenly revived due to work by Szent-Györgi &
Hadju, and it may turn out to be a way to penetrate the profound
problems of the relation between stimulus and response'. Actually, a study
of the physiological literature of the late nineteenth century shows that
this statement is not quite correct, in that Bowditch's paper was discussed
by Aubert (1880), Landois (1900), Tigerstedt (1913), Höber (1922),
Trendelenburg & Loewy (1924), and especially Abderhalden (1925).
However, the staircase phenomenon itself is only marginally mentioned
in all these discussions. A detailed historical analysis of the reasons why
Bowditch did not take up the results of his paper of 1871 in his next
publication (Bowditch, 1872), and why the work of Luciani (1872) gained
more importance would be of great interest to the scientific community.

During our intensive involvement with this 120-year-old text, we were
surprised by the wealth of original observations and experimental findings,
as well as by the careful methodological work, which was included. Some
of the principal findings are summarised in Table 1.

Thus Bowditch's observations, and the assessment he offered of factors
that characterise the force–interval relation, anticipated modern concepts
of electromechanical coupling and contractility. In approaching the 1871
paper with today's knowledge, therefore, one cannot help asking the
question: 'Why did the force–interval relationship, as described by
Bowditch, not receive recognition for so long, or, what are the reasons
why the force–interval relationship disappeared from light for so long?'

We would like to deal with these questions in the form of four theses:

Thesis 1: *The objects of scientific inquiry with which Bowditch was
occupying himself did not fit into the general system of work and thought
of his time.*

This does not seem to have been the case. When Bowditch writes in the
introduction to his publication that he is interested 'to study the
conditions under which the excitable and stimulatable pieces of heart
fatigue and recover', he is in complete accord with the research efforts
of Ludwig's laboratory in Leipzig (the list of publications from
Ludwig's laboratory studying the activity of the heart have been
elegantly summarised by Schröer, 1967). Many other researchers in

Table 1. *Contents of Bowditch's 1871 paper*

(*a*) *Main interval–force contributions*

Staircase (Treppe) phenomenon

Post-extrasystolic potentiation

Definition of the 'optimum interval' (a prequisite for the concept of mechanical
 restitution)

Description of accumulating positive and negative inotropic processes with
 different time constants during artificial stimulation of the heart (precursors
 of the PIEA and NIEA concepts of Koch-Weser & Blinks, 1963)

(*b*) *Other important contributions*

Differentation between artificial and endogenous excitation of the heart and
 their different pathways

The use of toxicological and pharmacological interventions as tools to study
 the relationship between interval and force

Establishment of the relationship between excitation and contraction as a
 determinant of physiological function

All-or-none law

(*c*) *Aspects which were alluded to*

Problems caused by the isolation of tissues

Difficulties in the extrapolation of results from isolated tissues to the intact
 organism

Differences between blood and serum perfusion versus perfusion with artificial
 solutions

The limitations which are imposed by apparatus, and which have to be
 respected by experimenters

---

cardiac physiology at that time, and for some years afterwards, were
preoccupied with relating changes in cardiac rhythm to alterations in
the force of contraction. In the period from 1866 (Cyon & Ludwig) to
1902 (Woodworth), a variety of research approaches dealing with the
relationship between stimulation and activity of the heart were pursued,
and a great deal of knowledge about the relationship between
stimulation of the heart and the developed contractile force was gained.
However, from the point of view of the philosophy and history of
science, the impact of these findings has not been adequately analysed.
All the prerequisites for the recognition of the principle of
electro-mechanical coupling seem to have been available, but no-one
seems to have taken this step. Perhaps further work on the question
was limited by methodological difficulties. Recording equipment and

methods of calibration were at an early stage of development, and each scientist had to make or develop his own apparatus to tackle a specific question (Schröer, 1967). In addition, it became more and more difficult to form a coherent picture of the activity of the heart from the increasing but fragmented body of knowledge which was accumulating. As Abderhalden (1925) pointed out '... a study of this discipline [physiology] which is so fundamental for the understanding of medicine, can only be successful if logical reasoning and the tying together of the innumerable individual facts will lead to a vivid picture of the whole organism'. A limiting factor may also have been that this research seemed to offer relatively few insights into the importance of the activity of the heart for the body (as relevant then as today).

Thesis 2: _Bowditch's work suffered under the influence of contemporary controversies._

Langendorff (1885, 1898) explained the increased force of contraction of the beat following a premature beat as a 'compensatory effect', i.e. compensating for the weaker premature beat and the missed regular beat. He postulated that the heart strives to conserve both its rhythm and the force of the contraction. This kind of explanation was quite popular during the next few decades (see Kaiser, 1892; Botazzi, 1896; Cushny & Matthews, 1897; Bornstein, 1906; Cushny, 1912), although they were rejected by Woodworth (1902), who in 1897 began to work systematically on the effects that had been described by Bowditch and to restudy them in both the amphibian and mammalian heart. He came to the conclusion that 'the great force of the beat following the extra contraction is dependent, in the frog's ventricle, mostly on the prolonged compensatory pause. It is not directly dependent, as Langendorff supposes on the weakness of the extra contraction'. In addition he confirmed the staircase phenomenon, as well as Bowditch's observations on the 'all-or-none' law, in the mammalian heart. He further observed that the spontaneous beat following an extra contraction of the apex was much stronger than the regular beat, and that the 'hastened' extra contraction had a stimulating effect which was proportonal to its prematurity, and persisted on average for about eight subsequent beats. He noted too that there was an optimal interval between beats which was shorter in the dog than in the frog. However, even though these observations were reproduced (Rihl, 1906), they were not regarded as important.

One should also note that surrounding much of this research was a controversy between the myogenic and neurogenic schools concerning the origin of the heart beat. We would like to suggest that preoccupation with this controversy, and the dominance of the concept of 'compensation' made it difficult for researchers to accept other determinants of the force of contraction.

Thesis 3: *New concepts in cardiovascular physiology began to displace other approaches.*

This indeed seems to have happened. The concept of regulation of the work of the heart through the end-diastolic fibre length (Starling's Law of the heart; Starling, 1918) dominated cardiovascular research in the first half of the twentieth century. Starling's concept incorporated an intrinsic myocardial response as one feature of a highly complex control system (Chapman, 1975), and seemed, at least to the community of scientists interested in the cardiovascular system, to explain practically all important phenomena which characterised the regulation of cardiac force. It thus gained lasting importance in the practice of medicine (Fye, 1983). Preoccupation with Starling's concept led to new ways of viewing the role of the activity of the heart for the body, thus influencing the 'Denkstil' (way of thinking) of the community of scientists ('Denkkollektiv', Fleck, 1935), which narrowed new research approaches. This is vividly illustrated in textbooks of physiology and cardiology from 1920 to the present day. There was a tendency to explain *all* changes in myocardial contraction in terms of changes in the initial length of the fibre, including the dependence of the force of contraction in the interval between beats. Wiggers (1925) for example, studied the ineffectiveness of premature beats with great skill, but did not really seriously concern himself with post-extrasystolic potentiation (Cranefield, 1965), arguing that the post-extrasystolic beat was stronger because the ventricle was more distended at the end of the longer interval before the beat.

Thesis 4: *Realisation of the interdependence of cardiac electrical and mechanical phenomena allowed the re-assessment and re-discovery of Bowditch's findings.*

As it became increasingly evident that cardiac rhythm and cardiac contraction influence each other via electro-mechanical coupling, the

findings of Bowditch and Woodworth became relevant again, as they
still are today. Several factors contributed to this 're-discovery' and
're-assessment'. First, the development of pacemaking systems opened
up the possibility of inducing artificial alterations in rhythm of the
heart to treat cardiac arrythmias. The advent of cardiac pacing
renewed interest in the fundamental principles underlying the
relationship between interval and developed force.

Secondly, renewed interest in cardiovascular pharmacology made it
necessary to define the conditions under which drugs could be tested
and compared with each other. In a superb review Koch-Weser and
Blinks (1963) drew attention to the importance of the interval between
beats in the assessment of the inotropy of various substances and the
tremendous difference of effects in different species.

Finally, there was a renewed interest in what has been termed
'contractility'. A number of observations made prior to those of
Starling had indicated that cardiac muscle was able to alter its intrinsic
contractile properties. In 1977 Katz wrote '... the importance of these
early observations did not become apparent until a symposium on this
subject was organised in 1955 at which Sarnoff presented the concept of
a 'family of Starling curves', which clearly integrated knowledge of the
length-dependent changes in contractile performance, described half a
century before by Otto Frank & E. H. Starling, with scattered bits of
evidence pointing to a significant role for alterations in 'myocardial
contractility'. It was recognised that conditions quite apart from the
cellular environment, such as the experimental conditions chosen by
the investigator, partly determine the particular combination of force
and shortening that the muscle exhibits (Milnor, 1982). Milnor further
observed that this dichotomy – the division of factors that determine
myocardial function into two classes – has become a central concept in
cardiac physiology. In effect, it becomes a distinction between the
capability of the muscle and its actual performance in a given situation.
The first of these, the *potential* for contraction that the muscle possesses
by virtue of local physicochemical conditions, has become referred to as
contractility (another term which is a source of controversy). The
second is the actual *performance* of the muscle in a given setting. This is
attributable to the limitations imposed by external mechanical conditions
in the ability of the muscle to respond.

Aware of these approaches to the study of contraction and
performance, and of the emergent role of calcium in the contractile
process, scientists came to recognise the possibility of using the

force–interval relationship to extend their understanding of excitation–contraction coupling in the mammalian heart *in situ*. Thus Yue & Sagawa (1987) wrote: 'The beautifully ordered fashion in which the strength of contraction of mammalian cardiac muscle responds to changes in stimulation pattern has long engendered the hope that clarification of these phenomena, known as the interval–force relationship, would lead to understanding the fundamental mechanisms underlying cardiac contraction.'

Conclusion

The pattern which we have outlined, and which in essence shows a neglect of the important insights made available by Bowditch 120 years ago, is very familiar to philosophers of science. It is due to the fact that a certain way of thinking determines the extent to which scientific insights will be accepted, rejected or neglected. If researchers belong to a certain community then they will communicate according to the rules which have been developed in that community. Observations and hypotheses which do not fit into the pattern which dominates the contemporary research approach are either rejected, not acknowledged, or even forgotten. This seems to have happened to the knowledge of the force–interval relationship which had been accumulated up to 1902. With the emergence and general acceptance of Starling's concept a completely different approach to understanding the function of the heart was established.

References

Abderhalden, E. (1925). *Lehrbuch der Physiologie in Vorlesungen*. Teil II. Berlin: Urban.

Aubert, H. (1880). Innervation der Kreislauforgane. In: *Handbuch der Physiologie*, Band 4, hrsg. von L. Hermann, pp. 348–80. Leipzig: Vogel.

Bornstein, A. (1906). Die Postextrasystole. *Zentralblatt Physiologie*, **20**, 401–5.

Botazzi, F. (1896). Über die 'postcompensatorische' Systole. *Zentralblatt Physiologie*, **10**, 401–5.

Bowditch, H. P. (1870). Letter from Leipzig, March 8th 1870. *Boston Medical and Surgical Journal*, 305–7.

Bowditch, H. P. (1871). Über die Eigenthümlichkeiten der Reizbarkeit, welche die Muskelfasern des Herzens zeigen. *Berichte der Königlich-Sächsischen Gesellschaft der Wissenschaften, Mathematisch-physische Classe*, **23**, 652–89.

Bowditch, H. P. (1872). Über die Interferenz des retardirenden und beschleunigten Herznerven. *Arbeiten aus der Physiologischen Anstalt zu Leipzig mitgetheilt von C. Ludwig*, pp. 259–80. Leipzig: Hirzel.

Chapman, C. B. (1975). Ernest Henry Starling. In: *Dictionary of Scientific Biography*, vol. XII, ed. Gillespie, Ch. C., pp. 617–19. New York: Scribner.

Cranefield, P. F. (1965). The force of contraction of extrasystoles and the potentiation of force of the post-extrasystolic contraction. A historical review. *Bulletin of the New York Academy of Medicine*, **41**, 419–27.

Cushny, A. R. (1912). Stimulation of the isolated ventricle with special reference to the development of spontaneous rhythm. *Heart*, **3**, 257–78.

Cushny, A. R. & Matthews, S. A. (1897). On the effect of electrical stimulation of the mammalian heart. *Journal of Physiology*, **21**, 213–30.

Cyon, E. & Ludwig, C. (1866). Die Reflexe eines der sensiblen Nerven des Herzens auf die motorischen Blutgefäße. *Berichte über die Verhandlungen der Königlich-Sächsischen Gesellschaft der Wissenschaften zu Leipzig, Mathematische-physische Classe*, 307–29.

Fishman, A. P. & Richards, D. W. (1964). Circulation of the blood. *Men and Ideas*. New York: Oxford University Press.

Fleck, L. (1935). *Erfahrung und Tatsache*. Frankfurt: Suhrkamp, 1983.

Fye, W. B. (1983). Ernest Henry Starling, his law and its growing significance in the practice of medicine. *Circulation*, **68**, 1145–48.

Hadju, S. & Szent-Györgi, A. (1952). Action of DOC and serum on the frog heart. *American Journal of Physiology*, **168**, 159–63.

Höber, R. (1922). *Lehrbuch der Physiologie des Menschen*. 3. Auflage, Berlin: Springer.

Kaiser, K. (1892). Untersuchungen über die Rhythmicität der Herzbewegungen. *Zeitschrift für Biologie*. Neue Folge, **11**, 203–26.

Katz, A. M. (1977). *Physiology of the Heart*. New York: Raven Press.

Koch-Weser, J. & Blinks, J. R. (1963). The influence of the interval between beats on myocardial contractility. *Pharmacological Reviews*, **15**, 601–52.

Landois, L. (1900). *Lehrbuch der Physiologie des Menschen*. 10. vermehrte und verbesserte Auflage, Berlin: Urban.

Langendorff, O. (1885). Über die elektrische Reizung des Herzens. *Archiv für Physiologie, Leipzig*, **8**, 284–7.

Langendorff, O. (1898). Untersuchungen am überlebenden Säugethierherzen. III. Abhandlung: Unregelmäßigkeiten des Herzschlages und ihre Ausgleichung. *Pflügers Archiv für die gesamte Physiologie*, **70**, 473–86.

Luciani, L. (1872). Die periodische Function des isolirten Froschherzens. *Arbeiten aus der Physiologischen Anstalt zu Leipzig mitgetheilt von C. Ludwig*, pp. 113–96. Leipzig: Hirzel.

Milnor, W. R. (1982). *Hemodynamics*. Baltimore: Williams & Wilkins.

Rihl, J. (1906). Zur Erklärung der Vergrößerung der postextrasystolischen Systole des Säugethierherzens. *Zeitschrift für Experimentelle Pathologie und Therapie*, **3**, 1–18.

Schröer, H. (1967). Carl Ludwig. *Begründer der messenden Experimentalphysiologie: 1816—1895*. (Große Naturforscher, 33). Stuttgart: Wiss. Verlagsgesellschaft.

Starling, E. H. (1918). *The Linacre Lecture on the Law of the Heart given at Cambridge 1915.* London: Longmans and Green.

Tigerstedt, R. (1913). *Lehrbuch der Physiologie.* 7. Auflage. Leipzig: Hirzel.

Trendelenburg, W. & Loewy, A. (1924). *Lehrbuch der Physiologie des Menschen* 4. Auflage des Lehrbuches von Zuntz und Loewy. Leipzig: Vogel.

Wiggers, C. J. (1925). The muscular reaction of the mammalian ventricles to artificial stimuli. *American Journal of Physiology,* **73,** 346–78.

Woodworth, R. S. (1902). Maximal contraction, 'staircase' contraction, refractory period and compensatory pause of the heart. *American Journal of Physiology,* **8,** 213–49.

Yue, D. T. & Sagawa, K. (1987). Insight into excitation–contraction coupling of heart derived from studies of the force–interval relationship. In *Activation, Metabolism and Perfusion of the Heart,* ed. S. Sideman & R. Beyar, pp. 261–77, Dordrecht: Martinus Nijhoff.

Part 2

The general process

The interval–strength relationship of cardiac muscle: past, present and future

D. G. ALLEN

Introduction

'The interval between a contraction of the heart and the preceding beat is of such importance for the strength of the contraction that the study of this effect is a prime necessity.' This quotation from the classic study by Bowditch (1871) marks the start of investigation of this perennially fascinating topic. The early years of investigations of the interval–strength relation were primarily descriptive; only in the last two or three decades has enough detail emerged concerning the cellular physiology of the heart to make investigations of the mechanism worthwhile. In the present short review both the phenomenology and the current understanding of cellular mechanisms will be described from a broad historical perspective. The section on the past will primarily be concerned with the description of the interval–strength relation in some of its many manifestations, while the section on the present will discuss current ideas of the underlying mechanisms. Finally, the future section will consider unresolved issues and possible directions for further research.

Past

The fact that changes in the rhythm of the heart affect the stroke volume has been known for many centuries. For instance, Galen, writing in the third century AD, was aware that a premature beat produced a weak pulse and that this beat was followed by a stronger than normal pulse. Of course, such observations are complicated by the changes in diastolic filling and more detailed studies had to await the ability to isolate the heart. Bowditch's study in 1871 used the isolated ventricle of the frog heart, filled with a variety of solutions including serum, and measured the

43

developed pressure on stimulation. His study describes many of the now familiar interval–strength phenomena:

1. The steady-state developed pressure increased as the stimulus interval was decreased, but at the shortest intervals pressure again declined.
2. The influence of one isolated contraction on a second declined as the interval between the two increased.
3. After a long rest, the developed pressure was small and increased with repeated regular stimulation (treppe or staircase).
4. Application of different solutions and drugs could modify the interval–strength phenomena.

In Bowditch's study the heart was not perfused or oxygenated, so long periods of stimulation led to a decline of pressure, which he described as fatigue, and was probably due both to lack of oxygen and to the accumulation of products of metabolism, such as lactic acid.

Woodworth (1902) extended these studies to the isolated mammalian ventricle. The apex of a dog heart was supplied with oxygenated defibrinated blood and stimulated electrically. This preparation was usually spontaneously active, so the effects of additional stimuli were characterised. An interesting innovation was to record the timing of stimulation on the pen recorder by passing a spark from the tip of the pen, which left a hole in the paper at the moment of stimulation. The phenomena observed by Bowditch in the frog were confirmed in the mammalian heart and in addition the refractory period and the reduction in tension after a very short interval (extrasystole) were explored. This study also demonstrated both that a premature contraction was small and that the subsequent contraction was large (post-extrasystolic potentiation).

These two early studies describe the interval–strength relation of the ventricle in some detail and do not differ in any important respect from more modern accounts. Further technical developments came with the use of isolated strips of heart muscle (e.g. Cattell & Gold, 1938). With these preparations, muscle length can be controlled and the solution bathing the muscle can easily be changed. The simplicity of the experimental approach and the complexity and variety of the resulting tension responses has led to a very large number of investigations. The classic review of Koch-Weser & Blinks (1963) listed over 300 papers on this topic. Their review described the many phenomena associated with the interval–strength relation and gave particular attention to the variations between different regions of the heart and different species.

Some representative results from mammalian ventricular muscle are shown in Fig. 1. Panel (*a*) shows a steady-state interval–strength relation obtained from a thin (i.e. <0.4 mm diameter) cat papillary muscle. At very long intervals (>200 s) the tension is small and independent of interval and is known as the rested state contraction (RSC). The RSC has a prolonged time-to-peak and the accompanying action potential is also of increased duration. Reduction in interval leads to a monotonic increase in tension until the refractory period prevents shorter intervals. The maximum tension achieved is close to the maximum of which the muscle is capable under any conditions (Fisher, Lee, Marlon & Kavaler, 1967) and probably represents maximal activation of the contractile machinery. If thicker muscles are used, the tension at the shorter intervals tends to decline after some time at the new interval (dashed line in Fig. 1(*a*)). Thus the steady-state relation in thicker muscle is depressed at short intervals. This phenomenon has been attributed to an anoxic core, and cellular changes that accompany this depression of tension are now relatively well understood (see later section).

Although interval–strength relations of this monotonic variety are common in ventricular muscle, there are many exceptions (see chapter by Ravens in this book, (pp. 245–58). For instance, rat ventricular muscle usually displays a large rested state contraction and typically the tension declines as stimulus interval is reduced (e.g. Orchard & Lakatta, 1985). Such interval–strength relations are often described as 'negative', since they have a negative slope when plotted as in Fig. 1(*a*). Atrial muscle from most species also displays more complex relations with larger tension at both long and short intervals compared with intermediate intervals (e.g. Koch-Weser & Blinks, 1963).

However, the complexity of the cellular mechanisms which underly the interval–strength relationship is more readily appreciated when non-steady-states are observed. For instance, Fig. 1(*b*) shows an example of the classic 'treppe' or staircase when stimulation is resumed after a long rest. The first contraction is small and slow (i.e. a RSC) and there is a rapid recovery of tension for four to six contractions. Thereafter, tension returns towards the steady-state level with a slow and approximately exponential time course ($t_{1/2}$ 1–2 min). Such records strongly suggest that two independent mechanisms are involved in the potentiated tension at short intervals.

Another popular approach to investigating the transient properties is to interpose an additional stimulus after various delays in a regular train of contractions. Fig. 1(*c*) shows the kind of response seen in most cardiac

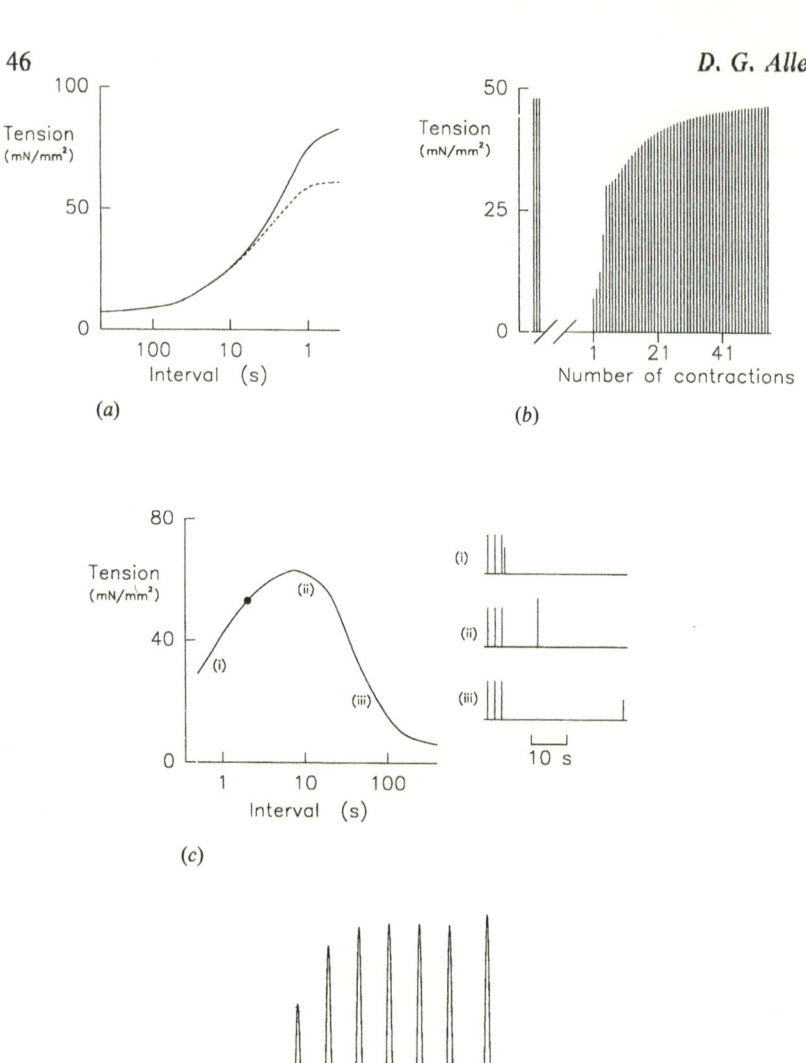

Fig. 1. Representative examples of the interval–strength relation in isolated mammalian ventricular muscle. Panels (a), (b) and (c) are modified from Allen, Jewell & Wood (1976) and show results from cat papillary muscle at 30 °C. Panel (d) is an unpublished record of pressure recorded from an isovolumic balloon in the left ventricle of a Langendorff-perfused rabbit heart at 37 °C. (a) Steady-state interval–strength relation in a thin papillary muscle (<0.4 mm diameter, solid line). In a thick preparation (>0.8 mm diameter, dashed line) the tension at short intervals is reduced. Note logarithmic scale on the abscissa.

(b) Recovery of tension after a long rest. Three control contractions at 3 s intervals preparations. When the interval is shorter than the refractory period there is of course no response. Once the stimulus interval exceeds the refractory period the interposed (premature) contraction is small. Increasing this interval leads to a recovery of tension known as rapid restitution (see chapter by Jóhannsson in this book, pp. 227–43). Once the stimulus interval exceeds the steady-state interval, there is nearly always an increase in tension (rest potentiation). At the temperature used in these experiments (30 °C), the largest contraction occurs after intervals of 5–20 s. Longer periods lead to a slow decline before the rested state contraction is achieved at very long intervals. The latter decline is known as rest decay.

Panel (*d*) of Fig. 1 shows a continuous record of pressure recorded from the left ventricle of an isolated perfused rabbit heart. The sino-atrial node had been destroyed and the heart was being stimulated at a rate which suppressed the remaining intrinsic pacemakers. After several control beats an extra stimulus was given 300 ms after the normal stimulus (paired pulsing) and resulted in a small premature contraction. The next normal contraction was greatly potentiated and this potentiation continued until a new steady state was reached after three to four pairs of contractions. The extra stimulus was then discontinued and the amplitude of single contractions returned to normal over three to four contractions. Paired pulse stimulation also leads to near maximal activation in many situations and is a more convenient way to establish maximal activation than high frequency stimulation because only a small number of contractions are required (Fisher *et al.*, 1967).

Present

As an oversimplification, the review by Koch-Weser and Blinks can be thought of as marking the end of the past era. In essence, the phenomena

Fig. 1 (*cont.*)

are shown; the preparation was then not stimulated for 8 minutes and stimulation then restarted at 3 s intervals. (*c*) Restitution and rest decay curve. The preparation was stimulated at 2 s intervals until tension was steady. The tension developed under these steady-state conditions is represented by the solid circle on the graph. Then a single stimulus was given after various delays and the tension developed is plotted as a function of the rest interval. Note the logarithmic scale on the abscissa. Panels (i), (ii) and (iii) show representative tension records when the interposed contraction occurred after 0.7 s (i), 10 s (ii) and 40 s (iii). (*d*) Paired pulse stimulation. Continuous pressure record; stimulus interval 2 s initially. After the third contraction an additional (paired) stimulus was added 0.3 s after the first stimulus and paired stimulation was continued for seven contractions before reverting to single stimuli.

were well known and had been described in considerable detail, but little was known of the cellular mechanisms involved. The development of understanding of the mechanism which underlies the interval–strength relation can for simplicity be considered in three periods.

Changes in intracellular [Ca^{2+}] cause the variations in tension

When Koch-Weser and Blinks reviewed the literature in 1963, the idea that changes in intracellular calcium might cause the variations in tension was discussed briefly, but understanding of calcium movements within the cardiac cell was in its infancy. In the early 1960s, acceptance of the role of Ca^{2+} as the intracellular messenger for contraction in muscle was not universal (see comments by Ebashi, 1980). However, as the decade progressed the identification of sarcoplasmic reticulum (SR) as the site into which Ca^{2+} was pumped during relaxation (Hasselbach, 1964) and the discovery of troponin (Ebashi & Kodama, 1966) meant that the role of Ca^{2+} gradually became firmly established.

An important difference between skeletal and cardiac muscle, which had long been appreciated, was that the tension developed in a tetanus of skeletal muscle was relatively insensitive to conditions under which it was stimulated, while the contraction of cardiac muscle was extremely variable and dependent on the conditions of stimulation. This variability has been given many names but is most often described as the contractility or inotropic state. As the role of Ca^{2+} became established as the link between excitation and contraction, an obvious possibility was that the variations in contractility arose from variations in the amount of Ca^{2+} released to activate contraction. Important evidence for this hypothesis came from measurements of radioactive Ca^{2+} influx and efflux. Thus both Ca^{2+} influx and efflux were shown to increase during inotropic interventions such as increased stimulus frequency (e.g. Winegrad & Shanes, 1962; Langer & Brady, 1963).

An important negative result in this period was the demonstration that levels of high energy phosphates, such as adenosine triphosphate (ATP) and phosphocreatine (PCr), were relatively insensitive to the inotropic state or the stimulation frequency (Furchgott & de Gubareff, 1958). This was important because it was already clear from skinned fibre studies that contraction could be elicited provided only that Ca^{2+} and ATP were present in the solution bathing the myofibrils. Thus, one possible modulator of tension production was the level of ATP available to the contractile proteins. This early work has been amply confirmed with recent NMR

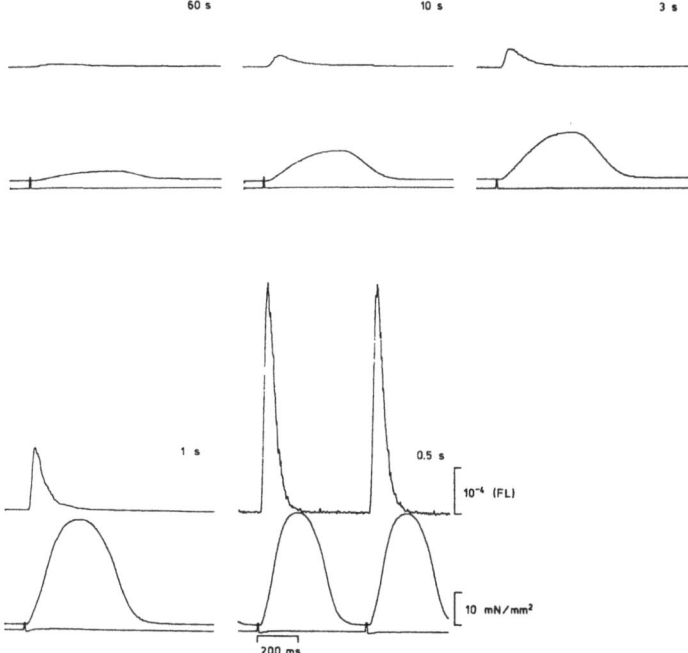

Fig. 2. Intracellular calcium in cat ventricular muscle at various stimulation intervals. From Allen & Kurihara (1980) with permission. Each panel shows aequorin light (upper trace) which indicates intracellular calcium concentration, developed tension (middle trace) and stimulus marker (lower trace). The preparation was in a steady state at each interval and the interval is shown above each panel. Light is measured in units of fractional luminescence (FL) and 10^{-4} represents $[Ca^{2+}]_i$ of about 1.8 µM. Temperature, 30 °C.

studies (e.g. Allen *et al.*, 1986; Elliott, 1987) and only at the highest stimulation frequencies are there detectable changes in ATP and PCr concentrations (see later section).

Final confirmation of the role of calcium came with the first measurements of intracellular calcium ion concentration $[Ca^{2+}]_i$ which showed that the major inotropic interventions (raised extracellular calcium concentration, increased frequency, catecholamines and cardiac glycosides) all lead to increases in the systolic $[Ca^{2+}]_i$ (Allen & Blinks, 1978). This analysis was made more quantitative when it was shown that a variety of interventions which caused the same degree of potentiation (raised Ca^{2+}, increased stimulus frequency, paired pulsing) each produced a similar rise in systolic $[Ca^{2+}]_i$ (Allen & Kurihara, 1980). Fig. 2, taken from this paper, shows the steady-state relation between aequorin light (representing intracellular $[Ca^{2+}]$) and tension as stimulus interval is decreased. These observations using the calcium indicator aequorin have now been confirmed in many cardiac tissues (e.g. Morgan & Blinks, 1981; Orchard & Lakatta, 1985) and have been extended to non-steady-state conditions and repeated with other Ca^{2+} indicators. For instance, Wier & Yue (1986) used aequorin to show that the rapid restitution of tension and post-extrasystolic potentiation were accompanied by comparable changes in $[Ca^{2+}]_i$. More recently the fluorescent indicator indo has been used in isolated cardiac cells to show that the increase in shortening when regular contractions are started after a rest are also associated with appropriate increases in $[Ca^{2+}]_i$ (Lee & Clusin, 1987; duBell & Houser, 1989).

In summary there is overwhelming evidence that both steady-state and transient changes in stimulus interval are associated with changes in $[Ca^{2+}]_i$ which parallel the changes in tension. Since the central role of Ca^{2+} in coupling of the action potential to contraction is now universally accepted, there seems no reason to doubt that these changes in $[Ca^{2+}]_i$ are actually the cause of the changes in tension.

Variations in intracellular $[Ca^{2+}]$ are a consequence of the degree of Ca^{2+} loading of the sarcoplasmic reticulum (SR)

A central question in cardiac physiology is the source of the Ca^{2+} which leads to the rise in $[Ca^{2+}]_i$ that causes contraction. While there is still debate on this issue, it is widely believed that the source of the majority of the Ca^{2+} is the SR and that it is variations in SR loading which cause the variations in tension associated with the interval–strength relation and many other inotropic interventions. In this section the evidence for this statement is briefly reviewed.

To consider this issue quantitatively, it is helpful to calculate the amount of Ca^{2+} required for activation of the contractile proteins. Cardiac muscle contains about 70 µmole troponin/kg tissue (Solaro *et al.*, 1974) and troponin has three Ca^{2+} binding sites (Holroyde *et al.*, 1980). Two of the sites, the Ca/Mg sites, are not thought to play a direct role in activation of acto-myosin activity because their affinity is so high that they are normally occupied by either a Ca^{2+} or Mg^{2+} ion and because they exchange Ca^{2+} very slowly. The other site (low affinity site) is thought to regulate acto-myosin activity. When this site is saturated with Ca^{2+} (70 µmole/kg tissue) the acto-myosin activity is maximal; intermediate levels of occupation lead to intermediate levels of activation. Thus the Ca^{2+} required for partial activation is in the middle part of this range, i.e. 30–40 µmole/kg tissue. In addition to this Ca^{2+} bound to troponin, a very small amount of Ca^{2+} will be free in the myoplasm (1–2 μmole/kg tissue). A further amount of Ca^{2+} will be required to bind to other Ca^{2+} binding sites in the cell; the most complete estimate of these is that of Fabiato (1983) whose measurements showed that a free $[Ca^{2+}]$ of 2.7 μM gave 50% tension and calculated a total of 114 μmole/kg tissue of bound Ca^{2+} under these conditions. Even under resting conditions there is some Ca^{2+} bound to these sites (7 μmole/kg tissue) so that the total Ca^{2+} which must be added to the myoplasm to achieve a 50% maximal twitch is (114–7) or roughly 100 μmole/kg tissue.

One approach to determining the source of this Ca^{2+} is to measure excitation-dependent uptake of radioactive Ca^{2+} or efflux of radioactive Ca^{2+} from loaded cells. Early estimates of influx and/or efflux were generally low, typically less than 2 μmole/kg tissue/contraction, e.g. Winegrad and Shanes (1962). However, Lewartowski (1983) has pointed out that in multicellular preparations contracting at normal rates, it is impossible to exclude the possibility that some of the Ca^{2+} taken up (or released) in one contraction is immediately released (or taken up) in the next. If this process occurs then the above values of influx/efflux will underestimate the true flux/contraction. To overcome this problem, Lewartowski has measured Ca uptake in isolated contractions and observed extremely high values of Ca^{2+} influx/contraction (230 μmole/kg tissue/contraction). When the preparations were stimulated at normal rates the above interpretative problems existed, but the results still suggested very high values of Ca^{2+} influx (105 μmole/kg tissue/contraction at 60 beats/minute). Another approach to this problem is to measure the changes in $[Ca^{2+}]$ in the extracellular space of an isolated multicellular preparation which is *not* perfused via its vascular bed. Because of diffusion restrictions to the bulk solution, the changes in extracellular $[Ca^{2+}]$ can give estimates of Ca^{2+} uptake and efflux, provided these do not overlap in time. Using this approach, several groups (Bers, 1983; MacLeod & Bers, 1987; Hilgemann & Langer, 1984) have estimated Ca^{2+} uptake to be in the range 10–30 μmole/kg tissue/contraction. Unfortunately the quantitative discrepancies between these various approaches are large; if the results from Lewartowski's group are correct, it is not necessary to postulate any intracellular Ca^{2+} release. However, the weight of physiological evidence (see below) suggests that the SR contributes most Ca^{2+} to the contractile process and suggests therefore that the lower estimates obtained by measurements of extracellular $[Ca^{2+}]$ are more likely to be correct. These matters are considered further in chapters by Langer (pp. 193–210) and by Lewartowski (pp. 173–92) in this book.

The best defined *trans*-sarcolemmal source of Ca^{2+} is the Ca^{2+} current. This can be measured reliably by integrating the component of inward current which is sensitive to Ca^{2+}-channel blockers. Most estimates are in the range 5–10 μmole/kg tissue/contraction (Reuter, 1974; Callewaert, Cleeman & Morad, 1988). However, from the earliest measurements of calcium current (i_{ca}) it has been clear that i_{ca} makes only a small contribution to the activator Ca^{2+}. First, as noted above, the quantity of Ca^{2+} involved is too small. Second, when a staircase of tension was produced by regular depolarisation after a rest, the tension showed the usual increase while the i_{ca} remained about the same size (Beeler & Reuter, 1970) or decreased (duBell & Houser, 1989). The constancy or decline of i_{ca} when tension and $[Ca^{2+}]_i$ increases shows very clearly that other sources of Ca^{2+} must be involved.

Where does the remaining Ca^{2+} come from? Most evidence suggests that the SR is the major source, but two other *trans*-sarcolemmal sources need some consideration. (i) The Na^+/Ca^{2+} exchanger. A provocative account by Mullins (1981) suggested a major role for Ca^{2+} influx on this carrier but recent analyses suggest a more circumscribed role. The stoichiometry of $3Na^+/1Ca^{2+}$ now seems established and this makes the exchanger both electrogenic and sensitive to the membrane potential (for a recent review see Eisner & Lederer, 1985). This influx of Ca^{2+} on the exchanger depends on both the membrane potential and $[Ca^{2+}]_i$. If the electrochemical equilibrium (units mV) of the exchanger is plotted on the same voltage and timescale as the action potential, e.g. Shattock & Bers (1989) then it is apparent that in most mammalian species, net influx of Ca^{2+} on the exchanger is confined to a brief period immediately after the depolarisation of the action potential and has a relatively small driving potential. In addition, recent measurements of Ca^{2+} influx via the exchanger (Crespo, Grantham & Cannell, 1990) suggest that the kinetics of the exchanger are too slow for the influx to make a major contribution. Furthermore, if Ca^{2+} entry on the Na^+/Ca^{2+} exchange is eliminated by removing Na^+ from the intracellular solution (Wier, 1990), the amplitude of contraction and the systolic $[Ca^{2+}]_i$ signal are not affected drastically. (For further discussion of Ca^{2+} entry on Na^+/Ca^{2+} exchange, see the review by Wier, 1990). (ii) Ca^{2+} bound to membrane sites. It has been proposed that Ca^{2+} bound to the sarcolemma makes a major contribution to contractile Ca^{2+} (Lüllmann & Peters, 1977; Langer, 1984). Unfortunately, while it is easy to show that substantial amounts of Ca^{2+} bind to the sarcolemma, no method of measuring that which is released during contraction has yet been devised, so the importance of this putative mechanism remains unknown.

In contrast, the contribution of SR Ca^{2+} has now been identified by a range of structural, physiological and pharmacological methods. The ability of the SR to sequester Ca^{2+} by pumping it out of the myoplasm was the first identified property (Hasselbach, 1964). Subsequently it was shown that caffeine causes the SR to release Ca^{2+} (Weber & Herz, 1968) and that this could trigger a variable-sized tension response in a fibre skinned in a way which removes the surface membrane but leaves the SR intact (Fabiato & Fabiato, 1977). Proof that a membrane-lined space is responsible for this Ca^{2+} release is easily obtained since the release is eliminated by brief treatment with detergent. Such studies in skinned fibres rapidly established that the SR has the capacity to store and release sufficient Ca^{2+} for full activation and to resequester it.

A variety of different techniques have now been utilised to show that the SR is the store of this labile component of Ca^{2+} in the intact cell. In principle the most direct technique would be the use of X-ray micro-analysis which can locate Ca^{2+} within the cell. Potentially this technique can measure the Ca^{2+} content of the SR and determine how much of this Ca^{2+} is transferred to the myofilaments during contraction. However, at present the resolution of the technique is restricted by the diameter of the ion probe and the thickness of the frozen section. Nevertheless, despite the current limitations, Wendt-Gallitelli (1985) has shown that a region of the cell which includes the SR has a high Ca^{2+} load during diastole and that this Ca^{2+} load declines during contraction. Furthermore, the diastolic loading varies with the inotropic state of the preparation, being low in a rested state contraction and high during paired pulse stimulation (Wendt-Gallitelli, Jacob & Wolburg, 1982).

Several methods of functional estimation of the SR Ca^{2+} content have also established that the SR is the site of this major Ca^{2+} store. The technique of sudden cooling to 5 °C produces a transient contracture presumably caused by sudden release of the SR Ca^{2+} content (Kurihara & Sakai, 1985). Bers (1989) has applied this approach to the interval–strength relation and shown a close relationship between the strength of an interposed contraction (see Fig. 1(c)) and the magnitude of cold contracture produced under the same conditions. The disadvantage of this technique is that there is no unequivocal evidence that SR, rather than some other intracellular store of Ca^{2+}, is the source of the Ca^{2+}. Caffeine is known to open Ca^{2+} channels in the SR (Rousseau &

Meissner, 1989) and can also produce a contracture if applied sufficiently rapidly. Smith, Valdeolmillos, Eisner & Allen (1988) have shown that the size of the caffeine contracture and the associated rise in $[Ca^{2+}]_i$ correlate well with the inotropic status of ventricular muscle. In addition, they showed that tension declined after a rest and that the caffeine contracture induced after a similar rest declined in a comparable way. Because the SR is the only Ca store known to be caffeine-releasable, this result points directly to the SR as the site of the labile Ca^{2+} store.

Finally, the use of ryanodine has also helped to clarify the role of SR in cardiac cells. Early experiments suggested that ryanodine blocked Ca^{2+} release from the SR (Jenden & Fairhurst, 1969) and led to a rapid decline in tension. Subsequently, it was shown that ryanodine selectively inhibited the potentiated tension associated with post-extra systolic potentiation (Wier & Yue, 1986), rest potentiation (Bers, 1985) and paired pulse stimulation (Sutko & Willerson, 1979). All these results are consistent with the idea that ryanodine prevents release of Ca^{2+} from a store which is loaded in an interval-dependent manner. Studies on the SR Ca^{2+} channel have now shown that ryanodine either increases the frequency of opening of these channels or, at higher concentrations, locks the channel in a partially open state (Rousseau, Smith & Meissner, 1987). Thus the most likely interpretation now seems to be that ryanodine prevents Ca^{2+} release by depleting the SR of its store of Ca^{2+}. Equally important from the point of view of localisation, it is now known that the protein to which ryanodine binds is both the structural foot protein which bridges the gap between T-tubules and SR and the SR Ca^{2+} channel (Inui, Saito & Fleischer, 1987).

Using these pharmacological tools, Wier (1990) has shown that when the Na^+/Ca^{2+} exchanger is eliminated and ryanodine is used to eliminate SR Ca^{2+} release, the measured intracellular $[Ca^{2+}]$ can be accurately predicted from the *trans*-sarcolemmal Ca^{2+} current (which was also measured) and the intracellular Ca^{2+} buffers. In the absence of ryanodine, the contraction and intracellular $[Ca^{2+}]$ were close to normal magnitude, which again suggests that the SR is the major Ca^{2+} source under normal conditions. The importance of these experiments is that they demonstrate that the Ca^{2+} current and a ryanodine-blockable component of Ca^{2+} release can account quantitatively for the observed increased in intracellular $[Ca^{2+}]$. Thus it is not necessary to postulate any additional sources of Ca^{2+}.

The pathways for SR loading
The final part of the story, as yet incompletely understood, concerns the details of the pathways by which SR is loaded to the appropriate levels.

In muscles in which the strength of contraction increases monotonically with decreasing interval, it is clear that the increased Ca^{2+} entry on the i_{ca} will lead to Ca^{2+} loading of the myoplasm and the SR and can explain an increase in tension. In addition, the periods of depolarisation will bias the Na^+/Ca^{2+} exchanger in the direction of increased influx or reduced efflux and will also lead to Ca^{2+} loading. Preparations with large RSC are more difficult to explain, and the complex changes of tension observed in the staircase and when extra contractions are interposed after various rests, represent the greatest challenge for mechanistic interpretations.

Staircase of tension

The four to six beat increase in tension which occurs when stimulation restarts is very characteristic of cardiac muscle (e.g. Fig. 1(b)) and has long been thought to represent the timecourse of reloading the SR Ca^{2+} store when Ca entry suddenly changes (Wood, Heppner & Weidmann, 1969). In this situation Ca^{2+} entry will occur by both i_{ca} and Na^+/Ca^{2+} exchanges. Measurements of radioactive Ca flux suggests a much enhanced Ca uptake on the first contraction compared with a steady-state uptake (Lewartowski, 1983). i_{ca} will make a contribution of 5–10 μmole/kg/ contraction but in most studies e.g. duBell & Houser (1989), its peak magnitude declines in repeated contractions presumably because of Ca^{2+}-dependent inactivation (Boyett, Kirby & Orchard, 1989). Further, Ca^{2+} entry on the Na^+/Ca^{2+} exchange may be substantially enhanced on the first contraction after a rest, both because the action potential is of greater amplitude and duration and because the systolic rise in $[Ca^{2+}]_i$ is much smaller. An interesting study by duBell & Houser (1989) compared Ca entry by these two routes. Single cells were rested and then regular voltage clamp pulses were applied and the changes in i_{ca} and systolic $[Ca^{2+}]_i$ transient were monitored during the positive staircase which resulted. One series of experiments was performed with pulses to $+10$ mV, the voltage at which peak i_{ca} is maximal. A second and third series were performed at -10 mV and $+30$ mV, voltages at which peak i_{ca} are similar and about 50% of that observed at $+10$ mV. At -10 mV there was little increase in the calcium transient or contraction, whereas at $+30$ mV there was a substantial increase in calcium transient and contraction over 10 beats. Furthermore, after 10 contractions the amplitude of contraction and the calcium transient were comparable at $+10$ and $+30$, suggesting that increased Ca entry on Na^+/Ca^{2+} exchange between $+10$ and $+30$ mV was comparable to the reduction in i_{ca}.

If Ca entry on the Na^+/Ca^{2+} exchange and i_{ca} are to increase the Ca^{2+} loading of the depleted SR, it is necessary to elevate the myoplasmic $[Ca^{2+}]$, since the only known route of entry into the SR is via the SR Ca pump. This rise in diastolic $[Ca^{2+}]$ during a staircase of tension following a rest has now been observed (Lee & Clusin, 1987; duBell & Houser, 1989).

The slow recovery of tension seems to require a different explanation. Most probably this phase represents the gradual accumulation of Na^+ entering with each action potential and reaching a steady state after several minutes. The resulting rise in $[Na^+]_i$ has now been measured in many studies (e.g. Cohen, Fozzard & Sheu, 1982; Boyett, Hart, Levi & Roberts, 1987). The link between $[Na^+]_i$ and contractility is also now well understood. Elevated $[Na^+]_i$ reduces Na^+ influx on the Na^+/Ca^{2+} exchange, reduces Ca^{2+} efflux and the myoplasmic $[Ca^{2+}]$ therefore rises (e.g. Eisner, Lederer & Vaughan-Jones, 1984). Finally the elevated diastolic $[Ca^{2+}]$ leads to increased SR Ca^{2+} loading and therefore to greater tension. The time course of the rise in $[Na^+]_i$ matches the slow increase in tension well. The magnitude of the $[Na^+]_i$ increase, however, is small and can only partly explain the observed rise in tension (Cohen *et al.*, 1982; Boyett *et al.*, 1987). Since these authors did not distinguish between the fast and slow phases of tension increase, it seems that the rise in $[Na^+]_i$ may explain the slow rise in tension fairly well.

Interposed beat

Rapid restitution The refractory period determines the earliest time at which an additional action potential can be stimulated. Action potentials at this time have reduced magnitude and duration because of incomplete recovery of the various currents involved (see Boyett & Jewell (1980) for review). It is possible that the reduced amplitude and duration of this action potential contributes to reduced Ca^{2+} release in this premature contraction. Several arguments, however, suggest that this effect is small. (i) Changes in action potential duration generally have little effect on the contraction in which the change is made (Beeler & Reuter, 1970; Drake-Holland *et al.*, 1983); the effect is usually observed on the subsequent contraction. (ii) Wier & Yue (1986) found that ryanodine generally eliminated the rapid restitution of tension except for the very shortest intervals. The latter result confirms the idea that it is variations in either loading or release of Ca^{2+} from the SR which causes rapid restitution. The traditional view (e.g. Wood *et al.*, 1969; Morad & Goldman, 1973; Allen *et al.*, 1976) was that the delay in recovery of tension observed in rapid restitution was caused by the time taken for Ca^{2+} to be transported from an uptake compartment to a release compartment. Operationally, this is an acceptable hypothesis. However the problem is that the likely uptake site is the longitudinal SR, where the SR pumps are located, while the release site is thought to be the terminal cisternae, where the release sites are located (for review, see Fleischer & Inui, 1989). Since the half-length of the longitudinal SR is only about 1 μm, it is easy to calculate that unobstructed diffusion of Ca^{2+} over a distance of 1 μm would be largely complete in ≈ 1 ms (e.g. Crank, 1975). Thus the contribution of this process to the time to the peak of rapid restitution (≈ 1–10 s) would appear to be negligible. Of course it is possible the diffusion is slowed by binding sites or other tortuosity factors, but it is hard to explain a factor of 10^4. An alternative possibility for the cause of this delay, raised by the work of Fabiato (1985) and discussed by Wier & Yue (1986), is that it is caused by slow reactivation of the SR Ca^{2+} channels following inactivation during systole. A third possibility is suggested by modelling of Ca^{2+} movements in skeletal muscle (e.g. Cannell & Allen, 1984). Skeletal muscle contains large amounts of an additional Ca^{2+} buffer, parvalbumin. This has kinetics of Ca^{2+} binding similar to the Ca/Mg site on troponin (Robertson, Johnson & Potter, 1981). When parvalbumin is loaded with Ca^{2+} during a tetanus, it subsequently releases its bound Ca^{2+} very slowly ($t_{1/2}$ of several seconds) and this is currently thought to be the cause of the delay observed by Winegrad (1968) and Somlyo *et al.* (1981) in the return of Ca^{2+} to the release site of the terminal cisternae of skeletal muscle. For this hypothesis to apply in cardiac muscle, it will be necessary to show that the unbinding of Ca^{2+} from some class of myoplasmic binding sites is sufficiently slow to explain the time course of restitution.

The decline in tension following long rests It is established that in preparations which show this property, the SR Ca^{2+} gradually declines with time (Smith *et al.*, 1988; Bers, 1989). It would seem that in these preparations the steady-state resting $[Ca^{2+}]_i$ is low and that Ca^{2+} can gradually leak out of the SR so that the SR Ca^{2+} loading reflects the decline in the myoplasmic $[Ca^{2+}]$. The steady-state resting $[Ca^{2+}]$ will depend on the mixture of inward leaks and outward pumps for both Ca^{2+} and Na^+. There is evidence that Ca^{2+} efflux via the Na^+/Ca^{2+} exchanger is substantially greater than that due to the surface membrane Ca^{2+} pump (Carafoli, 1985; Wier, 1990). If this is so, the $[Ca^{2+}]_i$ will be set principally by the level of $[Na^+]_i$ which, in turn, is set by the Na influx (channel, leaks and Na^+/H^+ exchanger) and the Na^+ pump (Eisner, Allen & Orchard, 1984).

Rested state contractions In most mammalian species the rested state contraction is small and slow and this has led to the suggestion that the SR is largely depleted of Ca^{2+} and that the contraction is mainly caused by *trans*-sarcolemmal Ca^{2+} entry (e.g. Allen *et al.*, 1976). This view is supported by the depletion of Ca^{2+} stores as measured by electron microprobe (Wendt-Gallitelli *et al.*, 1982). Depletion presumably occurs because during activity there is additional entry of Ca^{2+} which loads the myoplasm and then the SR. During a long rest the myoplasmic $[Ca^{2+}]_i$ returns to its stable level and Ca^{2+} gradually leaks out of the SR.

As noted earlier, rat ventricular muscle and many types of atrial muscle have a large RSC and their SR Ca^{2+} stores are relatively loaded with Ca^{2+} after a long rest. This result is surprising because repeated action potentials must allow additional Ca^{2+} through i_{ca} and bias the Na^+/Ca^{2+} exchanger in the direction of increased influx/decreased efflux; it is therefore puzzling that when this additional entry is stopped, Ca^{2+} stores become further loaded. An observation by Shattock & Bers (1989) goes some way to explaining the phenomenon. They found resting $[Na^+]_i$ to be higher in resting rat ventricular muscle compared to guinea pig (13 v 7 mM). On this basis, assuming a membrane potential of -80 mV in both cases, the Na^+/Ca^{2+} exchanger strongly favours Ca^{2+} extrusion in resting rabbit muscle whereas in rat muscle there is a small bias to Ca influx. Thus, a resting rat preparation will tend to have much higher resting $[Ca^{2+}]_i$ and its SR will be more loaded with Ca^{2+}. When stimulation in the rabbit ventricle starts, the depolarisation favours Ca entry, but this is minimised by the systolic elevation in $[Ca^{2+}]_i$ so that net influx will depend on the systolic $[Ca^{2+}]_i$. In rat muscle, however, the action potential is very short so that during the elevated systolic $[Ca^{2+}]_i$ there is a strong tendency for net efflux. Thus in rat ventricle, the combination of the short action potential and the high $[Na^+]_i$ means that after a rest SR Ca stores are elevated and activity leads to net efflux on the Na^+/Ca^{2+} exchanger. This interpretation is strongly supported by extracellular Ca measurements (Shattock & Bers, 1989) and by measurements of scattered light intensity fluctuations (Kort & Lakatta, 1988).

Paired pulse stimulation The potentiation of tension or pressure is often quite dramatic during paired pulse stimulation, a fivefold potentiation, as in Fig. 1(*d*), being not uncommon. It seems probable that at least two factors are involved. First, the paired pulse stimulation will double the number of action potentials per unit time. Because the second action potential is elicited just after the refractory period, it is usually of reduced amplitude and duration but nevertheless the proportion of time that the membrane potential is depolarised will increase substantially. This will increase Ca^{2+} entry by both i_{ca} and increase entry/reduce efflux on the Na^+/Ca^{2+} exchanger. It seems unlikely, however, that these factors alone can explain the potentiation since halving the stimulus interval would lead to an approximately similar change and the increase in tension on paired pulse stimulation is usually much greater than that achieved by halving the stimulus interval. The second factor is probably related to the timing of the stimuli. The second stimulus of the pair leads to a very small contraction, presumably because the Ca^{2+} released by the first stimulus has not yet returned to the release site (see discussion under interposed beats). Because of the low $[Ca^{2+}]_i$ during the second action potential, Ca^{2+} influx on the Na^+/Ca^{2+} exchanger may be much increased in this second action potential (Boyett, Kirby & Orchard, 1989). The first stimulus of the next pair, however, occurs at a time when Ca^{2+} released in both the previous pair of contractions is available for release. Detailed quantitative modelling will be required to establish whether these two factors are adequate to explain the potentiation of tension observed in paired pulse stimulation.

Other factors affecting tension at short intervals

Now that the role of $[Ca^{2+}]_i$ is established, there has been increasing interest in identifying situations in which factors other than $[Ca^{2+}]_i$ play a role. Of particular interest is the situation where metabolic demands exceed the available energy supply. This can occur in the intact heart either because of coronary atheroma with reduced blood supply or because, during intense cardiac activity, metabolic consumption exceeds energetic supply. In either of these situations, it is now known that products of metabolism accumulate within the cardiac cells (e.g. Bailey, Williams, Radda & Gadian, 1981; Allen, Morris, Orchard & Pirolo, 1985; Allen *et al.*, 1986) and specifically there is a fall of pH_i due, at least in part, to lactic acid accumulation, and a rise in inorganic phosphate (Pi). Skinned fibre studies have shown that both of these metabolites depress maximum Ca^{2+}-activated tension and reduce the Ca^{2+} sensitivity of the contractile proteins (Fabiato & Fabiato, 1978; Kentish, 1986). Thus the probable explanation for the fall of tension at very short intervals first noted by Bowditch (1871) is that the intracellular $[Ca^{2+}]$ is still elevated but the response of the contractile proteins to Ca^{2+} is reduced by the effects of pH and Pi on the proteins.

Future

From the above discussion of cellular mechanisms, it is clear that working hypotheses are available which are capable of explaining in a general way many of the phenomena observed in the interval–strength relation. What is now required is a more rigorous and quantitative test of the hypotheses involved.

One approach to this problem is more detailed quantitative modelling of the Ca^{2+} movements involved. Such a model needs to include all sources of Ca influx into the myoplasm, the various myoplasmic binding sites and the various pumps which remove Ca^{2+} from the cell. If all these elements are given the correct properties, then the intracellular Ca^{2+} in the model should be close to that measured and the various phenomena described when intervals are changed should be apparent. No model of this kind of complexity has yet been published, though the recent review by Wier (1990) represents the nearest approach so far.

The area of greatest uncertainty remains the magnitude and timecourse of Ca^{2+} release from the SR, although information about the SR Ca^{2+} channels and their coupling to T-tubules is growing very rapidly (for recent review, see Fleischer & Inui, 1989). It now seems certain that this is the source of most Ca^{2+} and that the release is triggered by a small rise in myoplasmic $[Ca^{2+}]$, but we do not yet know the details of this process. One difficulty which has long been apparent is the issue of how Ca^{2+} release is terminated. In its simplest form Ca^{2+}-induced release is a positive feedback process and once started would be expected to continue until either the SR was completely depleted or until the release process was inactivated. Fabiato (1985) found evidence for inactivation of release occurring in a Ca^{2+}-dependent manner in skinned preparations, which is clearly necessary to allow relaxation to occur in intact preparations. The extent to which the store is depleted in one contraction in the intact cell is not yet known. However, an important indication that the release from the store can vary comes from voltage clamp experiments. When the voltage of the clamp pulse is varied the calcium current is activated at about $-40\,mV$, peaks at about $0\,mV$ and is close to zero at $+60\,mV$ (e.g. Barcenas-Ruiz & Wier, 1987; Cannell, Berlin & Lederer, 1987; Callewaert *et al.*, 1988). However, the intracellular calcium transient has a much broader peak than the i_{ca} even when care is taken that the previous history of the cells is identical so that loading of the store with Ca^{2+} should be identical. This result implies that over a substantial range of amplitudes of i_{ca}, Ca^{2+} release is constant. However, when i_{ca} falls below a certain value the Ca^{2+} entry is no longer able to trigger the normal amount of Ca^{2+} release. It is not yet clear in the intact cells whether this mechanism (incomplete activation of Ca^{2+} release) contributes to contractility in addition to variations in filling of the Ca^{2+} store.

Another area in which it is likely that advances will occur is in the development of drugs which modify individual elements in the pathway of Ca^{2+} movements. For instance, a specific blocker of Na^+/Ca^{2+} exchange would be of immense value in the identification of the role of the exchanger, but extensive searches have only identified very non-specific blockers such as amiloride and dichlorobenzamil (e.g. Siegl, Cragoe, Trumble & Kaczorowski, 1984). The use of ryanodine and caffeine have been very important in defining the role of the SR and the advent of new drugs which affect the SR Ca^{2+} channel (e.g. Fleischer & Inui, 1989) is likely to lead to further increases in understanding.

In summary, after about a century of intensive investigation, understanding of the interval–strength relation is about to move into an era of specific hypothesis which can be tested quantitatively. A new era in which the techniques of molecular biology can be used to modify known proteins in the cell is just beginning, (e.g. Adams *et al.*, 1990) and will eventually lead to the ability to modify the interval–strength relation rather than simply understand it.

References

Adams, B. A., Tanabe, T., Mikami, A., Numa, S. & Beam, K. (1990). Intramembrane charge movement restored in dysgenic skeletal muscle by injection of dihydropyridine receptor cDNAs. *Nature*, **346**, 569–72.

Allen, D. G. & Blinks, J. R. (1978). Calcium transients in aequorin-injected frog cardiac muscle. *Nature*, **273**, 509–13.

Allen, D. G., Eisner, D. A., Morris, P. G., Pirolo, J. S. & Smith, G. L. (1986). Metabolic consequences of increasing intracellular calcium and force production in perfused ferret hearts. *Journal of Physiology*, **376**, 121–41.

Allen, D. G., Jewell, B. R. & Wood, E. H. (1976). Studies of the contractility of mammalian myocardium at low rates of stimulation. *Journal of Physiology*, **254**, 1–17.

Allen, D. G. & Kurihara, S. (1980). Calcium transients in mammalian ventricular muscle. *European Heart Journal*, **1**, 5–15.

Allen, D. G., Morris, P. G., Orchard, C. H. & Pirolo, J. S. (1985). A nuclear magnetic resonance study of metabolism in the ferret heart during hypoxia and inhibition of glycolysis. *Journal of Physiology*, **361**, 185–204.

Barcenas-Ruiz, L. & Wier, W. G. (1987). Voltage dependence of intracellular $[Ca^{2+}]_i$ transients in guinea pig ventricular myocytes. *Circulation Research*, **61**, 148–54.

Bailey, I. A., Williams, S. R., Radda, G. K. & Gadian, D. G. (1981). Activity of phosphorylase in total global ischaemia in the rat heart. A phosphorus-31 nuclear-magnetic-resonance study. *Biochemical Journal*, **196**, 171–8.

Beeler, G. W. & Reuter, H. (1970). The relation between membrane potential, membrane currents and activation of contraction in ventricular myocardial fibres. *Journal of Physiology*, 207, 211–29.

Bers, D. M. (1983). Early transient depletion of extracellular Ca during individual cardiac muscle contractions. *American Journal of Physiology*, **244**, H462–8.

Bers, D. (1985). Ca influx and sarcoplasic reticulum Ca release in cardiac muscle activation during postrest recovery. *American Journal of Physiology*, **248**, H366–81.

Bers, D. M. (1989). SR Ca loading in cardiac muscle preparations based on rapid-cooling contractures. *American Journal of Physiology*, **256**, C109–20.

Bowditch, H. P. (1871). On the peculiarities of excitability which the fibres of cardiac muscle show. *Berichte der Königlich-Sächsischen Gesellschaft der Wissenschaften*, **23**, 652–89.

Boyett, M. R., Hart, G., Levi, A. J. & Roberts, A. (1987). Effects of repetitive activity on developed force and intracellular sodium in isolated sheep and dog Purkinje fibres. *Journal of Physiology*, **388**, 295–322.

Boyett, M. R. & Jewell, B. R. (1980). Analysis of the effects of changes in rate and rhythm upon electrical activity in the heart. *Progress in Biophysics & Molecular Biology*, **36**, 1–52.

Boyett, M. R., Kirby, M. S. & Orchard, C. H. (1989). Paired pulse potentiation in isolated ferret ventricular muscle. *Journal of Physiology*, **410**, 66P.

Callewaert, G., Cleeman, L. & Morad, M. (1988). Epinephrine enhances Ca^{2+} current-regulated Ca^{2+} release and Ca^{2+} reuptake in rat ventricular myocytes. *Proceedings of the National Academy of Sciences, USA*, **85**, 2009–13.

Cannell, M. B. & Allen, D. G. (1984). Model of calcium movements during activations in the sarcomere of frog skeletal muscle. *Biophysical Journal*, **45**, 913–25.

Cannell, M. B., Berlin, J. R. & Lederer, W. J. (1987). Effect of membrane potential changes on the calcium transient in single rat cardiac muscle cells. *Science*, **238**, 1419–23.

Carafoli, E. (1985). The homeostasis of calcium in heart cells. *Journal of Molecular and Cellular Cardiology*, **17**, 203–12.

Cattell, M. & Gold, H. (1938). The influence of digitalis glucosides on the force of contraction of mammalian cardiac muscle. *Journal of Pharmacology and Experimental Therapeutics*, **62**, 116–25.

Cohen, C. J., Fozzard, H. A. & Sheu, S.-S. (1982). Increase in intracellular sodium ion activity during stimulation in mammalian cardiac muscle. *Circulation Research*, **50**, 651–62.

Crank, J. (1975). *The Mathematics of Diffusion*. 2nd edn., Oxford: Clarendon Press.

Crespo, L. M., Grantham, C. J. & Cannell, M. B. (1990). Kinetics, stoichiometry and role of the Na-Ca exchange mechanism in isolated cardiac myocytes. *Nature*, **345**, 618–21.

Drake-Holland, A. J., Noble, M. I. M., Pieterse, M., Schouten, V. J. A., Seed,

W. A., ter Keurs, H. E. D. J. & Wohlfart, B. (1983). Cardiac action potential duration and contractility in the intact dog heart. *Journal of Physiology*, **345**, 75–85.

duBell, W. H. & Houser, S. R. (1989). Voltage and beat dependence of Ca^{2+} transient in feline ventricular myocytes. *American Journal of Physiology*, **257**, H746–59.

Ebashi, S. (1980). Regulation of muscle contraction. *Proceedings of the Royal Society London*, B **207**, 259–86.

Ebashi, S. & Kodama, A. (1966). Interaction of troponin with F-actin in the presence of tropomyosin. *Journal of Biochemistry*, **59**, 425–6.

Elliott, A. C. (1987). Phosphorus nuclear magnetic resonance studies of metabolite levels and intracellular pH in muscle. PhD Thesis, University of London.

Eisner, D. A., Allen, D. G. & Orchard, C. H. (1984). The regulation of intracellular calcium concentrations in cardiac muscle. In *Control and Manipulation of Calcium Movements*, ed. J. R. Parratt, Plenum Press.

Eisner, D. A. & Lederer, W. J. (1985). Na-Ca exchange: stoichiometry and electrogenicity. *American Journal of Physiology*, **248**, C189–202.

Eisner, D. A., Lederer, W. J. & Vaughan-Jones, R. D. (1984). The quantitative relationship between twitch tension and intracellular sodium activity in sheep cardiac Purkinje fibres. *Journal of Physiology*, **355**, 251–66.

Fabiato, A. (1983). Calcium-induced release of calcium from the cardiac sarcoplasmic reticulum. *American Journal of Physiology*, **245**, C1–14.

Fabiato, A. (1985). Calcium-induced release of calcium from the sarcoplasmic reticulum. *Journal of General Physiology*, **85**, 189–320.

Fabiato, A. & Fabiato, F. (1977). Calcium release from the sarcoplasmic reticulum. *Circulation Research*, **40**, 119–29.

Fabiato, A. & Fabiato, F. (1978). Effects of pH on the myofilaments and the sarcoplasmic reticulum of skinned cells from cardiac and skeletal muscles. *Journal of Physiology*, **276**, 233–55.

Fisher, V. J., Lee, R. J., Marlon, A. & Kavaler, F. (1967). Paired electrical stimulation and the maximal contractile response of the ventricle. *Circulation Research*, **20**, 520–33.

Fleischer, S. & Inui, M. (1989). Biochemistry and biophysics of excitation–contraction coupling. *Annual Review of Biophysics & Biophysical Chemistry*, **18**, 333–64.

Furchgott, R. F. & de Gubareff, T. (1958). The high energy phosphate content of cardiac muscle under various conditions which alter contractile strength. *Journal of Pharmacology*, **124**, 203–18.

Hasselbach, W. (1964). Relaxing factor and the relaxation of muscle. *Progress in Biophysics & Molecular Biology*, **14**, 167–222.

Hilgemann, D. W. & Langer, G. A. (1984). Transsarcolemmal calcium movements in arterially perfused rabbit right ventricle measured with extracellular calcium-sensitive dyes. *Circulation Research*, **54**, 461–7.

Holroyde, M. J., Robertson, S. P., Johnson, J. D., Solaro, R. J. & Potter, J. D. (1980). The calcium and magnesium binding sites on cardiac troponin and their role in the regulation of myofibrillar adenosine triphosphatase. *Journal of Biological Chemistry*, **255**, 11688–93.

Inui, M., Saito, A. & Fleischer, S. (1987). Isolation of the ryanodine receptor from cardiac sarcoplasmic reticulum and identity with the feet structures. *Journal of Biological Chemistry*, **262**, 15637–42.

Jenden, D. J. & Fairhurst, A. S. (1969). The pharmacology of ryanodine. *Pharmacological Reviews*, **21**, 1–25.

Kentish, J. C. (1986). The effects of inorganic phosphate and creatine phosphate on force production in skinned muscles from rat ventricle. *Journal of Physiology*, **370**, 585–604.

Koch-Weser, J. & Blinks, J. R. (1963). The influence of the interval between beats on myocardial contractility. *Pharmacological Reviews*, **15**, 601–52.

Kort, A. A. & Lakatta, E. G. (1988). Spontaneous sarcoplasmic reticulum calcium release in rat and rabbit cardiac muscle: relation to transient and rested-state twitch tension. *Circulation Research*, **63**, 969–79.

Kurihara, S. & Sakai, T. (1985). Effects of rapid cooling on mechanical and electrical responses in ventricular muscle of guinea pig. *Journal of Physiology*, **361**, 361–78.

Langer, G. A. (1984). Calcium at the sarcolemma. *Journal of Molecular and Cellular Cardiology*, **16**, 147–53.

Langer, G. A. & Brady, A. J. (1963). Calcium flux in the mammalian ventricular myocardium. *Journal of General Physiology*, **46**, 703–19.

Lee, H.-C. & Clusin, W. T. (1987). Cytosolic calcium staircase in cultured myocardial cells. *Circulation Research*, **61**, 934–9.

Lewartowski, B. (1983). Calcium exchange. In *Cardiac Metabolism*, ed. A. J. Drake-Holland & M. I. M. Noble, pp. 101–16. Chichester: John Wiley.

Lüllmann, H. & Peters, T. (1977). Plasmalemmal calcium in cardiac excitation–contraction coupling. *Clinical & Experimental Pharmacology & Physiology*, **4**, 49–57.

MacLeod, K. T. & Bers, D. M. (1987). Effects of rest duration and ryanodine on changes of extracellular [Ca] in cardiac muscle from rabbits. *American Journal of Physiology*, **253**, C398–407.

Morad, M. & Goldman, Y. (1973). Excitation–contraction coupling in heart muscle: membrane control of development of tension. *Progress in Biophysics & Molecular Biology*, **27**, 257–313.

Morgan, J. P. & Blinks, J. R. (1981). Intracellular Ca^{2+} transients in the cat papillary muscle. *Canadian Journal of Physiology & Pharmacology*, **60**, 524–8.

Mullins, L. J. (1981). *Ion Transport in Heart*. New York: Raven Press.

Orchard, C. H. & Lakatta, E. G. (1985). Intracellular calcium transients and developed tension in rat heart muscle. *Journal of General Physiology*, **86**, 637–51.

Reuter, H. (1974). Exchange of calcium ions in the mammalian myocardium: mechanisms and physiological significance. *Circulation Research*, **34**, 599–605.

Robertson, S. P., Johnson, J. D. & Potter, J. D. (1981). The time-course of Ca^{2+} exchange with calmodulin, troponin, parvalbumin, and myosin in response to transient increases in Ca^{2+}. *Biophysical Journal*, **34**, 559–69.

Rousseau, E. & Meissner, G. (1989). Single cardiac sarcoplasmic reticulum Ca^{2+}-release channel: activation by caffeine. *American Journal of Physiology*, **256**, H328–33.

Rousseau, E., Smith, J. S. & Meissner, G. (1987). Ryanodine modifies conductance and gating behaviour of single Ca^{2+} release channels. *American Journal of Physiology*, **253**, C364–8.

Shattock, M. J. & Bers, D. M. (1989). Rat vs. rabbit ventricle: Ca flux and intracellular Na assessed by ion-selective microelectrodes. *American Journal of Physiology*, **256**, C813–22.

Siegl, P. K. S., Cragoe, E. J., Jr., Trumble, M. J. & Kaczorowski, G. J. (1984). Inhibition of Na^{+}/Ca^{2+} exchange in membrane vesicle and papillary muscle preparations from guinea pig heart by analogs of amiloride. *Proceedings of the National Academy of Sciences USA,* **81,** 3238–42.

Smith, G. L., Valdeolmillos, M., Eisner, D. A. & Allen, D. G. (1988). Effects of rapid application of caffeine on intracellular calcium concentration in ferret papillary muscles. *Journal of General Physiology,* **92,** 351–68.

Solaro, R. J., Wise, R. M., Shiner, J. S. & Briggs, F. N. (1974). Calcium requirements for cardiac myofibrillar activation. *Circulation Research,* **34,** 525–30.

Somlyo, A. V., Gonzalez-Serratos, H., Shuman, H., McClellan, G. & Somlyo, A. P. (1981). Calcium release and ionic changes in the sarcoplasmic reticulum of tetanised muscle: an electron probe study. *Journal of Cell Biology,* **90,** 577–94.

Sutko, J. L. & Willerson, J. T. (1979). Ryanodine alteration of the contractile state of rat ventricular myocardium. *Circulation Research,* **46,** 332–43.

Weber, A. & Herz, R. (1968). The relationship between caffeine contracture of intact muscle and the effect of caffeine on reticulum. *Journal of General Physiology,* **52,** 750–9.

Wendt-Gallitelli, M. F. (1985). Presystolic calcium-loading of the sarcoplasmic reticulum influences time to peak force of contraction. X-ray microanalysis on rapidly frozen guinea-pig ventricular muscle preparations. *Basic Research in Cardiology,* **80,** 617–25.

Wendt-Gallitelli, M. F., Jacob, R. & Wolburg, H. (1982). Intracellular membranes as boundaries for ionic distribution. *In situ* elemental distribution in guinea-pig heart muscle in different defined electromechanical coupling states. *Zeitschrift für Naturforschung,* **37c,** 712–20.

Wier, W. G. (1990). Cytoplasmic $[Ca^{2+}]$ in mammalian ventricle: dynamic control by cellular processes. *Annual Review of Physiology,* **52,** 467–85.

Wier, W. G. & Yue, D. T. (1986). Intracellular calcium transients underlying the short-term force–interval relationship in ferret ventricular myocardium. *Journal of Physiology,* **376,** 507–30.

Winegrad, S. (1968). Intracellular calcium movements of frog skeletal muscle during recovery from tetanus. *Journal of General Physiology,* **51,** 65–83.

Winegrad, S. & Shanes, A. M. (1962). Calcium flux and contractility in guinea pig atria. *Journal of General Physiology,* **45,** 371–94.

Wood, E. H., Heppner, R. L. & Weidmann, S. (1969). Inotropic effects of electric currents. *Circulation Research,* **24,** 409–45.

Woodworth, R. S. (1902). Maximal contraction, 'staircase' contraction, refractory period, and compensatory pause of the heart. *American Journal of Physiology,* **8,** 213–49.

A model for interval–force phenomena: unresolved issues

I. C. COOPER and M. I. M. NOBLE

Introduction

Ringer (1883) showed that calcium ions exchanged rapidly between intracellular and extracellular space in myocardium and that they were essential for contractility. Now Rich *et al.* (1988) have shown that the exchange and the effect on contractility occurs within one diastole. Many ideas on this subject have grown from the experience of studies of the force–interval relationship. These studies are relevant to the study of calcium release because it has been shown that with changes in interval between myocardial contractions, the tension and rate of rise of tension are linearly related to the calcium release, as measured with aequorin (Wier & Yue, 1986; see chapter by Yue in this book, pp. 95–109).

Another fundamental observation that is crucial to the understanding of calcium handling by myocardial cells is that of Antoni *et al.* (1969). They showed that modification of a single action potential did not affect the contraction of that beat, but affected the contraction of the subsequent beat. This shows that calcium entering the system during systolic depolarisation does not reach the contractile proteins, but enters an internal store. It is released from this store on the following depolarisation. From this it follows that any analysis of calcium handling must always take this lag into account. Throughout this review, *effects on calcium are searched for during a particular beat by observing the following beat*. This lag has led to the development of models of cellular calcium that can explain both the lag and other interval–force phenomena (for references see Wohlfart & Noble, 1982). A common feature of the models is the separation of the store into uptake and release compartments. In this chapter the same approach is adopted, but attempts are also made to assign to the functional compartments, anatomical possibilities and postulates of the role of subcellular organelles.

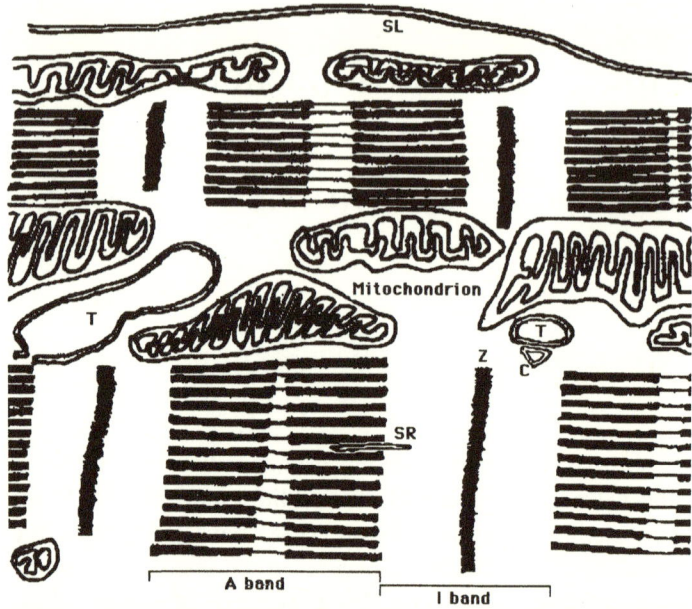

Fig. 1. Diagram to show relations of the various subcellular components in dog ventricular muscle. The proportions were obtained by computer scanning an electronmicrograph of a longitudinal section of cardiac muscle. The dimensions may be gauged from the A band which consists of myosin filaments 1.6 μm in length. SL = sarcolemma. Most of the SL exists as invaginations into the cell at each Z disc – the T-tubules. These are represented in section, marked T. SR = longitudinal sarcoplasmic reticulum, C = cisternae, or junctional SR; these have been drawn in to show their location and the distance of separation, but were not visible in the electronmicrograph. Mitochondria are plentiful and present a much greater surface area to the cytosol.

Anatomical considerations with respect to the myocardial calcium handling system

The ultrastructural anatomy of the myocardial cell has mostly been observed from the study of electronmicrographs. A schematic diagram made from a computer scan of such an electronmicrograph is presented in Fig. 1.

This shows the important structures and their special relationships. The sarcoplasmic reticulum (SR) is very difficult to see on plain observation of such pictures; in this case its components have been drawn in to illustrate their locations.

Sarcolemma (SL)

The characteristic feature of the sarcolemma of most working contractile myocardial cells is the extensive T-tubular system which is prominent in electronmicrographs. This poses a problem in deciding the relevance to force–interval effects of studies of excitation–contraction coupling with mechanically skinned preparations (Fabiato & Fabiato, 1975; Fabiato, 1983; Fabiato, 1985*a,b,c*). These studies require the use of a tissue lacking T-tubules, e.g. Purkinje fibres. It is difficult at the moment to relate the results from such studies to overall force–interval characteristics in ventricular muscle and intact heart. These studies are, however, important in establishing that calcium-induced calcium release occurs in the absence of sarcolemma.

A more extensively used method of skinning sarcolemma away from myocardial preparations is to use a detergent, but this unfortunately also removes the SR membranes. Thus, at the present time, there are no convincing data on force–interval relationships with and without the presence of sarcolemma.

That SL has properties for calcium binding and release has been shown by the studies of Langer (e.g. Langer, 1985). They show that there are calcium binding phospholipids which are located anatomically on the inner leaflet (Post *et al.*, 1988). The binding and release of calcium from these anionic lipids is dependent on proton activity (Langer, 1985), and therefore on transmembrane potential. Thus the idea of potential-dependent direct calcium release from the SL has developed a firm anatomical location, as with calcium-dependent calcium release from junctional SR.

Subsarcolemmal cisternae – junctional SR

That the sarcoplasmic reticulum is involved in calcium handling is well accepted. There seems good reason now to postulate anatomically separate parts. These are the longitudinal SR, located next to the contractile proteins and therefore apparently ideally placed anatomically for calcium uptake during relaxation, and the junctional SR close to the sarcolemma and therefore ideally placed for calcium release upon depolarisation of the sarcolemma. In both cardiac and skeletal muscle, the junctional SR is closely apposed to the sarcolemma at the cell surface and at the T-tubule membrane. The ryanodine receptor (see below) appears in the 'foot' structure which spans the gap between the T-tubule and the adjacent junctional SR. The SL-independent calcium-induced calcium release mechanism appears to be located within junctional SR, since it can be characterised in this subcellular fraction (see below). There are, however, some problems involved in assessing the relative contribution of junctional SR and SL to calcium binding and release. Electron microscopy shows that much of the surface area of the sarcolemma does not have junctional SR below it. However, calcium is distributed equally over the cell and Z-disc, i.e. T-tubule surfaces (Wendt-Gallitelli, 1986).

Longitudinal SR

The longitudinal component that is in apposition to the contractile filaments varies very much between species. The rat epitomises the type of myocardium which is densely provided with SR and has a high level of activation with calcium in systole. It has a force–frequency relationship unlike that of most species. Of particular note is the inverse relationship between steady state twitch force and frequency (Hadju, 1969), and the greatly prolonged mechanical restitution. Excitation–contraction coupling also differs in that there is a very short action potential with no plateau. Ryanodine (which is regarded as a reasonably specific inhibitor of the calcium-induced calcium release mechanism of SR, see chapter by Allen in this book, p. 43–65), has a major effect in this species. This could all be summarised by saying that rat heart is much more like skeletal muscle than the cardiac muscle of species like rabbit, guinea-pig, dog and man.

These latter species have relatively sparse SR anatomically, long action potentials with prominent plateaux, and a positive steady state force–frequency relationship; ryanodine has much smaller effects of overall contraction. There are intermediate species like the ferret, which behaves more like dog and man than the rat. These species show rest potentiation (see chapters by Ravens and Lewartowski in this book, pp. 245–58 and pp. 173–92), i.e. after a long rest they show a potentiated beat upon the first stimulus. This feature, which ferret shares with the rat, is also associated with moderately prominent SR development anatomically. One may postulate from these variations between species that force–frequency relations vary depending on the relative amount of SR present. A similar conclusion with regard to the rat has been reached by Jóhannsson (see his chapter in this book, pp. 227–43).

Mitochondria

Mitochondria are abundant in ventricular myocardium with its high metabolic rate. There is therefore a large surface area available on mitochondria for calcium binding; that this happens at high calcium ion concentrations has been demonstrated (Wendt-Gallitelli, 1986). From first principles, it follows that this large adsorption area will contribute to the removal of free calcium from the cytosol during the calcium transient, but the subsequent fate of this calcium is uncertain. This tissue is discussed in greater detail in the chapter by Lewartowski, pp. 173–92). The authors postulate that this calcium would be translocated back to release sites during diastole. However, the dynamics of such a process remains unclear.

Isolation and characterisation of subcellular organelles involved in calcium handling

Much work on the function of subcellular organelles has been inferred from studies in which heart tissue is homogenised and centrifuged. This permits separation of the fractions of lipid membranes which can form into vesicles. Subfractionation of these can be achieved by resuspension in carefully constituted media followed by centrifugation through sucrose gradients and layering over salt solutions. Further cycles of resuspension and centrifugation may be necessary before one can obtain reasonably pure fractions of SL, longitudinal SR and junctional SR (Meissner & Henderson, 1987).

These isolation procedures have been of great value in enabling investigators to characterise the functional properties of the various fractions using radiolabelled calcium, and other tracers. However, it is not surprising that the yields of these fractions can be variable. The problem of the quantitative contribution of the various subfractions to overall excitation–contraction behaviour remains.

Calcium release membranes

A particularly elegant way of studying the properties of the junctional SR fraction is to incorporate it into a lipid bilayer which can be voltage clamped. Thus, under the influence of applied electrical potentials, the opening and closing of single release channels can be recorded (Sitsapesan & Williams, 1990). Ryanodine binds specifically to the calcium-release channels of both cardiac and skeletal muscle SR. This has led to the use of ryanodine as a molecular probe in purifying and characterising the calcium-release channel (the so-called 'ryanodine receptor'). However, there are problems with its use as a tool, and variations in its effect from batch to batch emphasise this. In particular, the use of ryanodine has led to divergent results, e.g. it fully opens the channel reversibly, it irreversibly locks the channel into a subconductance open state, or it closes the channel completely in different experiments.

The single channel studies have shown that the primary activating ligand is calcium in nanomolar and micromolar concentrations. Further activation of the channel can be obtained with ATP and agents such as caffeine and the anthraquinones, e.g. doxorubicin (Holmberg & Williams, 1990). Cooling the channel also increases the open probability of the channel (Sitsapesan *et al.*, 1991). The effects of pH changes are not fully resolved, nor is the importance of the rate of change of calcium concentration at the cytosolic channel face. (In skeletal muscle, luminal calcium appears to be important.) A fundamental difference from skeletal muscle is that in the latter, the ryanodine receptor appears to be directly linked to the nifedipine binding site of the T-tubule via the 'foot'. Calcium release does not occur (as in heart) through calcium-induced calcium release.

Sarcolemmal calcium release was the subject of a previous controversy arising from the work of Lüllmann & Peters (1977), who proposed calcium binding to proton-dependent anionic phospholipids placed exclusively on the inner leaflet. These authors postulated that *all* the calcium released in heart muscle comes from the sarcolemmal site; this seems now to be wrong as judged from knowledge of junctional SR (above) and the various ryanodine experiments described in this chapter. However, the hypothesis can be retained for the ryanodine-independent behaviour. Evidence that calcium release can occur from sarcolemma is just as convincing as for junctional SR. Calcium exchange has been measured in cultured cells by Langer (1985) and the measurement repeated after gas dissection of the cells to remove all the cell contents including SR – only the sarcolemma remains. Repeat measurements show almost identical calcium exchange and pH dependence, indicating that there is an exchangeable calcium store located in sarcolemmal phospholipids. Treatment of cardiac tissue with phosphate-buffered fixative and precipitation of calcium as an electron-dense antimony complex shows that almost all of the tightly bound calcium is located in the sarcolemma. None is found in the SR (Borgers *et al.*, 1984). The prediction by Lüllmann & Peters of asymmetry of phospholipid composition between inner and outer sarcolemmal leaflets (with calcium binding phospholipid on the inner), has now been proved

(Post *et al.*, 1988). Such complete fulfilment of a hypothetical prediction is remarkable.

A fairly obvious point that is not often mentioned is that cisternae are close to the SL (Fig. 1) and that calcium released from the SL will obviously trigger release from the junctional SR, possibly more quickly and readily than calcium entering the cell from the extracellular space.

Physiological behaviour of the myocardial calcium handling system

Contraction and relaxation

It is well established that contraction results from a reaction between the contractile proteins, adenosine triphosphate (ATP) and calcium ions released into the myocardial cell cytoplasm, and the relationship between tension produced and calcium ion concentration (a non-linear sigmoid relationship), has been accurately defined (Kentish *et al.*, 1986). Changes in calcium release upon activation can be monitored (Allen & Kurihara, 1980; see also chapter by Allen in this book, pp. 43–65), using the relationship between calcium ion concentration and light emitted by aequorin (also non-linear).

The use of tension as a calcium ion transducer is limited by the fact that the entire relationship between calcium ion concentration and tension is altered by sarcomere length (Kentish *et al.*, 1986) and intracellular cyclic adenosine monophosphate (Herzig *et al.*, 1981), resulting from the action of catecholamines (Allen & Kurihara, 1980). If these two variables are kept constant and calcium release is altered only by changing the interval between excitations, tension and the rate of rise of tension turn out to be remarkably linearly related to calcium ion concentration as assessed with aequorin (Wier & Yue, 1986; and see chapter by Yue in this book, pp. 95–109).

Relaxation occurs through removal of calcium from the contractile proteins. To a certain extent this can occur through diffusion into the cytoplasmic space and adsorption on to the surfaces of organelles. This follows from the fact that some relaxation still occurs if depolarisation is prolonged, and if the SR is paralysed with ryanodine or caffeine. The rise of intracellular calcium ion concentration in systole will also result in some extrusion through calcium removal systems (see below). However, active removal of some calcium from the cytosol occurs through the action of the SR (England, 1983). What happens to the calcium after it has been taken up into the SR or been bound in this way?

The time course of calcium availability after relaxation

Just after the end of the refractory period, a premature excitation elicits a weak contraction. The contraction gains in strength as the interval prior to excitation is prolonged. The resulting positive curvilinear relationship between contractile tension and interval between excitations (Allen *et al.*, 1976; Edman & Jóhannsson, 1976) called 'mechanical restitution' has appeared within the last few years to provide important clues to the understanding of cellular calcium handling. (This phenomenon is reviewed in the chapter by Jóhannsson in this book, pp. 227–43).

The most popular idea is that calcium, as well as being taken up by the SR during relaxation, is released again by the SR upon excitation (Fabiato, 1985*a,b,c*). One might well ask at this point the following questions: 'If all the activator calcium is already in the SR after relaxation, why should there be a delay before it can be released again?', and 'What biochemical process within the SR is involved?'

As far as the authors are aware, no answers to these questions are to be found in the literature. One possibility is that the uptake site is the longitudinal SR and that the sarcolemmal cisternae (junctional SR) and subsarcolemma are the release sites. One could then postulate that the delay in releasability could be due to the diffusion time required for calcium to move from longitudinal ST to surface cisternae.

Upon repolarisation, it is postulated that the calcium affinity of one or other of the cisternae or sarcolemma (see chapter by Langer in this book, pp. 193–210) becomes maximal in the cell, so that calcium diffuses from other sites back to the cell surface and T tubules. An accumulation of calcium in the superficial release sites as a function of time would result in mechanical restitution. This diffusion must occur across calcium concentration gradients within the cell in which the absolute level of concentration never exceeds threshold for the contractile proteins (i.e., 10^{-7} to 10^{-11} M), so that the tissue remains relaxed. Thus the concentration gradient for diffusion during diastole will be less than for diffusion in the reverse direction upon activation, and the time taken will therefore be longer. As will be discussed below, this mechanism can only be postulated for the fast initial phase of mechanical restitution.

Other possible explanations (see chapter by Allen in this book, pp. 43–65) do not seem to explain the fact that hypertrophy prolongs this phase of mechanical restitution (Cooper, 1990). This is consistent with the idea of a diffusion distance, since the principal effect of hypertrophy is to increase cell size, i.e. increase the distance required for calcium to diffuse from the contractile proteins to the surface sites. Another phenomenon that is consistent with this idea is that the initial speed of restitution is similar between species (chapter by Jóhannsson in this book, pp. 227–43) even though the normal beat to beat interval in life is very different. For instance, full mechanical restitution in man takes approximately one second and a typical heart rate is 60 beats/min. By contrast the same order of interval is required for mechanical restitution in small rodents with prevailing heart rates of 300 beats/min. A biochemical process might be expected to adapt to optimise the interval for restitution and prevailing heart rate. The lack of such adaptation seems to speak for an anatomical basis for mechanical restitution related to cell size (which is relatively constant between species).

Cisternal calcium release is a popular idea now because of the discovery of ryanodine-sensitive calcium release channels in this 'junctional' or 'heavy' SR fraction (see above, and chapter by Allen in this book, pp. 43–65). An idea of the contribution of the junctional SR can be obtained by looking at mechanical restitution in isolated muscle strips before and after ryanodine (Cooper & Fry, 1990; Cooper, 1990). It is found that the time course of mechanical restitution can be characterised by a series of time constants, the number of which varies according to species. Thus the increase in contractility with increasing diastolic interval has time constants τ_1 and τ_2, which are followed by a decaying component with time constant τ_3 as shown in Fig. 2.

The second component of mechanical restitution characterised by τ_2 is

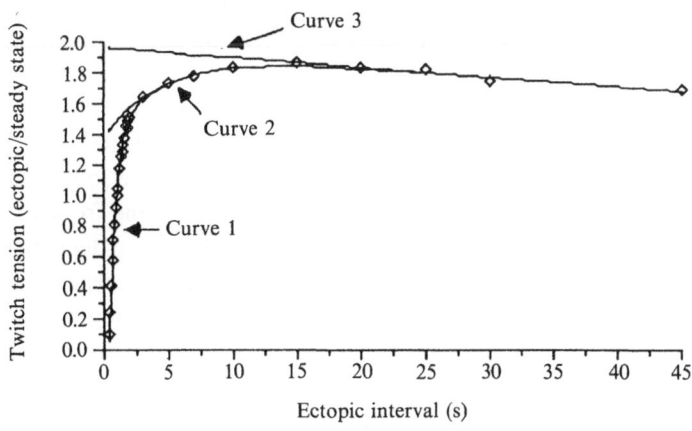

Fig. 2. Time course of mechanical restitution in human ventricular muscle at 37 °C. Three exponential curves extrapolated over data from a single experiment. Curves 1, 2 and 3 have time constants τ_1, τ_2 and τ_3 respectively.

not discernible in guinea-pigs, or in other species after ryanodine (Cooper, 1990). One could speculate that the second component represents the contribution of diastolic calcium accumulation in junctional SR, leaving the first component to represent diastolic calcium accumulation by sarcolemma (SL). The species differences in the rising phase of mechanical restitution are largely absent after ryanodine, which removes phase 2 (Cooper, 1990). The prominence of phase 2 is the reason why there is rest potentiation in some species (e.g. rat) and rest decay in others (e.g. guinea-pig) – see chapters by Lewartowski and by Ravens in this book, pp. 173–92 and pp. 245–58)

Ryanodine speeds up the first phase (reduces τ_1), suggesting that junctional SR accumulation of calcium is relatively slow and its removal reveals the faster SL accumulation.

Does mechanical restitution start with relaxation or repolarisation?

In recent meetings on excitation–contraction coupling, this question has appeared crucial because, if calcium merely requires time to become releasable within the SR and merely needs second inward current calcium to trigger release, the time course of mechanical restitution should begin with relaxation, whereas if trigger calcium has to accumulate at the polarised sarcolemma (Lüllmann, Peters & Preuner, 1983) to be released upon depolarisation, the time course of mechanical restitution should begin with repolarisation.

Pacing experiments suggested the latter (Franz *et al.*, 1983), but the variation in repolarisation time achieved (dependent on action potential duration) was sufficiently small for this result to be unconvincing.

In order to test this point more critically, Arlock, Noble & Wohlfart (1990) varied the duration of the diastolic interval between depolarisations using voltage clamp methods. They recorded the force of the following depolarisation as a function of (a) the total test interval (time from the moment of depolarisation of previous clamp until the moment of depolarisation of the subsequent clamp) and (b) the test diastolic interval (time from *repolarisation* of the previous clamp until the moment of depolarisation the subsequent clamp). They obtained the usual positive curvilinear relationship between the previous interval between clamps and the force elicited by the second depolarisation (mechanical restitution). They then studied this for two durations of the previous clamp, namely 200 and 500 ms. If mechanical restitution depends on a biochemical process within SR, or on transfer from longitudinal to junctional SR, the time course

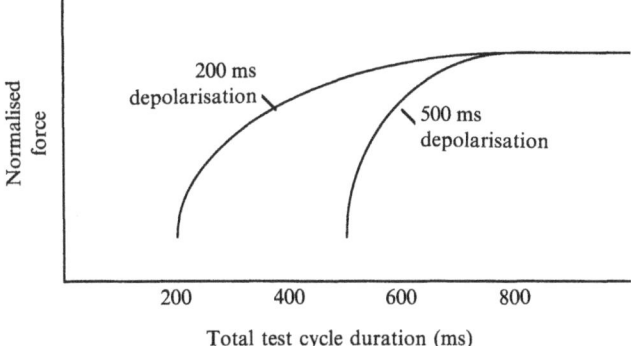

Fig. 3. Schematic diagram of results of Arlock, Noble & Wohlfart (1990). The test cycle (length plotted on the abscissa) consisted of a depolarisation lasting 200 or 500 ms, followed by a variable diastolic interval. The relationship of force to interval (mechanical restitution) was measured. The onset of mechanical restitution was delayed by 300 ms in the case of the 500 ms depolarisation, i.e. mechanical restitution is initiated by repolarisation.

should begin with calcium release and re-uptake, elicited by the first depolarisation. However, if trigger calcium (to trigger calcium release from SR) has to accumulate near the polarised sarcolemma to be released upon depolarisation, the time course of mechanical restitution should begin with repolarisation, i.e. the test diastolic interval determines mechanical restitution. The result points clearly to the latter, in that mechanical restitution was delayed 300 ms for a first clamp of 500 ms compared to a clamp of 200 ms when test interval was the independent variable (Fig. 3). The onset of mechanical activity was identical for the two test clamp durations when test *diastolic* interval was the independent variable.

These results arc capable of different interpretations if considered in isolation. The second inward current also restitutes over the first phase of mechanical restitution, and declines over the second (SR dependent) phase. Thus, in the intact preparation, one could simply conclude that the first phase is accompanied by a proportional calcium induced calcium release from junctional SR. However, such an interpretation could not be sustained if similar results were to be obtained in the presence of ryanodine; experiments addressed to this point are clearly required.

Calcium recirculation

That calcium recirculates within the internal store is argued from the fact that calcium released on a particular stimulus is proportional to the calcium released on the preceding beat, as long as each of these stimuli occur after a constant interval. This phenomenon is also the basis for explanations of the time course of decay of contractility from a potentiated state (ter Keurs *et al.*, 1990 and chapter by ter Keurs in this book, pp. 259–76). Recirculation of calcium is an old idea that was persuasively advocated by Morad & Goldman (1972). Does this recirculation take place within the longitudinal SR, or does the recirculated calcium have to move to superficial sites to be released on the subsequent beat (a postulate that follows from the study of mechanical restitution, above)? The former proposition implies that SR is the release as well as the uptake site (Fabiato & Fabiato, 1975; Fabiato, 1983); the latter suggestion implies a separate release site, e.g. subsarcolemmal cisternae – junctional SR (Kaufmann *et al.*, 1974) or sarcolemma (Lüllmann *et al.*, 1983). The authors are not aware of any simple experiments of the effect of ryanodine on recirculation; such experiments should shed some light on this unresolved issue. In their opinion, the inhibition of post-extrasystolic potentiation by ryanodine points to recirculation probably occurring via the SR. On the other hand, frog displays post-extrasystolic potentiation despite a poorly developed internal store (Morad & Goldman, 1972).

The proportionality of calcium release on one beat to that of the previous beat has been shown in a number of studies (Wohlfart & Noble, 1982). With other variables held constant, it is found that the tension (or rate of tension, or aequorin light signal) of one beat is linearly related to the tension of the preceding beat. The slope of this linear relationship is the proportion of calcium released on one beat which is recirculated to the next – the 'recirculation fraction'.

Potentiation induced by voltage-clamping (Wood, Heppner & Weidmann, 1969) allows this relationship to be explored over a much wider range of values than previous methods. Much prolongation of a depolarisation causes enormous potentiation of the force of the contraction caused by the next depolarisations. Recirculation was studied in this way by Arlock & Wohlfart (1990) who plotted the force of the second potentiated beat against that of the first potentiated beat. Non-linearity was shown up at the extreme edge of the range, and linearity confirmed in the physiological range previously studied. Some interventions which would obviously be expected to have an effect on recirculation fraction (e.g. adrenaline) have not been explored with this methodology. Such experiments would seem to be of great importance in future research. The determinants of recirculation fraction remain unknown. A major uncertainty is the relative importance of the avidity of the SR for calcium (e.g.

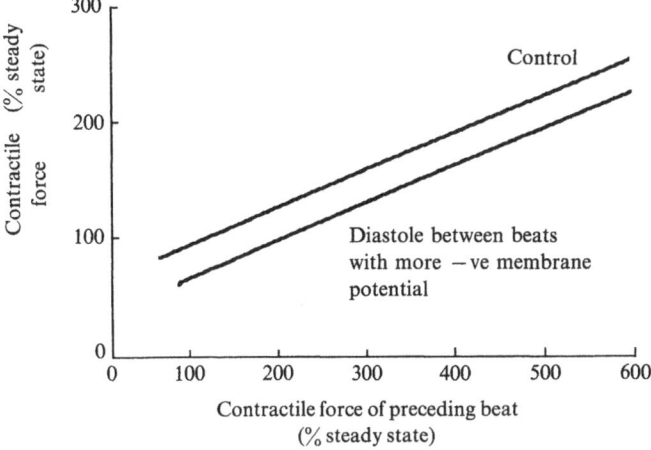

Fig. 4. Schematic diagram of results reported by Arlock, Noble & Wohlfart (1991). The preceding contraction was potentiated by a prolonged voltage clamp depolarisation (pre-preceding depolarisation). The contractile force was proportional to this potentiated preceding contraction with a slope of the relationship equal to the recirculation fraction (RF). When one diastole between the beats was clamped to a more negative potential, to increase diastolic extrusion by Na/Ca exchange, contractile force was reduced at all levels of potentiation, i.e. a fixed amount of calcium extrusion was achieved without a change in the fraction of Ca extruded (which is equal to 1-RF).

as enhanced by cyclic AMP) versus the avidity of extrusion routes for calcium (affecting recirculation fraction as the 'left over' intracellular calcium).

Calcium extrusion

Extrusion will occur in systole when calcium is released and the increased intracellular calcium ion concentration would be expected to drive calcium extrusion in proportion to that concentration. The contribution of diastolic Na/Ca exchange was recently investigated in experiments by Arlock, Noble & Wohlfart (1991) shown schematically in Fig. 4.

They were able to increase calcium extrusion for a single diastole by lowering diastolic potential, presumably by altering sodium/calcium exchange. Following a prolonged potentiating depolarisation, beats at equal intervals were initiated by further control depolarisations. The resting potential between these was the steady-state potential of −40 mV. The force of the second potentiated beat was plotted against that of the first potentiated beat to obtain an almost linear relationship with a slope equal to the recirculation fraction. When the resting membrane potential between the first and second potentiated beats was changed to $-70\,\text{mV}$ a parallel downward shift of the relationship occurred, indicating no change in recirculation fraction, but a fixed amount of calcium extrusion.

These results are compatible with the idea of calcium extrusion being divided into (a) an amount in diastole dependent on membrane potential but not on the amount released in the previous systole and (b) an amount in systole proportional to the amount released. Which of the known extrusion methods – Na/Ca exchange and Ca pumping (Caroni & Carafoli, 1981) – could be responsible for each of these components? Clearly both could be responsible for (b) because both would be expected to increase Ca extrusion when intracellular Ca increases. However, there are good reasons (below) for postulating that the Na/Ca exchange mechanism works in the calcium in/sodium out mode during depolarisation. If this is substantiated, it leaves calcium pumping as the remaining known possibility for systolic calcium extrusion. Property (a) is clearly dependent on diastolic membrane potential in a manner compatible with Na/Ca exchange.

Thus a major question mark remains over the cellular mechanism responsible for calcium recirculation and extrusion which is proportional to calcium release.

Potentiation

The phenomenon whereby a premature depolarisation is followed by a strong beat may also provide clues to the mechanisms of cellular calcium handling.

This phenomenon occurs whether the action potential of the extra-systole is prolonged (rabbit) or shortened (dog, man) and the potentiation

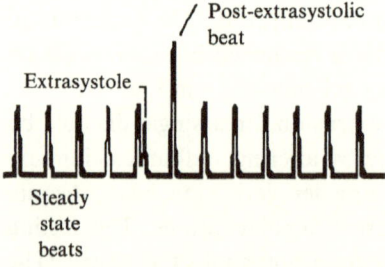

Fig. 5. Schematic diagram of post-extrasystolic potentiation.

can produce more than double the force of the control beats. A similar phenomenon is the potentiation caused by a previous prolonged depolar-isation (Wood *et al.*, 1969; Arlock & Wohlfart, 1990), in which a more than doubling of force is easily achieved. This suggests an excess of calcium entry on the premature beat over and above any calcium 'saved' because of incomplete calcium release on the extrasystole (see discussions of mechanical restitution above). This excess calcium entry implies a negative feedback control of released calcium on calcium inflow rate during the action potential, i.e. a premature beat which is weak and associated with a small calcium release lets in more calcium ions (Wohlfart & Noble, 1982). There is a negative feedback effect of released calcium upon second inward current (Bassingthwaite, Fry & McGuigan, 1976); this current, which is inhibited by calcium ions (Hess & Tsien, 1984), is a possible means of extra Ca ion entry on the weak beat (but see discussion below).

The other possible mechanism for negative feedback control of Ca ion entry by intracellular calcium is Na/Ca exchange, but this requires that this is a mechanism for Ca ion *entry* during depolarisation, thus excluding it as a mechanism for systolic calcium extrusion.

Calcium release

It is currently thought that calcium is released from the sarcoplasmic reticulum, when a little calcium entering through the calcium channel on the second inward current triggers the main release from the SR calcium store by the process of calcium-induced calcium-release, a phenomenon that can be demonstrated when sarcolemma is removed (Fabiato, 1983, 1985*a,b,c*; see also chapter by Allen in this book, pp. 43–65). Does it logically follow that calcium entering by the calcium channel is the trigger for normal calcium release? That this is the case has been argued from the effects of calcium antagonists such as nifedipine which have negative inotropic effects, but it is uncertain whether these are pure pharmacologi-cal tools. There are at least three different proteins which separately bind verapamil, diltiazem and the dihydropyridines; there is also lipid binding, and the effects of calcium antagonists on contractility are variable. Indeed, some dihydropyridines are positively inotropic.

The role of the second inward current is also called into question by voltage clamp experiments in which potentiation (by a preceding prolonged depolarisation) is associated with suppression of the second inward current (Bassingthwaite *et al.*, 1976). Furthermore, an inverse relationship

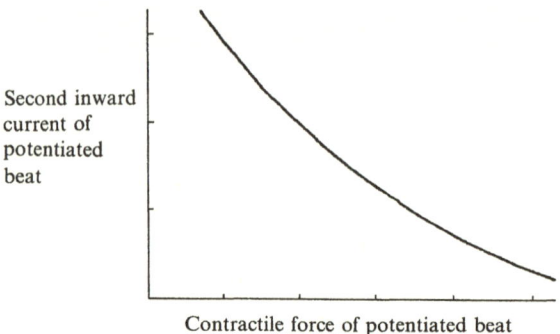

Second inward
current of
potentiated
beat

Contractile force of potentiated beat

Fig. 6. Schematic diagram of results of Arlock & Wohlfart (1990). Contractile force was potentiated by a prolonged preceding voltage clamp depolarisation. The relationship of second inward current to contractile force of the potentiated beats was inverse.

between current and force has been confirmed by Arlock and Wohlfart in both multicellular (1990) and unicellular (unpublished) preparations – see Fig. 6.

This is apparently discordant with the idea that calcium release from the SR is proportional to the trigger calcium entering through the second inward current (Fabiato, 1985a,b,c). It is still possible to retain this idea as long as one postulates rather extreme changes in the gain of the calcium-induced calcium release process. The result is more consistent with calcium release being dependent on the amount in the SR, which is then released by a threshold amount of calcium in an all-or-none manner.

There are some other discordant facts. External calcium can rapidly exchange with the calcium of the internal store (e.g. Rich et al., 1988). This group has identified the fast pool of contractile calcium in both rat and rabbit (with evidence that it is sarcolemmal) and also a slower pool in the rat, which they identify as being located in sarcoplasmic reticulum. The fast pool of calcium is not extracellular because it is rapidly affected (full effect within one diastole) by change in extracellular sodium ion concentration via Na–Ca exchange (Rich et al., 1988); the very rapid time course for complete exchange confirms a sarcolemmal site for the fast calcium pool.

Important facts are (1) that ryanodine does not abolish the fast phase of mechanical restitution, and (2) that the onset of mechanical restitution requires repolarisation of the sarcolemma. These considerations seem to lend some credence to the idea that the ryanodine-independent calcium release could be derived from the sarcolemma as postulated by Lüllman

& Peters (1977), and Langer (1985). Such calcium could act as the trigger for calcium-induced calcium release. There is obviously a requirement for more definition of which features of the many phenomena described are ryanodine sensitive, accepting the reservations given about this tool above.

'*Dead time*'

Variation in the duration of the action potential affects the following beat rather than the concomitant beat, i.e. extra calcium entering in a particular depolarisation does not contribute to the concomitant reaction of calcium with the contractile elements but enters the internal calcium store and is released on the subsequent depolarisation. In intact dog experiments Drake *et al.* (1982) found no correlation between action potential duration (recorded monophasically) and contractility of the concomitant beat, but did find a correlation with contractility of the subsequent beat (Drake-Holland *et al.*, 1983). However, there was a residual negative constant after correlation, so that a constant time had to be subtracted from the action potential duration of the first beat when expressing the proportionality with contractility of the subsequent beat. This was called 'dead time'. The dead time averaged 120 ms and implied that the first 120 ms of depolarisation was 'dead' for calcium entry. Clearly, the second inward current begins during this time. How could it not be carrying calcium inward?

Arlock and Wohlfart (1990) tested this point more formally by recording contractile force as a function of the duration of preceding clamped depolarisation.

The well known potentiating effect of duration of depolarisation upon subsequent force is illustrated in Fig. 7. However, there is a clear time delay before this potentiation begins. This point has been emphasised by drawing a line to the data which intercepts the time axis. F2 does not exceed the control force (100%) for about 120 ms. This is remarkably similar to the results obtained in dogs.

Further experiments are required to test this finding. However, at the moment it appears that the first 100 ms of depolarisation is neutral for calcium entry. This is most easily explained on the basis of a balance between calcium entry during this time from the second inward current and calcium exit via sodium/calcium exchange (Powell & Noble, 1989). In early systole with a high intracellular calcium (during the intracellular calcium release), such sodium/calcium exchange has a positive equilibrium potential favouring sodium entry and calcium exit generating an inward current.

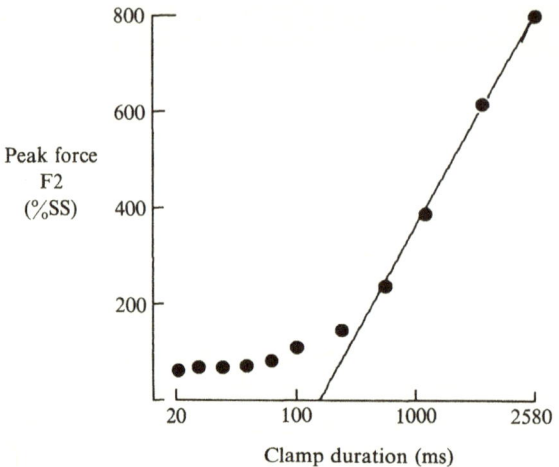

Fig. 7. The force of a beat following a prolonged voltage clamp depolarisation expressed as a function of the duration of that depolarisation. Note that there is little effect for 100 ms.

Calcium entry

If the mechanism of calcium entry during a prolonged depolarisation causing potentiation is not the second inward current, we must postulate that it occurs through the remaining known mechanism–systolic Na/Ca exchange. Evidence on this question was obtained in voltage clamp experiments (e.g. Arlock & Wohlfart, 1990).

The dependence of second inward current upon membrane potential is a bell-shaped function (Fig. 8) with a maximum at around zero. If this is the mode of calcium entry, the force of the following contraction should have a similar relationship to the (preceding) systolic membrane potential. In contrast, Na/Ca exchange at low (late systolic) intracellular calcium favours Ca extrusion more and more as membrane potential goes from about -10 mV to more negative potential, and favours calcium entry more and more as membrane potential goes from about -10 mV to more positive potentials. The force of the subsequent contraction is less than control with depolarisations to less than -10 mV, and rises progressively with depolarisations to more and more positive potentials. Thus the force of the subsequent contraction closely mirrors the calcium entry via Na/Ca exchange of the (preceding) depolarisation. It should be noted that the increasing potentiation with increasing systolic membrane potential is accompanied by a decreasing second inward current amplitude (Fig. 8),

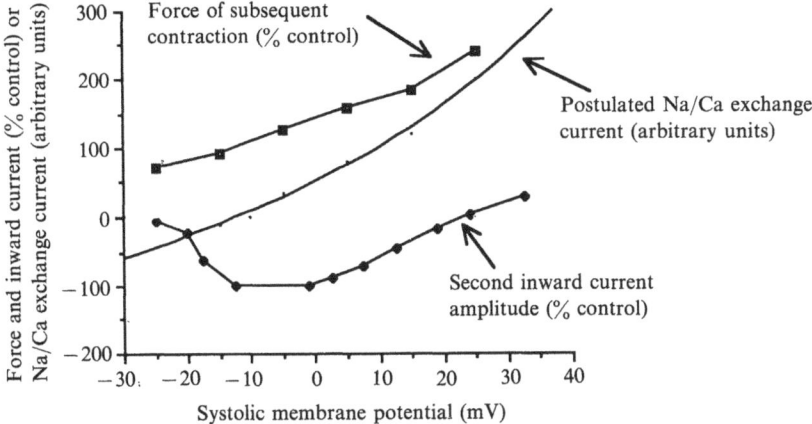

Fig. 8. Data for second inward current and force replotted from Arlock & Wohlfart (1990). Inward currents are plotted with negative sign. As the calcium entry (assessed from force of the subsequent beat) increases, second inward current increases and then declines. Over most of the negative membrane potential range, these two variables change in opposite directions. Calcium entry assessed from the force of the subsequent beat provides an estimate of Na/Ca exchange current. This current is assumed to have an equilibrium potential in late systole (after decay of the calcium transient) at $-10\,\mathrm{mV}$, and outward current (positive) is associated with calcium entry (three Na^+ for one Ca^{2+}) at more positive potentials. See also Fig. 6 in the chapter by Boyett *et al.*, p. 120.

again emphasising the dichotomy between late systolic calcium entry and second inward current, together with the consonant changes in Na/Ca exchange and calcium entry.

Clearly much further research will be required in the future to clarify these problems.

Mechanism of the Bowditch effect

Thus far, the force–interval phenomena of mechanical restitution and post-extrasystolic potentiation has been concentrated on. What of Bowditch's staircase?

In Bowditch's original experiments, the change from rest to beating was accompanied by a rising increase in contractility from beat to beat until a plateau value was reached (see translation of his paper in this book pp. 3–30). In intact hearts this phenomenon is seen as a similar build-up in contractility after a decrease on the first beat when the frequency of contraction is increased (Fig. 9) (the PIEA of Blinks & Koch-Weser, 1961).

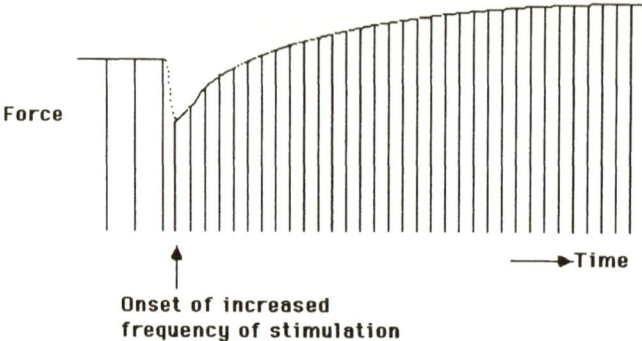

Force

→Time

↑
**Onset of increased
frequency of stimulation**

Fig. 9. Typical effect of an increase in stimulation frequency on force in mammalian ventricular muscle. When the frequency of stimulation is increased, the first beat is weaker (incomplete mechanical restitution or negative inotropic effect of activation); contractility builds up over time during subsequent beats (Bowditch effect, frequency potentiation or positive inotropic effect of activation).

The phenomenon is also responsible for the increase in contractility of the optimum contractile response with priming frequency (Edman & Jóhannsson, 1976; Pidgeon *et al.*, 1980).

There is still doubt about the mechanism whereby released calcium is increased by a higher prevailing frequency of contraction. Edman and Jóhannsson's idea was that the increase in number of depolarisations per minute, which they quantified as the total time the membrane was depolarised, implies increased time for calcium entry. Such an increased entry would lead to continuously increasing contractility, so that one must assume that calcium extrusion 'catches up' after a lag time, leading to the plateau of the response and the new steady state (Noble, 1978). Edman and Jóhannsson were thinking at that time about second inward current as the means of entry because there was no reason then to doubt that this was a 'calcium current'. Doubt must now be cast on this idea in view of the finding of 'dead time' (above) which (if it is a correct observation), indicates that second inward current is neutralised as a calcium entry pathway by calcium extrusion mediated by sodium/calcium exchange (Powell & Noble, 1989).

The same kind of reasoning can, however, be applied to sodium. The increase in number of depolarisations per minute does lead to an increase in intracellular sodium. This, and its consequences, are fully explored in the chapter of this book by Boyett *et al.*, pp. 111–72. One consequence of the increase in intracellular sodium is an increase in Na/K ATP-dependent sodium pumping. Na/K exchange is electrogenic, so that increased frequency causes diastolic hyperpolarisation and increased background outward current causing shortening of the action potential (Drake *et al.* 1982; Seed *et al.*, 1987).

Another consequence of increased intracellular sodium is increased systolic calcium entry and decreased diastolic calcium extrusion via Na/Ca exchange. This will lead to an accumulation of calcium in the internal store, and increased released calcium, i.e. a Bowditch effect. Boyett & Harrison (1992–see below), have indeed successfully simulated this with their model. Also, in view of our present hypothesis for Na/Ca exchange as a mechanism for systolic calcium entry (above), we can return to the Edman and Jóhannsson idea, but with Na/Ca exchange as the mechanism of calcium entry, i.e. an increased number of depolarisations per minute leading to increased time for calcium entry by Na/Ca exchange. Thus a Bowditch effect would occur by this means even without the assistance offered by increased intracellular sodium.

What is the most appropriate model for force–interval relationships, calcium handling and excitation–coupling in 1992?

The previous neglect of sarcolemmal properties has led to the postulation of models that have veered towards that extreme (e.g. Noble & Drake-Holland, 1990) or towards previously more generally accepted ideas (Fabiato & Fabiato, 1975; Fabiato, 1983, 1985*a,b,c*). Present working hypotheses are required to retain the essential features of previous models (see chapter by Allen in this book, pp. 43–65), and also take into consideration some of the new information presented in this chapter.

It is desirable that the function of the model be formalised by equations so that predictions can be made for experimental testing. This has been done for rabbit atrium by Hilgemann & Noble (1987). In this chapter, we have confined ourselves to ventricular muscle which can also be modelled by a modified version (Boyett & Harrison, 1992), which is elaborated in the chapter by Boyett *et al.* in this book. One particular interesting feature of this model is calcium entry via Na/Ca exchange during a premature stimulus, similar to that postulated above (Fig. 8) for prolonged depolarisation.

There is of course, no doubt that such a model will prove inadequate in the future. There are clearly a number of unresolved issues which we have attempted to highlight, together with others that we have not gone into. The purpose of this, as with previous models, is to stimulate necessary future research. It seems that Bowditch, force–interval and excitation/contraction coupling research is now at a very exciting stage.

Acknowledgements

M. I. M. Noble is supported by the Garfield-Weston Trust as Weston Professor of Cardiovascular Medicine. We are grateful to Rebecca Sitsapesan for assistance and criticism.

References

Allen, D. G., Jewell, B. R. & Wood, E. H. (1976). Studies of the contractility of mammalian myocardium at low rates of stimulation. *Journal of Physiology*, **254**, 1–17.

Allen, D. G. & Kurihara, S. (1980). Calcium transients in mammalian ventricular muscle. *European Heart Journal*, 1 Suppl A, 5–15.

Antoni, H., Jacob, R. & Kaufmann, R. (1969). Mechanische Reaktionen des Frosch- und Säugetiermyocards bei Veränderung der Aktionspotential-Dauer durch konstante Gleichstromimpulse. *Pflügers Archiv*, **306**, 33–57.

Arlock, P., Noble, M. I. M. & Wohlfart, B. (1990). Cardiac cell membrane repolarization is required for the onset of mechanical restitution in isolated ferret ventricular muscle. *Journal of Physiology*, **420**, 87P.

Arlock, P., Noble, M. I. M. & Wohlfart, B. (1991). Effect of diastolic membrane potentials on twitch force in isolated ferret papillary muscle. *Journal of Physiology*, **438**, 19P.

Arlock, P. & Wohlfart, B. (1990). Force production following transient transmembrane potential changes in ferret and guinea pig papillary muscles. *Acta Physiologica Scandinavica*, **140**, 63–72.

Bassingthwaite, J. B., Fry, C. H. & McGuigan, J. A. S. (1976). Relationship between internal calcium and outward current in mammalian ventricular muscle; a mechanism for control of the action potential duration? *Journal of Physiology*, **262**, 15–37.

Blinks, J. R. & Koch-Weser, J. (1961). Analysis of the effects of changes in rate and rhythm upon myocardial contractility. *Journal of Pharmacology and Experimental Therapeutics*, **134**, 373–89.

Borgers, M., Thone, F., Verheyen, A. & ter Keurs, H. E. D. J. (1984). Localisation of calcium in skeletal and cardiac muscle. *Histochemical Journal*, **16**, 295–309.

Boyett, M. R. & Harrison, S. M. (1992). The control of cardiac contractility by Na–Ca exchange; a study using a computer model of excitation–contraction coupling in the heart. *Journal of Physiology*, in press.

Caroni, P. & Carafoli, E. (1981). The Ca^{2+}-pumping ATPase of heart sarcolemma. Characterisation, calmodulin dependence, and partial purification. *Journal of Biological Chemistry*, **236**, 3263–70.

Cooper, I. C. (1990). Mechanical restitution in isolated human myocardium. MD Thesis, University of London.

Cooper, I. C. & Fry, C. H. (1990). Mechanical restitution in isolated mammalian myocardium: species differences and underlying mechanisms. *Journal of Molecular and Cellular Cardiology*, **22**, 439–52.

Drake, A. J., Noble, M. I. M., Schouten, V., Seed, A., ter Keurs, H. E. D. J. &

Wohlfart, B. (1982). Is action potential duration of the intact dog heart related to contractility or stimulus rate? *Journal of Physiology*, **331**, 499–510.

Drake-Holland, A. J., Noble, M. I. M., Pieterse, M., Schouten, V. J. A., Seed, W. A., ter Keurs, H. E. D. J. & Wohlfart, B. (1983). Cardiac action potential and contractility in the intact dog heart. *Journal of Physiology*, **345**, 75–85.

Edman, K. A. P. & Jóhannsson, M. (1976). The contractile state of rabbit papillary muscle in relation to stimulation frequency. *Journal of Physiology*, **254**, 565–81.

England, P. J. (1983). Phosphorylation of cardiac muscle contractile proteins. In *Cardiac Metabolism*, ed. A. J. Drake-Holland & M. I. M. Noble, pp. 365–90. Chichester: J. Wiley & Sons.

Fabiato, A. (1983). Calcium-induced release of calcium from the cardiac sarcoplasmic reticulum. *American Journal of Physiology*, **245**, C1–14.

Fabiato, A. (1985a). Rapid ionic modifications during the aequorin-detected calcium transient in skinned canine cardiac Purkinje cell. *Journal of General Physiology*, **85**, 189–246.

Fabiato, A. (1985b). Time and calcium dependence of activation and inactivation of calcium-induced release of calcium from sarcoplasmic reticulum of a skinned canine cardiac Purkinje fibre. *Journal of General Physiology*, **85**, 247–89.

Fabiato, A. (1985c). Stimulated calcium current can both cause calcium loading in and trigger calcium release from the sarcoplasmic reticulum of a skinned canine cardiac Purkinje cell. *Journal of General Physiology*, **85**, 291–320.

Fabiato, A. & Fabiato, F. (1975). Contractions induced by a calcium-triggered release of calcium from the sarcoplasmic reticulum of single skinned cardiac cells. *Journal of Physiology*, **249**, 469–95.

Franz, M. R., Schaefer, J., Schoettler, M., Seed, W. A. & Noble, M. I. M. (1983). Electrical and mechanical restitution of the human heart at different rates of stimulation. *Circulation Research*, **53**, 815–22.

Hajdu, S. (1969). Mechanics of the Woodworth staircase phenomenon in heart and skeletal muscle. *American Journal of Physiology*, **216**, 206–14.

Herzig, J. W., Kohler, G., Pfizer, G., Ruegg, J. C. & Woffle, G. (1981). Cyclic AMP inhibits contractility of detergent-treated glycerol extracted cardiac muscle. *Pflügers Archiv*, **391**, 208–12.

Hess, P. & Tsien, R. W. (1984). Mechanism of ion permeation through calcium channels. *Nature*, **309**, 453–6.

Hilgemann, D. W. & Noble, D. (1987). Excitation–contraction coupling and extracellular calcium transients in rabbit atrium: reconstruction of basic cellular mechanisms. *Proceedings of the Royal Society B*, **230**, 163–205.

Holmberg, S. R. M. & Williams, A. J. (1990). Patterns of interaction between anthraquinone drugs and the calcium release channel from sarcoplasmic reticulum. *Circulation Research*, **67**, 272–83.

Kaufmann, R., Bayer, R., Furniss, T., Krause, H. & Tritthart, H. (1974). Calcium-movement controlling cardiac contractility – II. Analog computation of cardiac excitation–contraction coupling on the basis of calcium kinetics in a multi-compartment model. *Journal of Molecular and Cellular Cardiology*, **6**, 543–59.

Kentish, J. C., ter Keurs, H. E. D. J., Ricciardi, L., Bucx, J. J. & Noble, M. I. M. (1986). Comparison between the sarcomere length–force relations of intact and skinned trabeculae from rat right ventricle. *Circulation Research*, **58**, 755–68.

Langer, G. A. (1985). The effect of pH on cellular and membrane calcium binding and contraction of myocardium. A possible role for sarcolemmal phospholipid in EC coupling. *Circulation Research*, **57**, 374–82.

Lüllmann, H. & Peters, T. (1977). Plasmalemmal calcium in cardiac excitation–contraction coupling. *Clinical Experimental Pharmacology and Physiology*, **4**, 49–57.

Lüllmann, H., Peters, T. & Preuner, J. (1983). Role of plasmalemma for calcium homeostasis and for excitation–contraction coupling in cardiac muscle. In *Cardiac Metabolism* ed. A. J. Drake-Holland and M. I. M. Noble, pp. 1–18. Chichester: J. Wiley & Sons.

Meissner, G. & Henderson, J. S. (1987). Rapid calcium release from cardiac sarcoplasmic reticulum vesicles is dependent on Ca^{2+} and is modulated by Mg^{2+}, adenine nucleotide, and calmodulin. *Journal of Biological Chemistry*, **262**, 3065–73.

Morad, M. & Goldman, Y. (1972). Excitation–contraction coupling in heart muscle: membrane control of development of tension. *Progress in Biophysics and Molecular Biology*, **27**, 257–313.

Noble, M. I. M. (1978). *The Cardiac Cycle*. Oxford: Blackwell Scientific Publications.

Noble, M. I. M. & Drake-Holland, A. J. (1990). A cellular calcium model for the second inward channel, calcium release, uptake, sequestration, recirculation and restitution. In *Imaging Analysis and Simulation of the Cardiac System*, ed. S. Sideman & R. Beyar, pp. 525–43, London: Freund Publishing House.

Pidgeon, J., Lab, M., Seed, W. A., Elzinga, G., Papadoyannis, D. & Noble, M. I. M. (1980). The contractile state of cat and dog heart in relation to the interval between beats. *Circulation Research*, **47**, 559–67.

Post, J. A., Langer, G. A., Op den Kamp, J. A. F. & Verkleij, A. J. (1988). Phospholipid asymmetry in cardiac sarcolemma. Analysis of intact cells and 'gas-dissected' membranes. *Biochimica et Biophysica Acta*, **943**, 256–66.

Powell, T. & Noble, D. (1989). Calcium movements during each heart beat. *Molecular and Cellular Biochemistry*, **89**, 103–8.

Rich, T., Langer, G. A. & Klassen, M. G. (1988). Two components of coupling calcium in single ventricular cells of rabbits and rats. *American Journal of Physiology*, **254**, 937–46.

Ringer, S. (1883). A further contribution regarding the influence of the different constituents of the blood on the contraction of the heart. *Pflügers Archiv*, **308**, 91–110.

Seed, W. A., Noble, M. I. M., Oldershaw, P., Wanless, R. B., Drake-Holland, A. J., Redwood, D., Pugh, S. & Mills, C. (1987). Relationship of human cardiac action potential duration to the interval between beats; implications for the validity of rate corrected QT interval (QTc). *British Heart Journal*, **57**, 32–7.

Sitsapesan, R. & Williams, A. J. (1990). Mechanisms of caffeine activation of single calcium-release channels of sheep cardiac sarcoplasmic reticulum. *Journal of Physiology*, **423**, 425–39.

Sitsapesan, R., Montgomery, R., MacLeod, K. T. & Williams, A. J. (1991). Sheep cardiac sarcoplasmic reticulum calcium-release channels: modification of conductance and gating by temperature. *Journal of Physiology*, **434**, 469–88.

ter Keurs, H. E. D. J., Gao, W. D., Bosker, H., Drake-Holland, A. J. & Noble,

M. I. M. (1990). Characterisation of the decay of frequency induced potentiation and of post-extrasystolic potentiation. *Cardiovascular Research*, **24**, 903–10.

Wendt-Gallitelli, M. F. (1986). Ca-pools involved in the regulation of cardiac contraction under positive inotropy. X-ray microanalysis on rapidly-frozen ventricular muscles of guinea-pig. *Basic Research in Cardiology*, **81** (Suppl), 25–32.

Wier, W. G. & Yue, D. T. (1986). Intracellular calcium transients underlying the short-term force–interval relationship in ferret ventricular myocardium. *Journal of Physiology*, **376**, 507–30.

Wohlfart, B. & Noble, M. I. M. (1982). The cardiac excitation–contraction cycle. *Pharmacology & Therapeutics*, **16**, 1–43.

Wood, E. H., Heppner, R. L. & Weidmann, S. (1969). Inotropic effects of electric currents. *Circulation Research*, **24**, 409–45.

Part 3

Cellular processes underlying interval–force behaviour and their control

Relationships between intracellular free calcium and force with changes of interval

DAVID T. YUE

Early investigators of the force–interval relation (FIR) held in common one clairvoyant hunch (e.g. Woodworth, 1902; Braveny & Kruta, 1958); that the FIR reflected accumulation and depletion of some 'activator substance' as a function of stimulus rate. The process of grounding this notion in experimental reality began with the discovery that calcium binding to troponin regulates tension development (Ebashi & Endo, 1968); calcium ions then became suspect as the mysterious activator substance. Direct observations of parallel fluctuations of tension and calcium followed with the use of aequorin as an indicator of intracellular free $[Ca^{2+}]$ ($[Ca^{2+}]_i$) (Allen & Kurihara, 1980; Wier, 1980). The latter observations brought to fruition the current consensus that the FIR actually provides a look at the interrelation between cytoplasmic calcium and stimulus rate, as viewed through the 'lens' of a calcium-tension relation. This chapter focuses upon the elementary properties of this important lens, in particular the relation between $[Ca^{2+}]_i$ and tension during twitch contraction of heart muscle.

Steady-state relation between $[Ca^{2+}]_i$ and tension: relevant to physiological twitch contraction?

The majority of our knowledge about the relation between $[Ca^{2+}]_i$ and tension in heart has been limited to that obtained at steady state in preparations with disrupted surface membranes (e.g. the review by Fabiato, 1982). Yet physiological twitch contractions, those relevant to the FIR, arise from phasic $[Ca^{2+}]_i$ transients that rise and fall on the timescale of 100 ms or less. This consideration raises a first, and crucial question: do steady-state relations between $[Ca^{2+}]_i$ and tension pertain to physiological twitch contractions?

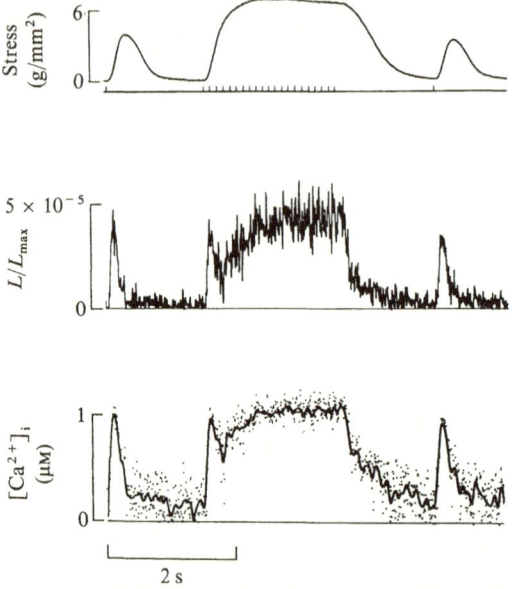

Fig. 1. Original records of tension (stress), aequorin luminescence (L/L_{max}), and $[Ca^{2+}]_i$ (calculated from luminescence) obtained from a rapidly stimulated ferret papillary muscle in 6 mM extracellular [Ca] and 5 μM ryanodine. The unfiltered $[Ca^{2+}]_i$ record appears as points in the bottom trace. The filtered $[Ca^{2+}]_i$ record (10 Hz lowpass filter) is the solid curve in the bottom trace. Stimuli were delivered at the times indicated by the marks displayed below the upper trace. Records obtained at 30 °C here, and in all subsequent figures except Fig. 6. Further details of the methods have been described at length (Yue, Marban, & Wier, 1986; Yue, 1987). From Yue *et al.* (1986) with the permission of the Rockefeller University Press.

To investigate this point, one needs to produce steady levels of $[Ca^{2+}]_i$ and tension in intact muscle. Such a requirement for steady levels in intact tissue had long been considered to be difficult or impossible to achieve. However, Fig. 1 demonstrates the finding that, after exposure to ryanodine, an inhibitor of normal calcium release from sarcoplasmic reticulum (Imagawa *et al.*, 1987; Rousseau, Smith & Meissner, 1987), nearly steady levels of $[Ca^{2+}]_i$ and tension could be produced upon rapid 10 Hz stimulation of a cardiac papillary muscle microinjected with the photoprotein aequorin. Furthermore, Figs. 2(*a*) and 2(*b*) show that by varying extracellular $[Ca^{2+}]$ the levels of $[Ca^{2+}]_i$ and tension could be graded from rest (trace 1) to an apparently saturating level (trace 5), thus enabling the determination of the steady-state relation between $[Ca^{2+}]_i$ and tension in intact muscle (Fig. 2(*c*)).

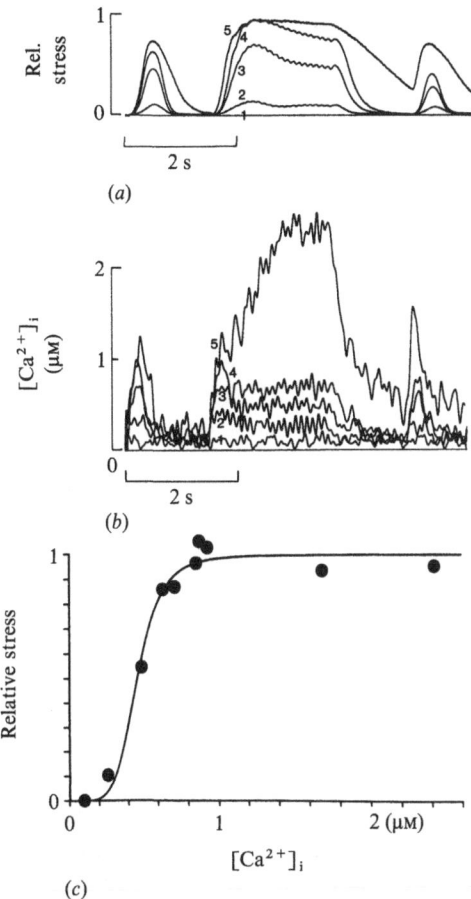

Fig. 2. Different steady levels of force and $[Ca^{2+}]_i$ obtained at various extra-cellular [Ca] in ferret papillary muscle. (a) Tension normalised by the maximum achieved. (b) $[Ca^{2+}]_i$ after lowpass filtering at 10 Hz, corresponding to extra-cellular [Ca] of: (1) 1 mM, unstimulated; (2) 1 mM; (3) 3 mM; (4) 5 mM; (5) 15 mM and 300 nM Bay K 8644. (c) Tension (normalised relative to the maximum achieved) plotted as a function of $[Ca^{2+}]_i$. Points are plotted from records 1–5 and from five other tetani (not shown). The solid curve is a best-fitting Hill function with $n = 5.6$ and half-saturation at 0.46 μM. From Yue *et al.* (1986) with the permission of the Rockefeller University Press.

How does the interrelation between $[Ca^{2+}]_i$ and tension during physiological contractions compare with such a steady-state relation? Fig. 3 plots peak tension as a function of peak $[Ca^{2+}]_i$ from physiological contractions (before exposure to ryanodine), and compares this with the plot of steady-state $[Ca^{2+}]_i$ and tension (circles and solid curve) obtained

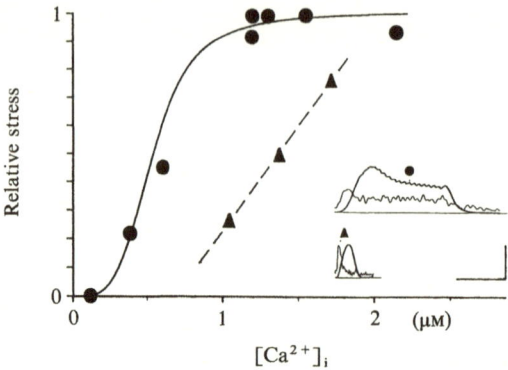

Fig. 3. Relationship between $[Ca^{2+}]_i$ and tension obtained during rapid stimulation and during physiological contractions in ferret papillary muscle. The filled circles represent the relationship between steady force and $[Ca^{2+}]_i$ obtained during rapid stimulation as in Fig. 1. The solid triangles are the relationship between peak force and peak $[Ca^{2+}]_i$ for physiological contractions. The inset shows representative tension (thick trace) and $[Ca^{2+}]_i$ (thin trace) signals from which the two relations were constructed. Horizontal calibration was 1 s, and vertical calibration was 1.5 µM or 50% maximal force. Adapted from Yue *et al.* (1986).

during rapid stimulation. The inset displays representative records of tension and $[Ca^{2+}]_i$ of the sort used to construct the two relations. That the dashed relation, representing the physiological contractions, is substantially right-shifted with respect to the solid, steady-state relation indicates that $[Ca^{2+}]_i$ and tensions are clearly not at steady state.

This result cautions against extrapolating from the steady state to explain changes in the behaviour of physiological contractions. One pertinent example is that current understanding of the Frank–Starling relation is based largely upon observed shifts of the steady-state $[Ca^{2+}]_i$-tension relation along the $[Ca^{2+}]_i$ axis with variations in muscle length (Babu, Sonnenblick, & Gulati, 1988). Such an explanation now conspicuously requires refinement, since Fig. 3 demonstrates clearly that the steady-state relation does not apply to the physiological heartbeat.

Empirical relationships between tension and $[Ca^{2+}]_i$ during physiological twitch contraction

If tension and $[Ca^{2+}]_i$ are not at steady state during physiological contractions, how then are these two variables interrelated under the conditions used to determine the FIR? This issue is addressed in Fig. 4,

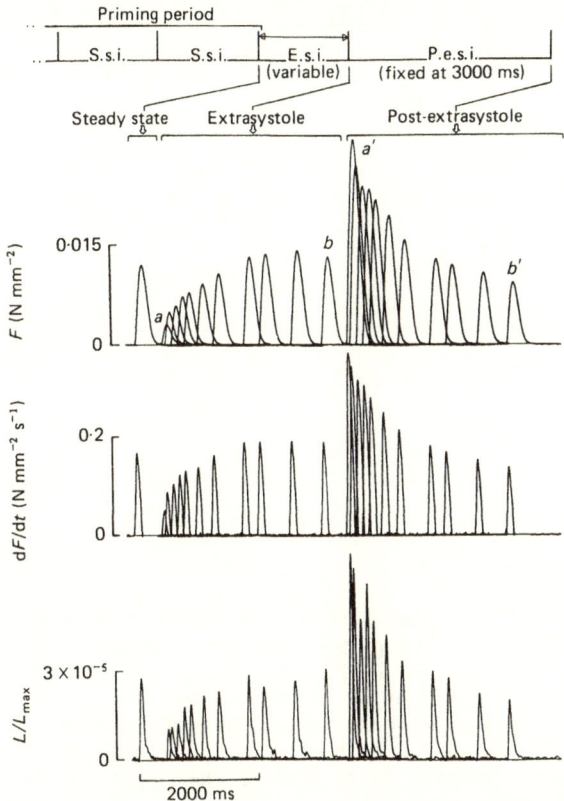

Fig. 4. Original records illustrating restitution and post-extrasystolic potentiation in ferret papillary muscle, with the stimulation protocol at top. Traces show tension (top); rate of tension development (middle), and aequorin luminescence (bottom) from steady-state, extrasystolic, and post-extrasystolic beats. Records have been aligned in time to superimpose steady-state responses. Responses a and a′ are from an extrasystole and subsequent post-extrasystole obtained with e.s.i. = 50 ms; b and b′ correspond to e.s.i. = 3000 ms. S.s.i. was 1500 ms, and extracellular [Ca] = 0.7 mM. Traces average 16–32 sweeps. From Wier & Yue (1986), with the permission of the *Journal of Physiology*. In this and the following figures, the term force is used interchangeably with tension per unit cross-sectional area of the muscle.

which shows force (F), the derivative of force (dF/dt) and $[Ca^{2+}]_i$-regulated luminescence (L/L_{max}) arising from a multitude of variably restituted and potentiated contractions that span nearly the entire range of contractility of which the muscle was capable. The stimulus protocol used to elicit the responses is shown at top. Fig. 5 correlates the strength

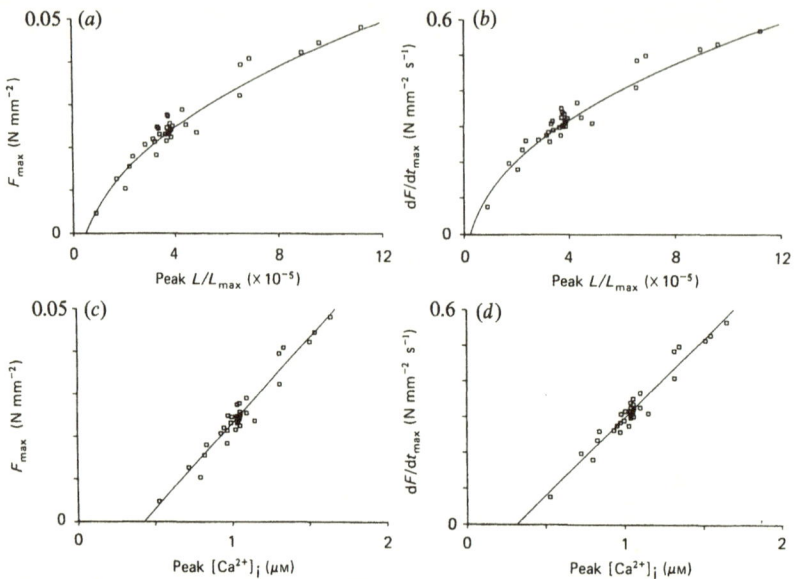

Fig. 5. Relation of L/L_{max} to F_{max} (*a*), and to dF/dt_{max} (*b*) derived from variably restituted and potentiated beats in ferret papillary muscle. The continuous curves in (*a*) and (*b*) are of the form F_{max} or $dF/dt_{max} = G(L/L_{max})^{1/2.37} + H$ ($G =$ 2.965 N mm^{-2} and $H = 0.017$ N mm^{-2} in (*a*); $G = 32.4$ N mm^{-2} s^{-1} and $H =$ 0.134 N mm^{-2} s^{-1} in (*b*). (*c*) and (*d*) show the same relations after peak L/L_{max} has been calibrated to peak $[Ca^{2+}]$. The continuous lines in (*c*) and (*d*) were fitted to the data by linear regression. From Wier & Yue (1986), with the permission of the *Journal of Physiology*.

of contraction and $[Ca^{2+}]_i$ for these responses. Panels (*a*) and (*b*) plot peak F (F_{max}) and peak dF/dt (dF/dt_{max}) as a function of peak L/L_{max}, respectively; these show curvilinear relations. However, when luminescence is calibrated to $[Ca^{2+}]_i$, both F_{max} and dF/dt_{max} correlate linearly with peak $[Ca^{2+}]_i$ in panels (*c*) and (*d*). The results indicate that, although tension and $[Ca^{2+}]_i$ are not at steady state during twitch contraction, both F_{max} and dF/dt_{max} nevertheless bear an intimate, and perhaps linear relation to peak $[Ca^{2+}]_i$. Although the observed linearity may be considered to be an entirely empirical finding, this characteristic is highly reproducible. In fact, later on in the chapter, it will be argued that the linear relation between dF/dt_{max} and peak $[Ca^{2+}]_i$ may derive from a more fundamental property of cardiac muscle.

So far conclusions have drawn heavily upon estimates of $[Ca^{2+}]_i$ derived from muscles microinjected with aequorin. As with any Ca

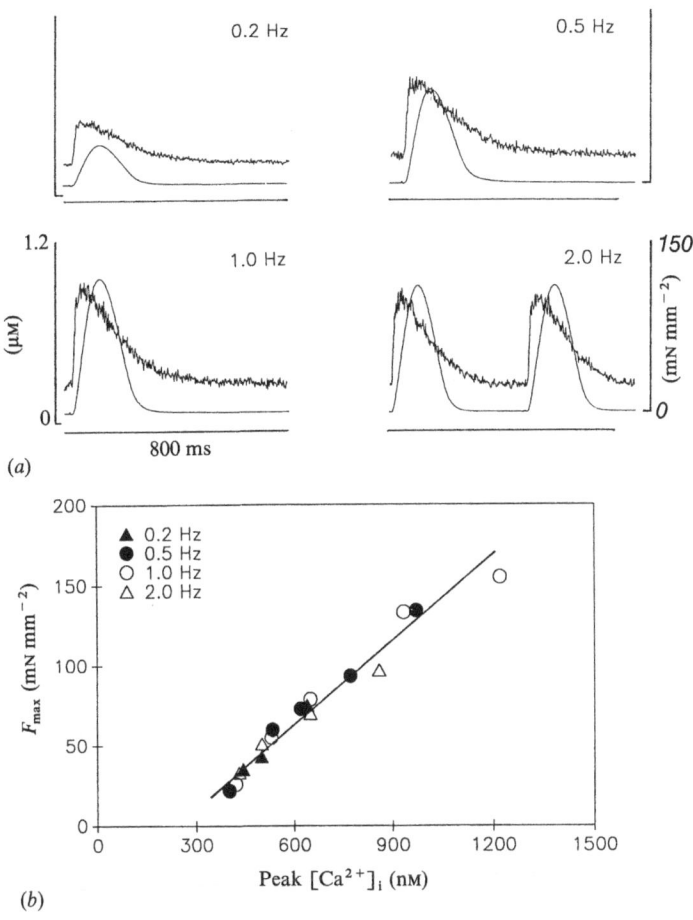

Fig. 6. Relation between Ca and tension during various frequencies of stimulation in a rat trabecula at 22 °C. (a) Tension (noise-free) and $[Ca^{2+}]_i$ (after calibration of Fura-2 ratios) records obtained with extracellular $[Ca] = 1$ mM. (b) F_{max} and peak $[Ca^{2+}]_i$ from records in (a), and others obtained at different extracellular $[Ca]$. Adapted from Backx *et al.* (1990).

indicator, the aequorin methodology is subject to potential errors (see, e.g. Yue & Wier, 1985). Fig. 6 summarises results from an elegant study by Backx, Lamont, and ter Keurs (1990) that uses Fura-2, a fluorescent Ca indicator, to estimate $[Ca^{2+}]_i$ from a cardiac trabecula loaded iontophoretically with the indicator. Here, F_{max} and peak $[Ca^{2+}]_i$, monitored in contractions elicited at various rates of stimulation, also correlate quite linearly. Because the potential errors of Fura-2 are opposite to those of aequorin (Yue & Wier, 1985), the concordance of results with the two methodologies provides strong support for the intimate relation between F and $[Ca^{2+}]_i$ during twitch contraction of heart muscle.

Relation between peak $[Ca^{2+}]_i$ and *amount* of Ca released from sarcoplasmic reticulum (SR)

To this point the interrelation between tension and $[Ca^{2+}]_i$ has been considered. Yet, mechanistic models developed to explain the FIR (e.g. Wohlfart, 1979, and his chapter of this book) reason in terms of the amount of calcium released from SR as a function of stimulus interval. Hence, although strength of contraction and peak $[Ca^{2+}]_i$ are closely, and perhaps linearly related, there may still be considerable distortion in the relationship between peak $[Ca^{2+}]_i$ and amount of calcium released from SR on a given beat. Because of this concern, this section develops a model that relates free intracellular $[Ca^{2+}]$ to total myoplasmic $[Ca]$ (free $[Ca^{2+}]$ + $[Ca]$ bound by intracellular buffers). This sort of analysis provides a first-order assessment of how total $[Ca]$ released from SR relates to resulting $[Ca^{2+}]_i$.

Fig. 7 summarises the Ca-buffering model used here. It is identical to that of Robertson *et al.* (1981), except that: (a) more recently determined rate constant values (Pan & Solaro, 1984), were incorporated, and (b) the

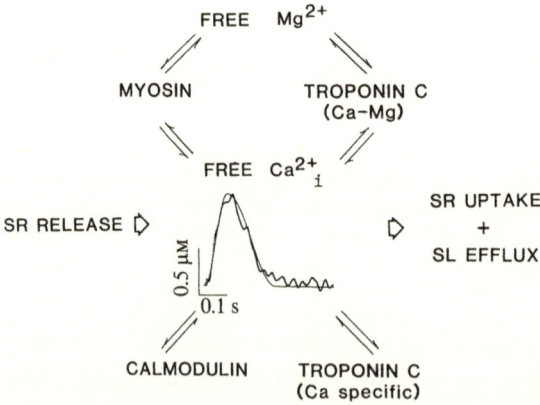

Fig. 7. Schematic diagram of calcium buffering model for heart muscle. The noisy trace in the centre is an experimentally determined $[Ca^{2+}]_i$ signal obtained from an aequorin-injected preparation; the superimposed smooth trace is the assumed $[Ca^{2+}]_i$ transient for the model. SR and SL refer to sarcoplasmic reticulum and sarcolemma, respectively. Adapted from Yue, Wier & Sagawa (1984).

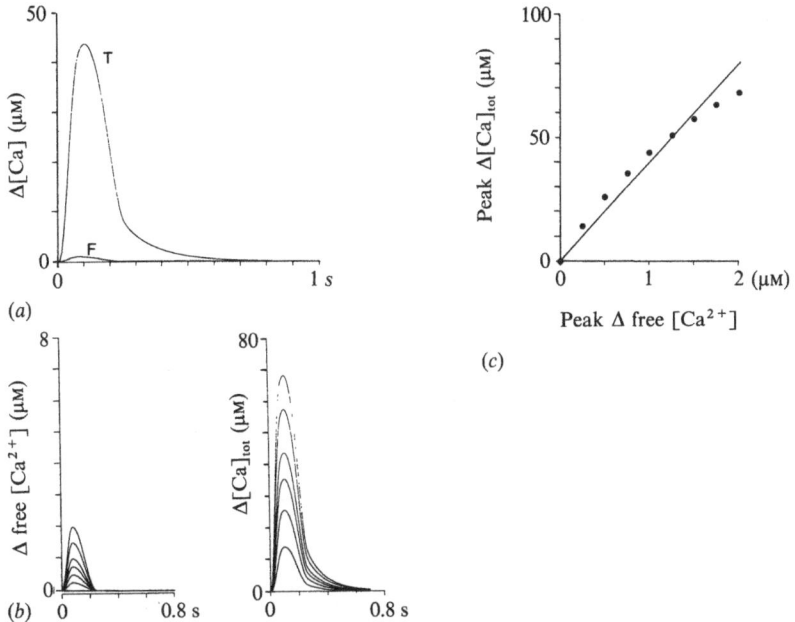

Fig. 8. Kinetic model analysis of the relationship between $[Ca^{2+}]_i$ and total $[Ca]$. (a) Trace F is the change in $[Ca^{2+}]_i$ ($[Ca^{2+}]_i$ – resting $[Ca^{2+}]_i$) assumed for a twitch. Trace T is the total change (increase) in $[Ca]$ (bound and free) calculated from the model. (b) Left; set of developed $[Ca^{2+}]_i$ transients applied as an input to the model. Developed $[Ca^{2+}]$ is the net change in free intracellular $[Ca^{2+}]$ ($[Ca^{2+}]_i$ – resting $[Ca^{2+}]_i$). Right: corresponding set of traces representing the net increase in total $[Ca]$ ($\Delta[Ca]_{tot}$) calculated from the model in response to the developed $[Ca^{2+}]_i$ transients at left. (c) Relationship between peak $\Delta[Ca]_{tot}$ and peak Δfree $[Ca^{2+}]$ (filled circles) derived from the kinetic buffering model. Line is a visual fit. Adapted from Yue *et al.* (1984).

$[Ca^{2+}]_i$ transients used as the input to the binding model were chosen to approximate our experimentally determined $[Ca^{2+}]_i$ transients according to the following equation (eqn. 1):

$$[Ca^{2+}]_i \, (\mu M) = 0.1 + (A/2)(1 - \cos[\pi t/0.08]) \qquad :0 < t < 0.08 \text{ s}$$

$$= 0.1 + (A/2)(1 - \cos[\pi(t + 0.09)/0.17]) \quad :0.08 < t < 0.25 \text{ s}$$

$$= 0.1 \qquad\qquad\qquad :0.25 \text{ s} < t$$

where A is the peak developed $[Ca^{2+}]_i$. For a given $[Ca^{2+}]_i$ transient (trace F in Fig. 8(a)), the net increase in total myoplasmic $[Ca]$, defined as $\Delta[Ca]_{tot}$ ($[Ca^{2+}]_i$ + $[Ca]$ bound to buffers – resting $[Ca^{2+}]_i$ – resting $[Ca]$ bound to buffers), could be calculated for any instant during the contraction cycle (trace T in Fig. 8(a)) by numerical integration of the model. The net increase in $\Delta[Ca]_{tot}$ must have been equal to the $[Ca]$ that entered the myoplasmic space by SR release minus that which departed by SR uptake and sarcolemmal efflux. Ca influx by sarcolemmal Ca channels is considered to be too small to figure in this calculation. If one assumes that very little $[Ca]$ has left the myoplasm by the time of peak $\Delta[Ca]_{tot}$, then the peak increase in $\Delta[Ca]_{tot}$ would be a good estimate of the total $[Ca]$ released from SR on a given beat. To mimic the experiment-ally-observed changes in developed $[Ca^{2+}]_i$, Δ free $[Ca^{2+}]$, the variable A was varied while other factors in eqn. 1 were kept constant. This is in keeping with the experimental result that variably restituted and potenti-ated $[Ca^{2+}]_i$ transients are very close to being differently scaled versions of each other. Fig. 8(b) shows the various Δ free $[Ca^{2+}]$ and $\Delta[Ca]_{tot}$ transients produced by such variation. Fig. 8(c) plots the peak values of these transients as a function of each other, thereby establishing the relation between amount of $[Ca]$ released and peak developed $[Ca^{2+}]_i$. The relation is slightly curved and concave to the x-axis. This is a manifestation of the progressive saturation of the buffers as the total released $[Ca]$ is increased. However, as suggested by the hand-fitted line in the figure, the relationship is approximated rather well by a linear relation passing through the origin. Hence, not only is the relation between F_{max} (or dF/dt_{max}) and peak $[Ca^{2+}]_i$ close to linear, so too may be the relation between amount of $[Ca]$ released from SR and peak $[Ca^{2+}]_i$. Indeed, the FIR appears to be quite a good lens through which to view the Ca handling of heart muscle.

Fundamental implications of a linear relation between dF/dt_{max} and peak $[Ca^{2+}]_i$?

Why should F_{max} (or dF/dt_{max}) correlate linearly with peak $[Ca^{2+}]_i$? Is this relationship merely fortuitous, or does it provide important mechanis-tic clues as to how F and $[Ca^{2+}]_i$ are related under transient conditions? This section raises tantalising evidence favouring an affirmative response to this question.

Fig. 9(a–d) shows experimental records obtained from a physiological contraction before exposure to ryanodine. The portion of these records during which $[Ca^{2+}]_i$ is expected to be spatially uniform, and therefore most suitable for rigorous kinetic analysis, is indicated by the computer model estimates of the spatial variance of $[Ca^{2+}]_i$ in Fig. 9(e) (from Wier & Yue, 1986). The convergence of the solid trace in the middle (spatial-average $[Ca^{2+}]_i$) and the dashed traces (bracketing spatial standard

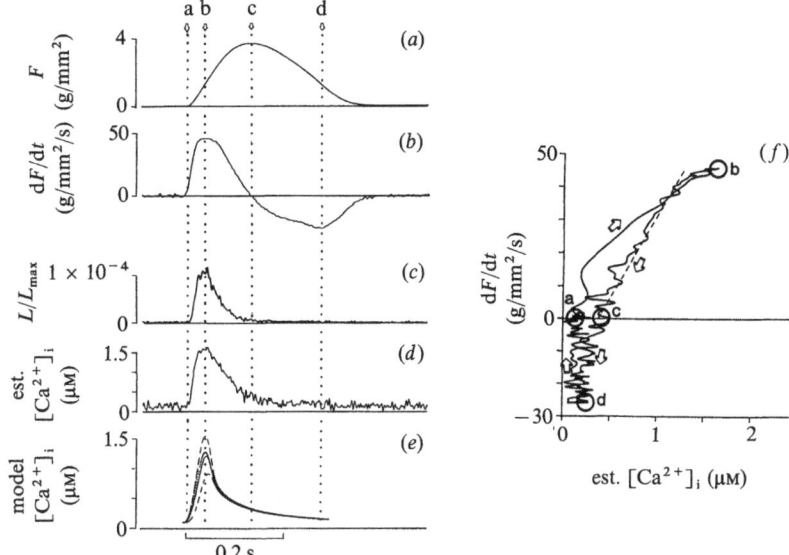

Fig. 9. Experimental records and model analysis of physiological contraction in ferret papillary muscle: (a) Developed tension (F); (b) Rate of rise of tension (dF/dt); (c) Aequorin luminescence (L/L_{max}); (d) $[Ca^{2+}]_i$ calculated from luminescence; (e) Computer model estimates of spatial distribution of $[Ca^{2+}]_i$. Solid trace of (e) is spatial average $[Ca^{2+}]_i$, dashed traces are bracketing spatial standard deviations of $[Ca^{2+}]_i$, and dotted curve is $[Ca^{2+}]_i$ expected to be reported from aequorin luminescence. (f) Moment to moment plot of dF/dt vs. $[Ca^{2+}]_i$ derived from (b) and (d). Arrows show direction in which plot was traced. Open circles and labels a–d indicate points in plot corresponding to various points in contraction defined as onset (a); dF/dt_{max} (b); peak tension (c); and maximum negative dF/dt (d). Adapted from Yue (1987).

deviations of $[Ca^{2+}]_i$) indicate that $[Ca^{2+}]_i$ should become spatially uniform shortly following the peak of the $[Ca^{2+}]_i$ transient and onward (instant b and thereafter).

Examination of these records demonstrates a striking resemblance between the positive portion of the dF/dt trace (Fig. 9(b)) and the $[Ca^{2+}]_i$ trace (Fig. 9(d)), especially in the interval where $[Ca^{2+}]_i$ tends towards greater spatial homogeneity (instants b–c). To examine this similarity more closely, Fig. 9(f) plots dF/dt vs. $[Ca^{2+}]_i$ for every instant throughout an entire cardiac cycle. The resultant trajectory forms a loop which is traversed as indicated by the arrows; the points in the loop corresponding to the instants a–d are circled and labelled accordingly. The portion of the trajectory shortly following b and onward through c closely follows the

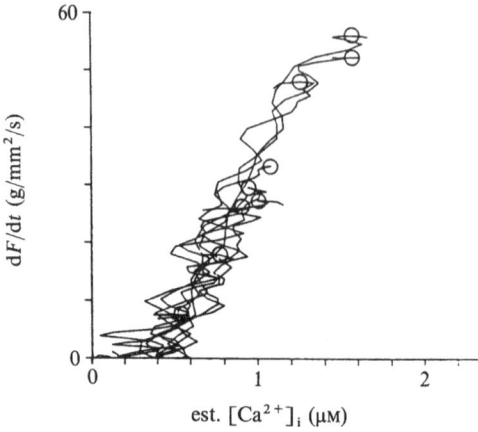

Fig. 10. Plots of dF/dt vs. $[Ca^{2+}]_i$ from physiological contractions of different strength before exposure to ryanodine. Plots were derived from between points b and c of nine contractions in ferret papillary muscle. Open circles indicate points at which maximal dF/dt was reached. Adapted from Yue (1987).

dashed linear line. The contrasting deviation from the linear path of the early portion of the trajectory (a–b) can probably be attributed to artefacts derived from the condition of spatial heterogeneity of $[Ca^{2+}]_i$ (Yue, 1987).

Fig. 10 tests whether the linear correlation between positive dF/dt and $[Ca^{2+}]_i$, obtained between points b and c in a single contraction (Fig. 9(f) dashed line), might predict the relation between dF/dt and $[Ca^{2+}]_i$ during the analogous phase of contractions of different strength. The figure plots dF/dt vs. $[Ca^{2+}]_i$ measured between points b and c in nine physiological contractions of vastly different strength. That all the traces here in Fig. 10 superimpose to form a unique, approximately linear trajectory raises the hypothesis that positive dF/dt relates to $[Ca^{2+}]_i$ on an instantaneous basis according to a single, linear relationship, so long as $[Ca^{2+}]_i$ is spatially uniform.

Further support for this hypothesis is provided in Fig. 11(a) which demonstrates a unique trajectory traced by dF/dt and $[Ca^{2+}]_i$ for contractions with not only different strength, but also with markedly slowed time course produced by exposure to ryanodine. The plus symbols in Fig. 11(a) represent the trajectory derived from between b and c of a physiological contraction before exposure to ryanodine (derived from topmost set of records in panel (b) inset). The solid traces in Fig. 11(a)

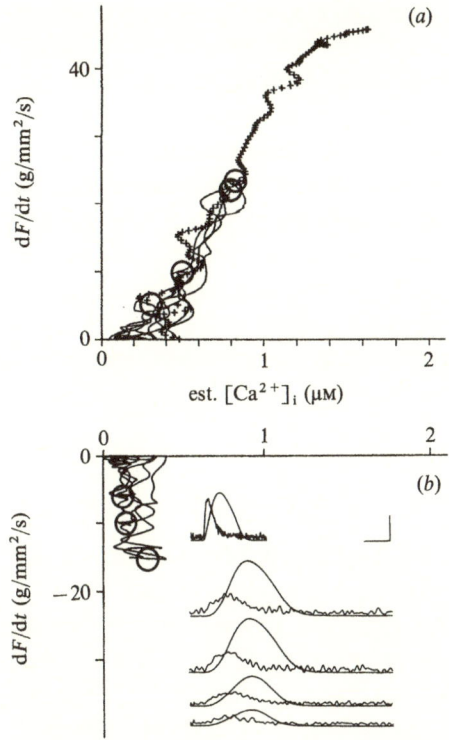

Fig. 11. Plots of dF/dt vs. estimated $[Ca^{2+}]_i$ from physiological contractions and contractions slowed by 5 μM ryanodine in ferret papillary muscle. (*a*) Positive dF/dt expressed as a function of $[Ca^{2+}]_i$. Plus symbols comprise a trace derived from between points b and c of a physiological contraction before exposure to ryanodine. Solid traces are derived from between points a and c of four slowed contractions of different strength. Open circles in (*a*) indicate points at which dF/dt_{max} was reached in slowed contractions. (*b*) Negative dF/dt expressed as function of $[Ca^{2+}]_i$. Traces are derived from points c onward of three of four slowed contractions shown in (*a*). Open circles in (*b*) indicate points at which maximum negative dF/dt was reached. (*b*) inset: Records of tension and $[Ca^{2+}]_i$ of a single physiological (top) and four slowed contractions from which plots in (*a*) and (*b*) were derived. Vertical calibration bar corresponds to 2 g mm^{-2} or 1 μM. Horizontal calibration bar is 200 ms long. From Yùe (1987), with permission from the American Physiological Society.

are the trajectories derived from the entire rising phase of tension (a–c) of four contractions with time course slowed by ryanodine (derived from bottom four sets of records in panel (*b*) inset). That the instantaneous correlation applies not only to physiological contractions of enormously different strength, but also to contractions with substantially slowed $[Ca^{2+}]_i$ transients provides cogent evidence that this relation is not merely fortuitous, but represents a fundamental kinetic property of muscle activation.

This instantaneous relationship provides us with an attractive quantitative approach to describing the rising phase of physiological contractions: $dF/dt \propto [Ca^{2+}]_i$. Thus, $F \propto \int [Ca^{2+}]_i \, dt$, or tension integrates $[Ca^{2+}]_i$. This formulation suggests that the linear correlations between F_{max} (or dF/dt_{max}) and peak $[Ca^{2+}]_i$ are but subphenomena of this more general property. Mechanistically speaking, the existence of a linear, instantaneous relationship between a substrate ($[Ca^{2+}]_i$) and the first derivative of a subsequent product (F) gives reason to postulate a first-order, rate-limiting step in the chemical reactions linking calcium ions to force.

Conclusion

Mechanistic interpretation of the FIR requires the transduction of [Ca] release from SR to contraction to be understood. Measurements based on aequorin and Fura-2 reveal a particularly simple (perhaps linear) link between $[Ca^{2+}]_i$ and tension. This empirical observation may be an important clue as to the molecular mechanism of activation in heart muscle. Computer modelling further suggests that peak $[Ca^{2+}]_i$ and the amount of [Ca] released from SR are correlated by a slightly sublinear relationship. Taken together, these results point to an intimate and almost linear relationship between strength of contraction and amount of [Ca] released from SR.

References

Allen, D. G. & Kurihara, S. (1980). Calcium transients in mammalian ventricular muscle. *European Heart Journal*, 1 (suppl A), 5–15

Babu, A., Sonnenblick, E. & Gulati, J. (1988). Molecular basis for the influence of muscle length on myocardial performance. *Science*, 240, 74.

Backx, P. H., Lamont, C. & ter Keurs, H. E. D. J. (1990). Calcium measurements in rat cardiac trabeculae using Fura-2. *Biophysical Journal*, 57, 346a.

Braveny, P. & Kruta, V. (1958). Dissociation de deux facteurs: Restitution et potentiation dans l'action de l'intervalle sur l'amplitude de la contraction du myocarde. *Archives of International Physiology and Biochemistry*, 74, 169–78.

Ebashi, S. & Endo, M. (1968). Calcium ion and muscle contraction. *Progress in Biophysics and Molecular Biology*, 18, 123–83.

Fabiato, A. (1982). Calcium release in skinned cardiac cells: variations with species, tissues, and development. *Federation Proceedings*, 1, 2238–44.

Imagawa, T., Smith, J. S., Coronado, R. & Campbell, K. P. (1987). Purified ryanodine receptor from skeletal muscle sarcoplasmic reticulum is the Ca^{2+}-permeable pore of the calcium release channel. *Journal of Biological Chemistry*, **262**, 16636–43.

Pan, B. & Solaro, R. (1984). Characterization of Ca binding sites of troponin-c in chemically skinned cardiac muscle fibres. *Biophysical Journal*, **45**, 393a.

Robertson, S., Johnson, J. & Potter, J. (1981). The time-course of Ca exchange with calmodulin, troponin, parvalbumin, and myosin in response to transient increases in Ca. *Biophysical Journal*, **34**, 559–69.

Rousseau, E., Smith, J. S. & Meissner, G. (1987). Ryanodine modifies conductance and gating behavior of single Ca^{2+} release channel. *American Journal of Physiology*, **253**, C364–8.

Wier, W. G., (1980). Calcium transients during excitation–contraction coupling in mammalian heart: aequorin signals of canine Purkinje fibers. *Science* **207**, 1085–87.

Wier, W. G. & Yue, D. T. (1986). Intracellular calcium transients underlying the short-term force–interval relationship in ferret ventricular myocardium. *Journal of Physiology*, **376**, 507–30.

Wohlfart, B. (1979). Relationship between peak force, action potential duration and stimulus interval in rabbit myocardium. *Acta Physiologica Scandinavica*, **106**, 395–409.

Woodworth, R. S. (1902). Maximal contraction, 'staircase' contraction, refractory period, and compensatory pause of the heart. *American Journal of Physiology*, **8**, 213–49.

Yue, D. T. (1987). Intracellular $[Ca^{2+}]$ related to rate of force development in twitch contraction of heart. *American Journal of Physiology*, **252**, H760–70.

Yue, D. T. & Wier, W. G. (1985). Estimation of intracellular $[Ca^{2+}]$ by nonlinear indicators: a quantitative analysis. *Biophysical Journal*, **48**, 533–7.

Yue, D. T., Wier, W. G. & Sagawa, K. (1984). Direct measurement of the intracellular $[Ca^{2+}]$ transients underlying the cardiac force–interval relationship. *VIth Proceedings of the Cardiovascular Systems Dynamics Society*, pp. 1–4.

Yue, D. T., Marban, E. & Wier, W. G. (1986). Relationship between force and intracellular $[Ca^{2+}]$ in tetanized mammalian heart muscle. *Journal of General Physiology*, **87**, 223–42.

The role of intracellular calcium, sodium and pH in rate-dependent changes of cardiac contractile force

M. R. BOYETT, J. E. FRAMPTON,
S. M. HARRISON, M. S. KIRBY, A. J. LEVI,
E. McCALL, D. R. MILNER & C. H. ORCHARD

Introduction

Since the time of Bowditch (1871) it has been recognised that the force of contraction of cardiac muscle is dependent on the rate and rhythm of the heart beat (for review see Koch-Weser & Blinks, 1963). After an increase in the rate of stimulation, or when stimulation is commenced after a rest, there is often (but not always) an immediate decrease in force as a result of the so-called negative inotropic effect of activation (NIEA – Koch-Weser & Blinks, 1963), and this is usually followed by a progressive increase in force over several minutes as a result of the positive inotropic effect of activation (PIEA). In general, the slow increase in force, known as a positive staircase, is greater than the initial decrease and as a result the heart beats more strongly at higher rates. This chapter is primarily concerned with the mechanisms underlying the slow increase in force during the staircase.

The staircase is the result of an increase in the Ca^{2+} transient

Rate-dependent changes in force are the result of changes in the intracellular Ca^{2+} transient responsible for contraction (Allen & Blinks, 1978; Allen & Kurihara, 1980; Orchard & Lakatta, 1985; Wier & Yue, 1986). Fig. 1 shows changes in the contraction (measured optically) and the Ca^{2+} transient (measured with Fura-2) of a single rat ventricular myocyte on changing the stimulation rate. The contractions appear as downward-going deflections because a single cell *decreases* in length during a contraction. On increasing the rate (e.g. from 0.2 to 2 Hz), there was a progressive increase in the amplitude of the Ca^{2+} transient and this was

M. R. Boyett et al.

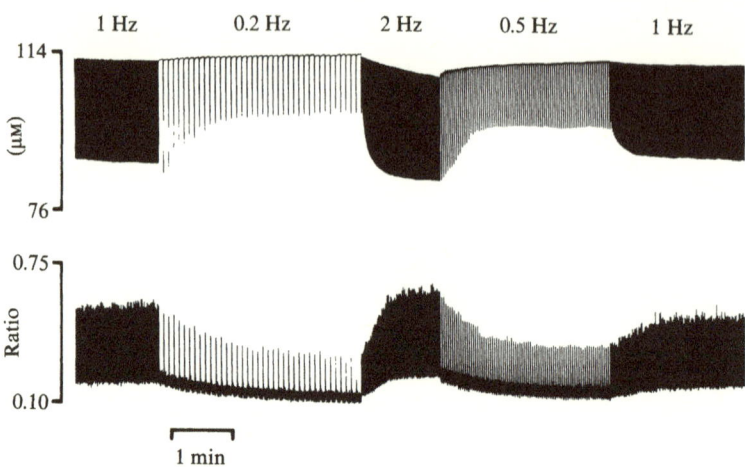

Fig. 1. Rate-dependent changes in the contraction and Ca^{2+} transient of a rat ventricular myocyte. The length of the cell was measured optically and is shown in the upper trace. During each contraction the cell shortened in length; the contractions therefore appear as downward-going deflections. The Ca^{2+} transient was measured using Fura-2 AM. The lower trace shows the ratio of the Fura-2 fluorescence in response to excitation at 340 nm to the fluorescence in response to excitation of 380 nm; this ratio is a measure of the intracellular Ca^{2+} concentration. The stimulation rate is shown above the records. Bathing Ca^{2+}, 1 mmol l^{-1}; temperature 25 °C.

accompanied by a progressive increase in the amplitude of the contraction during the staircase.[1] On decreasing the rate there was a progressive decrease in the amplitude of both the Ca^{2+} transient and the contraction. Fig. 2 shows superimposed records of individual Ca^{2+} transients (a) and contractions (b) from the experiment shown in Fig. 1 at the four different stimulation rates used. It shows clearly both the increase in the intra-cellular Ca^{2+} concentration at the peak of the Ca^{2+} transient and the greater shortening of the cell during the contraction at higher rates. In Fig. 3(a) the length of the cell at the peak of the contraction has been plotted against the Fura-2 fluorescence ratio (a measure of the intra-

[1] It may be a surprise that the rat ventricular myocyte used for Fig. 1 contracted more strongly at the higher rates of stimulation, because rat ventricular muscle is widely believed to contract less strongly at higher rates (e.g. Orchard & Lakatta, 1985). In the authors' laboratory single rat ventricular myocytes can show either type of behaviour (but not in the same cell) and rat papillary muscles can show either type of behaviour depending on the experimental conditions. An increase in the strength of contraction of rat ventricular muscle at high rates has also been noted by others (Henry, 1975; Capogrossi et al., 1986; see also Schouten & ter Keurs, 1986).

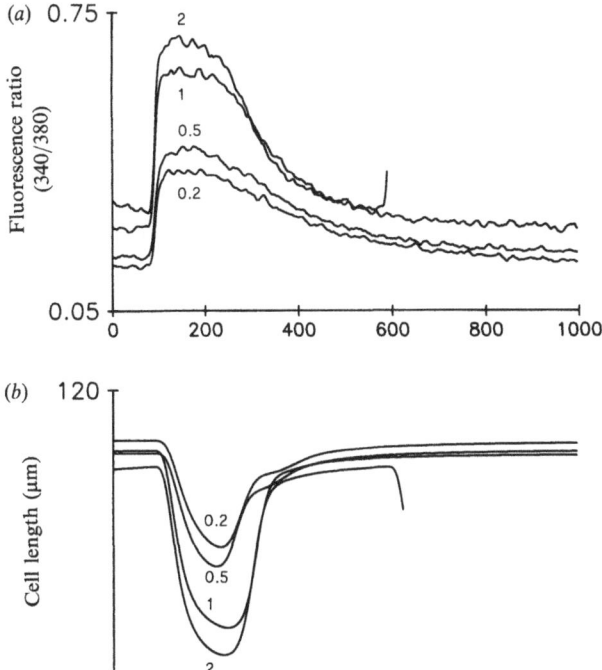

Fig. 2. Fast time base records of Ca^{2+} transients (*a*) and contractions (*b*) of a rat ventricular myocyte at different stimulation rates. The stimulation rate (in Hz) is shown next to each trace. Each trace is an average of 16 responses. From the experiment shown in Fig. 1.

cellular Ca^{2+} concentration) at the peak of the Ca^{2+} transient. The data are from the experiment shown in Fig. 1 and the different symbols correspond to the different stimulation rates used. Despite the wide range of stimulation rates used the data roughly fall along a common trajectory – this is evidence that the rate-dependent changes in the contraction are indeed the result of the changes in the Ca^{2+} transient.

The cause of the increase in the Ca^{2+} transient during the staircase

It is well accepted that the Ca^{2+} transient is the result of (a) Ca^{2+} influx across the cell membrane via the Ca^{2+} current, i_{Ca}, and (ii) Ca^{2+} release

(a)

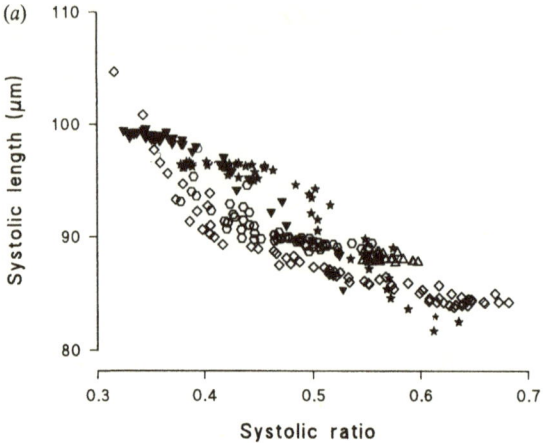

(b)

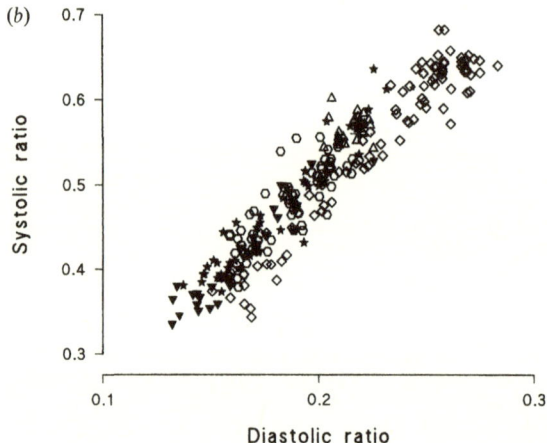

Fig. 3(a). The relationship between the contraction and intracellular Ca^{2+} of a rat ventricular myocyte on changing the stimulation rate. The length of the cell at the peak of the contraction is plotted on the ordinate and the Fura-2 fluorescence ratio at the peak of the Ca^{2+} transient is plotted on the abscissa. The different symbols correspond to the different stimulation rates used: open triangles, 1 Hz; closed triangles, 0.2 Hz; open diamonds, 2 Hz; closed stars, 0.5 Hz; open hexagons, second period of stimulation at 1 Hz. From the experiment shown in Fig. 1. (b). The relationship between systolic and diastolic Ca^{2+} of a rat ventricular myocyte on changing the stimulation rate. The Fura-2 fluorescence ratio at the peak of the Ca^{2+} transient is plotted on the ordinate, and the fluorescence ratio prior to the Ca^{2+} transient is shown on the abscissa. From the same experiment as panel (a). The symbols have the same meaning as in panel (a).

from the sarcoplasmic reticulum. Bers (1985) has suggested that the importance of the two sources of Ca^{2+} varies in different species and tissues.[2] This chapter is primarily concerned with tissues in which Ca^{2+} release from the sarcoplasmic reticulum is the most important source, although tissues in which Ca^{2+} influx dominates will also be considered. In tissues in which Ca^{2+} release from the sarcoplasmic reticulum is important, the increase in the Ca^{2+} transient is presumably the result of a progressive increase in Ca^{2+} release, which could occur for one of two reasons. Ca^{2+} release from the sarcoplasmic reticulum is thought to be triggered by i_{Ca} and Ca^{2+}-induced Ca^{2+} release (Fabiato, 1985). Because the amount of Ca^{2+} released is thought to be dependent on the size of the trigger (Fabiato, 1985), an increase in Ca^{2+} release could be the result of an increase in i_{Ca}. Alternatively, more Ca^{2+} could be released because of an increase in the Ca^{2+} content of the sarcoplasmic reticulum. The second of the two possibilities has received most attention. Lewartowski & Pytkowski (1987) reviewed various lines of evidence and concluded that there is an increase in the Ca^{2+} content of the sarcoplasmic reticulum at high stimulation rates (for an earlier review see Langer, 1968). For example, X-ray microanalysis has shown a stimulation-dependent increase in the Ca^{2+} content of the sarcoplasmic reticulum of guinea-pig ventricular muscle (Wendt-Gallitelli, 1985; Wendt-Gallitelli & Jacob, 1982; Isenberg & Wendt-Gallitelli, 1987). Evidence of an increase in the Ca^{2+} content of the sarcoplasmic reticulum of rat ventricular myocytes at high rates is shown in Fig. 4 (see also Frampton, Orchard & Boyett, 1990b) – the Ca^{2+} transient of rat ventricular muscle is thought to be largely dependent upon Ca^{2+} release from the sarcoplasmic reticulum (Bers, 1985). Fig. 4(a) once again shows superimposed Ca^{2+} transients at different rates; the increase in systolic Ca^{2+} at the peak of the Ca^{2+} transient at the higher rates is clear. To assess the Ca^{2+} content of the sarcoplasmic reticulum, caffeine was used (see also Smith et al., 1988); when the cell had reached a

---

[2] Bers' (1985) work is based on the use of ryanodine and caffeine to block function of the sarcoplasmic reticulum. In some tissues the application of these drugs has little effect on the contraction and Bers concluded that the Ca^{2+} transient is largely the result of Ca^{2+} influx, whereas in other tissues the drugs greatly reduce the contraction and Bers concluded that in these tissues the Ca^{2+} transient is largely the result of Ca^{2+} release from the sarcoplasmic reticulum. However, these conclusions rest on the assumption that the sarcoplasmic reticulum in all tissues is equally sensitive to ryanodine and caffeine. In addition, at high stimulus rates ryanodine may not effectively block sarcoplasmic reticulum function (Bers, Bridge & MacLeod, 1987). Therefore, although the classification by Bers (1985) is attractive, it cannot be considered proven.

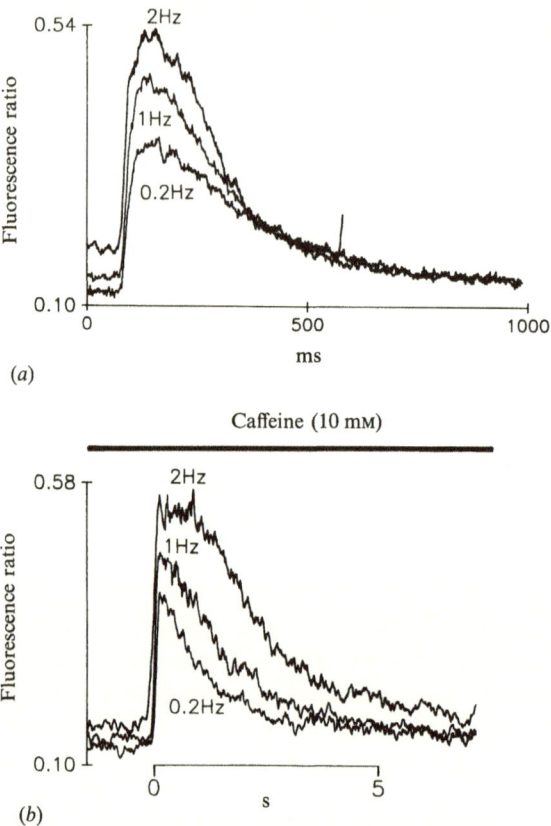

(a)

Caffeine (10 mM)

(b)

Fig. 4. The effect of the stimulation rate on the Ca^{2+} content of the sarcoplasmic reticulum, measured using caffeine, of a rat ventricular myocyte. (a) Superimposed Ca^{2+} transients at three different stimulation rates. Each trace is an average of 16 responses. (b) The caffeine-induced increase in intracellular Ca^{2+} following stimulation at the three rates. Traces superimposed. Caffeine, 10 mmol l^{-1}, was applied about 5 s after stopping stimulation in order to release Ca^{2+} from the sarcoplasmic reticulum. From the same cell as panel (a). The stimulation rate is shown next to each trace. Intracellular Ca^{2+} was measured using Fura-2 AM and the Fura-2 fluorescence ratio is plotted on the ordinate in both graphs. Bathing Ca^{2+}, 1 mmol l^{-1}; temperature, 25 °C

steady state at each stimulation rate, stimulation was stopped and about 5 s later caffeine, 10 mmol l^{-1}, was applied to release Ca^{2+} from the sarcoplasmic reticulum. Following the higher stimulation rates the Ca^{2+} content of the sarcoplasmic reticulum, as indicated by the amplitude of the caffeine triggered release of Ca^{2+}, was greater (Fig. 4(b)).

Although Fig. 4 suggests that the Ca^{2+} content of the sarcoplasmic reticulum is greater at higher stimulation rates, it does not prove that the sarcoplasmic reticulum is responsible for the increase in the Ca^{2+} transient and hence the strength of contraction at higher rates. Such proof is provided by Fig. 5. Fig. 5(a) shows the force developed by a ferret papillary muscle at different stimulation rates under control conditions and in the presence of ryanodine to block sarcoplasmic reticulum function (the Ca^{2+} transient of ferret ventricular muscle is largely the result of Ca^{2+} release from the sarcoplasmic reticulum – Bers, 1985). In Fig. 5(b) the force of contraction has been plotted against the stimulus interval before and after the application of ryanodine. Under control conditions the muscle generated greater force at the higher stimulation rates (shorter stimulus intervals) as expected, but after block of sarcoplasmic reticulum function the force of contraction was depressed and furthermore the increase in force at the higher rates was greatly reduced. Similar results were obtained from a total of four ferret papillary muscles, and have also been obtained using rat ventricular myocytes. These results suggest that the increase in the force of contraction at high rates is largely the result of the sarcoplasmic reticulum.

What is responsible for the increase in the Ca^{2+} content of the sarcoplasmic reticulum at high stimulation rates? Figs. 1 and 2 show that at high stimulation rates there is a rise of diastolic Ca^{2+} as well as systolic Ca^{2+}. A rise in diastolic Ca^{2+} at high rates has also been recorded in sheep Purkinje fibres by Lado, Sheu & Fozzard (1982) using Ca^{2+}-sensitive microelectrodes. In rat ventricular myocytes it has been noted that there is a unique and roughly linear relationship between diastolic and systolic Ca^{2+} on changing the stimulation rate or on varying the bathing Ca^{2+} concentration (Frampton, Orchard & Boyett, 1990a). For example, in Fig. 1 diastolic Ca^{2+} rises and falls along a similar time course to the rises and falls of systolic Ca^{2+} as the stimulation rate changes. The linear relationship between systolic and diastolic Ca^{2+} for the experiment in Fig. 1 is shown in Fig. 3(b). In seven experiments in which Fura-2 was calibrated the slope of the relationship (the ratio of the change in systolic Ca^{2+}, nmol l^{-1}, to the change in diastolic Ca^{2+}, nmol l^{-1}) varied from 4 to 9.

On the basis of the observations described so far, a hypothesis can be put forward. An increase in the stimulation rate leads to an increase in diastolic Ca^{2+}. This results in greater Ca^{2+} uptake by the sarcoplasmic reticulum, an increase in the Ca^{2+} content of the sarcoplasmic reticulum, greater Ca^{2+} release, an increase in the Ca^{2+} transient and finally an

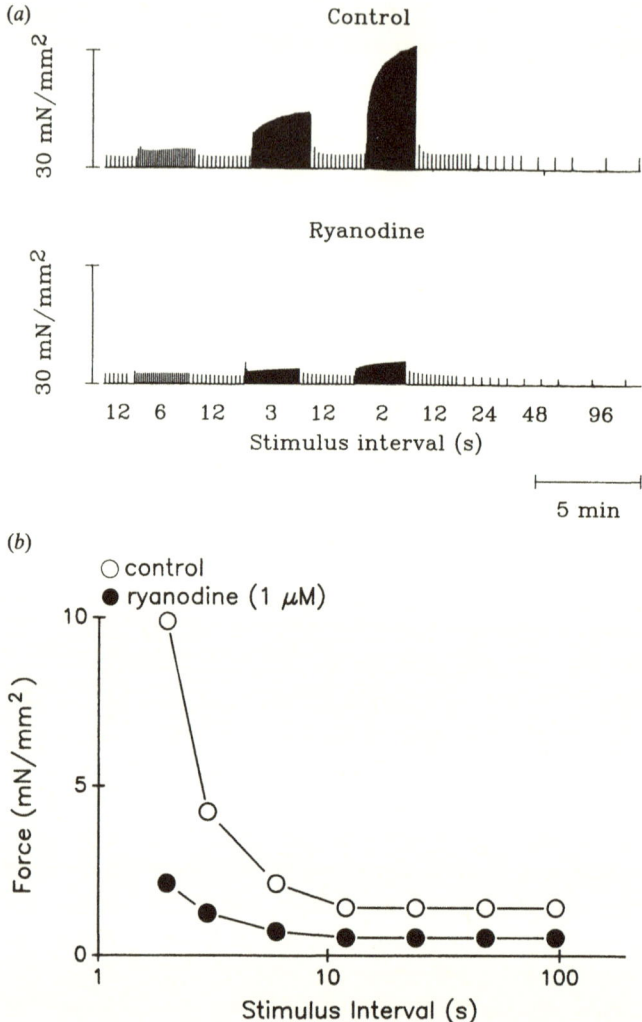

Fig. 5. The effect of block of sarcoplasmic reticulum function by ryanodine on the increase in the force of contraction of a ferret papillary muscle at high stimulation rates. (a) Chart records showing the changes in the force of contraction on changing the stimulation rate before (upper record) and after (lower record) the application of ryanodine, 1 μmol l^{-1}. The stimulus interval (the reciprocal of the stimulation rate in Hz) is shown below the records. Note that the contractions appear as upward-going deflections. (b) The relationship between the force of contraction at steady state and the stimulus interval before, and after, the application of ryanodine. From the same experiment as panel (a). Bathing Ca^{2+}, 2 mmol l^{-1}; temperature, 30 °C.

increase in the contraction of the muscle.[3] In this scheme the sarcoplasmic reticulum is acting as an amplifier, amplifying the changes in diastolic Ca^{2+} by a factor of 4 to 9.

In tissues in which Ca^{2+} influx is the most important source of Ca^{2+} for the Ca^{2+} transient, the increase in the Ca^{2+} transient during the staircase is presumably the result of a beat-to-beat increase in Ca^{2+} influx per beat. Noble & Shimoni (1981), Payett, Schanne & Ruiz-Ceretti (1981), Bers (1983), Boyett & Fedida (1984), Lee (1987) and Bers & Hess (1988) have obtained evidence of such beat-to-beat increases in Ca^{2+} influx (for a review of earlier evidence see Langer, 1968). For example, Bers (1983) monitored Ca^{2+} influx in rabbit ventricle during each beat by the depletion of extracellular Ca^{2+} (measured with a Ca^{2+} sensitive micro-electrode) during each beat. On resumption of stimulation after a rest interval, twitch tension and Ca^{2+} influx per beat increased to their steady-state values with a similar time dependence, except for the first beat. Furthermore, in voltage clamp experiments on guinea-pig ventricular myocytes Bers & Hess (1988) observed that the Ca^{2+} current, i_{Ca}, is reduced in amplitude after a rest and when stimulation is resumed i_{Ca} increases back to its steady-state amplitude over a few beats. Note that, even in tissues in which the sarcoplasmic reticulum is an important source of Ca^{2+} for the Ca^{2+} transient, a beat-to-beat increase in Ca^{2+} influx is expected to contribute or lead to an increase in the strength of contraction by direct activation of the myofilaments or by increasing the amount of Ca^{2+} released from the sarcoplasmic reticulum (Ca^{2+} release is proportional to the size of the trigger, i_{Ca}). However, this may not be a ubiquitous mechanism because in some tissues a *decrease* in i_{Ca} has been observed during the positive staircase (e.g. duBell & Houser, 1989).

The cause of the increase in the Ca^{2+} content of the myocyte at high stimulation rates

This section is of particular relevance to tissues in which the Ca^{2+} transient is largely the result of Ca^{2+} release from the sarcoplasmic reticulum.

---

[3] There are alternative hypotheses to explain the linear relationship between systolic and diastolic Ca^{2+} that should be mentioned. First, it is possible that the sarcoplasm and sarcoplasmic reticulum are loaded with Ca^{2+} independently but in parallel – this will lead to parallel rises in diastolic and systolic Ca^{2+}. Secondly, because of a Ca^{2+} leak from the sarcoplasmic reticulum into the sarcoplasm, diastolic Ca^{2+} may rise as the Ca^{2+} content of the sarcoplasmic reticulum rises – again this will lead to parallel rises in diastolic and systolic Ca^{2+}. Finally, raising diastolic Ca^{2+} may reduce the concentration of free Ca^{2+} buffer (i.e. Ca^{2+} buffer not bound to Ca^{2+}) in the sarcoplasm and consequently more Ca^{2+} from whatever source (i_{Ca} or Ca^{2+} release from the sarcoplasmic reticulum) will be available to trigger Ca^{2+} release or directly activate the myofilaments.

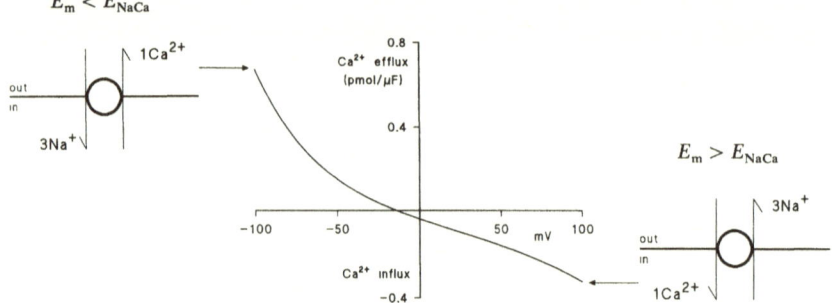

Fig. 6. The calculated relationship between the net Ca^{2+} flux via the Na–Ca exchanger and the membrane potential. At potentials less than E_{NaCa} the exchanger results in net Ca^{2+} efflux (left-hand schematic diagram) and at more positive potentials it results in net Ca^{2+} influx (right-hand schematic diagram). The Ca^{2+} flux was calculated by dividing i_{NaCa} (eq. 24) by $-F$. Constants used: k_{NaCa}, 20.7 A $(mol\,l)^{-4}\,\mu F^{-1}$; r, 0.34; $[Ca]_i$, $100 \times 10^{-9}\,mol\,l^{-1}$; T, 310 K; $[Na]_i$, 6×10^{-3} $mol\,l^{-1}$; $[Na]_b$, $[Ca]_b$, F, R – see Table 1, p. 147.

The increase in diastolic Ca^{2+} and the Ca^{2+} content of the sarcoplasmic reticulum at high rates is the result of a *net* increase in the Ca^{2+} content of the myocyte; Lewartowski & Pytkowski (1987), for example, have shown that the increase in force during the staircase of guinea-pig ventricular muscle is accompanied by an increase in the exchangeable ^{45}Ca content of the muscle (for further evidence see Langer & Brady, 1963; Langer, 1965; Langer, 1968; Sands & Winegrad, 1970). A net increase in the Ca^{2+} content of the cell can only be the result of an increase in Ca^{2+} influx or a decrease in Ca^{2+} efflux across the membrane. In this section various mechanisms that may be responsible for this increase in Ca^{2+} content will be considered.

Because each of the mechanisms involves the Na–Ca exchanger, the properties of the exchanger will first be considered. The stoichiometry of the exchanger is thought to be 3 Na^+:1 Ca^{2+}; it is therefore electrogenic and moves net positive charge across the membrane (e.g. Ehara, Matsuoka & Noma, 1989). Because the exchanger is electrogenic, it is affected by the membrane potential as shown in Fig. 6. At potentials negative to the reversal potential of the exchanger (E_{NaCa}), it operates in the Na^+ influx-Ca^{2+} efflux mode (Fig. 6, left), because the energy provided by the movement of Na^+ down its concentration gradient as well as the movement of charge down the electrical gradient (if the cell interior is negative) is sufficient to move Ca^{2+} out of the cell up its concentration gradient. Na–Ca exchange is thought to be the principal means for the extrusion of Ca^{2+} from the cell. At potentials positive to the reversal potential of the exchanger, the exchanger operates in the Na^+ efflux–Ca^{2+} influx mode (Fig. 6, right), because the energy provided by the movement of Ca^{2+} down its concentration gradient as well as the movement of charge down the electrical gradient (if the cell interior is positive) is sufficient to move Na^+ out of the cell up its concentration gradient. The value of the reversal potential is a function of the Na^+ and Ca^{2+} equilibrium potentials (E_{Na} and E_{Ca}):

$$E_{NaCa} = 3E_{Na} - E_{Ca} \qquad (1)$$

The equilibrium potentials are, of course, a measure of the concentration gradients of the ions and are dependent on the intracellular and extracellular concentrations of the ions.

Three possible mechanisms responsible for the increase in the Ca^{2+} content of the myocyte during the staircase will be considered:

1. At steady-state, Ca^{2+} efflux via the exchanger must equal Ca^{2+} influx if the cell is to be in a state of ionic balance. To achieve this, the exchanger acts as a negative feedback device and Ca^{2+} efflux via the exchanger is proportional to the intracellular Ca^{2+} concentration, $[Ca]_i$, (Fig. 7, curve (*a*)). Ca^{2+} influx occurs primarily as the Ca^{2+} current, i_{Ca}. At higher rates Ca^{2+} influx is expected to be greater, because there are more action potentials and thus Ca^{2+} currents per unit time. For example, Niedergerke, Page & Talbot (1969) using ^{45}Ca measured Ca^{2+} influx into frog ventricular muscle to be only $0.004\ pmol\ cm^{-2}\ s^{-1}$ at rest, whereas there was an extra Ca^{2+} influx of $0.13\ pmol\ cm^{-2}$ per beat.[4] On the basis of these data, Ca^{2+} influx during 1 Hz stimulation will be 33.5 times greater than at rest. At rest the cell will be in ionic balance and Ca^{2+} efflux will equal Ca^{2+} influx, but on commencing stimulation Ca^{2+} influx will exceed Ca^{2+} efflux[5]; as a result $[Ca]_i$ will rise, which in turn will stimulate Ca^{2+} efflux via the exchanger (Fig.

---

[4] Based on more recent measurements of i_{Ca} in isolated ventricular myocytes, the extra Ca^{2+} influx per beat may be higher than this. For example, it can be calculated from the measurements of Isenberg (1982) of i_{Ca} in bovine ventricular myocytes that the Ca^{2+} influx via i_{Ca} during a 100 ms voltage clamp pulse to $+5\ mV$ is $10\ pmol\ cm^{-2}$.

[5] There is an exception to this that should be noted. In some tissues such as rat ventricular muscle and rabbit atrial muscle, the first beat after a rest is usually large. It is possible that during a rest the sarcoplasmic reticulum (unlike that of other tissues, fails to empty of Ca^{2+}. There is evidence that the large first Ca^{2+} transient after the rest results in a large efflux of Ca^{2+} via the Na–Ca exchanger such that Ca^{2+} efflux via the exchanger is greater than Ca^{2+} influx via i_{Ca} (Hilgemann & Noble, 1987; see also Boyett *et al.*, 1989*a*). As a result of this the sarcoplasmic reticulum may be rapidly depleted of Ca^{2+} in the first few beats, and the contraction of the muscle declines. After this, however, the behaviour seen is the same as in other tissues, i.e. a slow increase in the strength of contraction. It is possible that after the first few beats, Ca^{2+} efflux is less than Ca^{2+} influx as in other tissues.

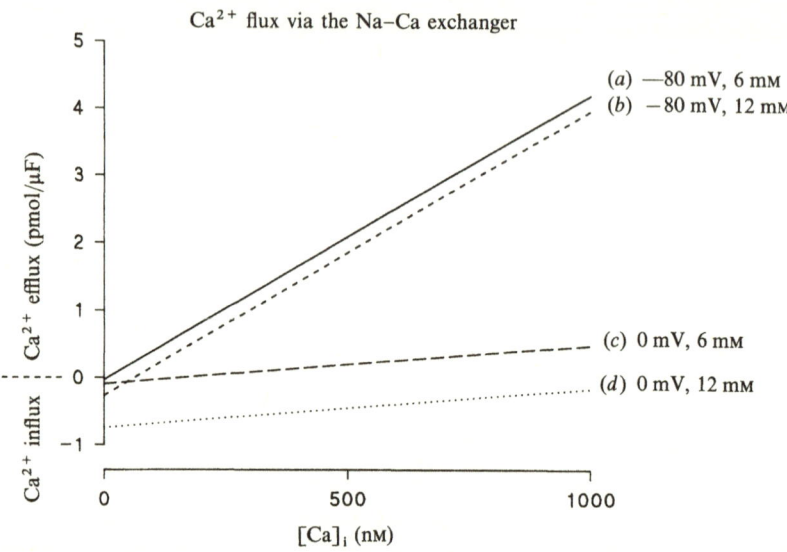

Fig. 7. The relationship between the calculated Ca^{2+} flux via the Na–Ca exchanger and the intracellular Ca^{2+} concentration for two membrane potentials (-80 and $0\,mV$) and two intracellular Na^+ concentrations (6 and $12\,mmol\,l^{-1}$). (See the legend to Fig. 6 for details of the calculations.)

7) until eventually it is once again equal to Ca^{2+} influx. Similar arguments apply to an increase in the stimulation rate. The increase in $[Ca]_i$ will ultimately lead to an increase in the strength of contraction and could be responsible for the staircase. This mechanism has been discussed by others (e.g. Kaufmann et al., 1974; Edman & Jóhannsson, 1976), although it has received little attention in recent years, because it has been eclipsed by the second of the two possible mechanisms.

2. At high rates, the intracellular Na^+ activity, a^i_{Na}, is elevated. Early evidence of the rise in a^i_{Na} was reviewed by Langer (1968). Since that time, evidence of a rise in a^i_{Na} at high stimulation rates has been obtained using Na^+-sensitive microelectrodes in Purkinje fibres (Cohen, Fozzard & Sheu, 1982; Lederer & Sheu, 1983; Boyett, Hart & Levi, 1987a; Boyett, Hart, Levi & Roberts, 1987b; Lee, Im & Sonn, 1987; Ellis, 1985; Bountra, Kaila & Vaughan-Jones, 1988a,b), ventricular muscle (Hotokebuchi et al., 1987; Wang et al., 1988) and atrial muscle (Ruch, Kennedy & Seifen, 1988). The rise in a^i_{Na} has also been simulated using a computer model (Boyett & Fedida, 1988). Bountra et al. (1988a), for example, observed that in sheep Purkinje fibres a^i_{Na} showed a linear dependence on the stimulation rate,

and on average rose by $0.57 \text{ mmol l}^{-1} \text{ Hz}^{-1}$. It is well known that a rise in intracellular Na^+ leads to an increase in the strength of contraction as a result of the Na–Ca exchange mechanism (e.g. Eisner, Lederer & Vaughan-Jones, 1981; Eisner, 1990). A rise in a^i_{Na} will reduce the Na^+ concentration gradient and thus the energy available for Ca^{2+} extrusion via the exchanger; in Fig. 7 a rise in a^i_{Na} can be seen to shift the relationship between Ca^{2+} extrusion and $[Ca]_i$ to the right (compare curves (a) and (b). As a result, Ca^{2+} efflux via the exchanger will decline, Ca^{2+} efflux via the exchanger will be less than Ca^{2+} influx via i_{Ca} etc, and $[Ca]_i$ (and thus the force of contraction) will rise until Ca^{2+} efflux is once again equal to Ca^{2+} influx. Langer (1968) was the first to suggest that the rate-dependent rise in a^i_{Na} could be responsible for the increase in the strength of contraction during the staircase (see also Langer, 1983).

3. At higher rates the membrane is depolarised for a greater proportion of the cardiac cycle. In relation to Fig. 6, the effect of potential on the exchanger has already been discussed. In Fig. 7 depolarisation can be seen to shift the relationship between Ca^{2+} efflux and $[Ca]_i$ to the right (compare curves (a) and (c)). In addition, depolarisation reduces the sensitivity of the exchanger to $[Ca]_i$ (i.e. the slope of the relationship is reduced) and increases its sensitivity to a^i_{Na} (the difference between curves (c) and (d) is greater than the difference between (a) and (b)). As a result of these changes, once again, $[Ca]_i$ must rise in order to stimulate Ca^{2+} efflux so that it matches Ca^{2+} influx.

Evidence will be presented to show that each of the mechanisms above may have an important role to play in the positive staircase.

Ca^{2+} influx via the Ca^{2+} current is important for the generation of the staircase

Lakatta & Spurgeon (1980) noted that a reduction of i_{Ca} by the Ca^{2+} antagonist verapamil slowed the rise in force during the staircase of cat ventricular muscle after a rest, whereas an increase in i_{Ca} by isoproterenol accelerated the rise in force. In guinea-pig (and also cat) ventricular muscle, the increase in force during the staircase occurs in two phases – during the fast phase there is a rapid increase in force during the first few beats and during the slow phase there is a progressive increase in force over a period of several minutes. Seibel (1986) concluded that the fast phase (but not the slow phase) in guinea-pig papillary muscle is closely related to i_{Ca} because both noradrenaline and dibutyryl-cAMP (which increase i_{Ca}) augment the fast phase of the staircase (Seibel et al., 1978).

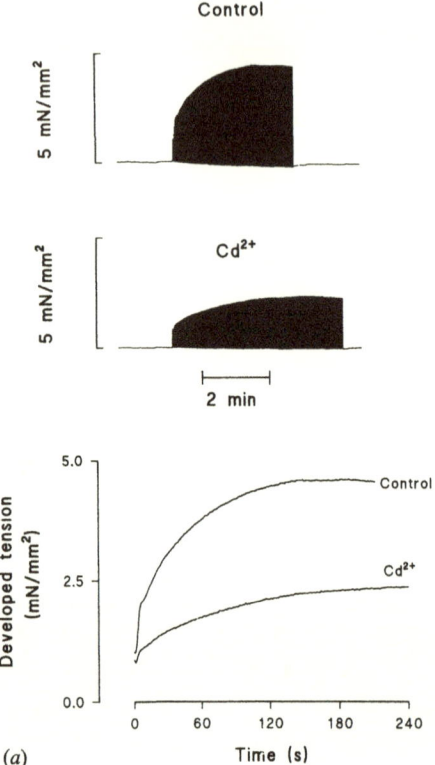

Fig. 8. The effect of Cd^{2+} (*a*) and BAY K 8644 (*b*) on the staircase of guinea-pig papillary muscle. The top two traces in each panel show the increase in tension during a staircase at 0.83 Hz after a 10 min rest under control conditions (first trace) and in the presence of either Cd^{2+}, 6.5 μmol l^{-1}, or BAY K 8644, 0.1 μmol l^{-1} (second trace). The staircases are superimposed in the graphs – the peak tension developed by each beat during the staircase is plotted against time.

Recently, the effects of interventions expected to either increase or decrease the amplitude of i_{Ca} on the staircase of guinea-pig papillary muscle have been investigated in more detail. Some of the results are shown in Fig. 8. Fig. 8(*a*) shows the effect of Cd^{2+}, 6.5 μmol l^{-1},[6] a blocker of i_{Ca} (Narahashi, Tsunoo & Yoshi, 1987), on the staircase when the muscle was stimulated at 0.83 Hz after a 10 min rest. During the control

[6] A Cd^{2+} concentration was chosen that was sufficient to approximately halve the tension produced during regular stimulation at 0.66 Hz. In seven muscles this ranged from 5 to 9.5 μmol l^{-1}. This concentration is sufficient to reduce but not fully block i_{Ca} – the concentration for half maximal block of L-type Ca^{2+} current has been reported to be 7 μmol l^{-1} (Narahashi *et al.*, 1987) and 3–13 μmol l^{-1} (Bryerly, Chase & Stimers, 1985). i_{Ca} could not be fully blocked because the contraction would be eliminated.

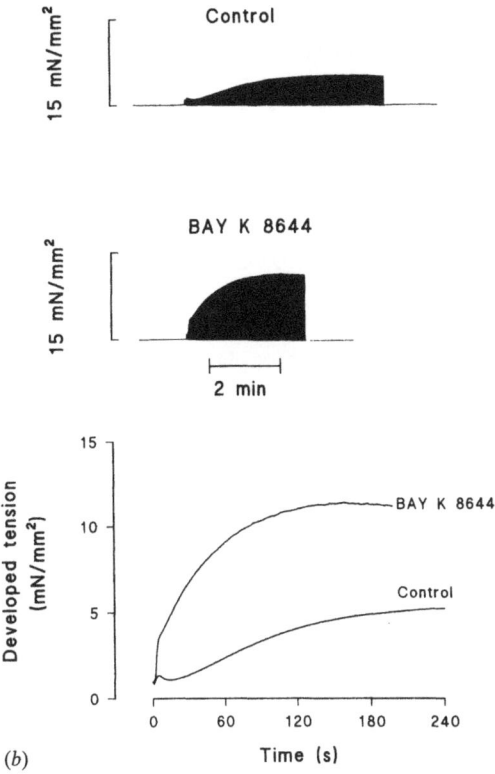

Fig. 8 (*contd*).

staircase the force of contraction increased in fast and slow phases as described above. After the addition of Cd^{2+} (second trace) the amplitude of the first beat after the rest was little affected, but the fast phase was almost completely eliminated and the slow phase was greatly reduced. This is best shown by the graph in Fig. 8(*a*) in which the two staircases are superimposed. In seven muscles, force increased 11.8 ± 2.4 times (mean $\pm$ s.e.m.) during a staircase at 0.83 Hz after a rest under control conditions, but only 3.3 ± 1.1 times ($p < 0.01$) after the addition of Cd^{2+}, 5–9.5 μmol$\,l^{-1}$. Similar findings were obtained when nifedipine was used to reduce the amplitude of i_{Ca}. Fig. 8(*b*) shows the effect of BAY K 8644, 0.1 μmol$\,l^{-1}$,[7] a Ca^{2+} channel agonist (Schramm *et al.*, 1983), on a

[7] A concentration of BAY K 8644 was chosen to approximately double the tension produced during regular stimulation at 0.66 Hz. In different muscles this ranged from 0.1 to 0.2 μmol$\,l^{-1}$. This is sufficient to increase i_{Ca} – the concentration to produce a half-maximal effect on i_{Ca} is 0.1 μmol$\,l^{-1}$ (Schramm *et al.*, 1983).

staircase at 0.83 Hz after a 10 min rest. Once again BAY K 8644 had little effect on the first beat, but it greatly increased the rise in force during both the fast and slow phases of the staircase. In four muscles force increased 9.3 ± 2.6 times during the staircase at 0.83 Hz after a rest under control conditions, but 17.4 ± 3.6 times ($p < 0.005$) after the addition of BAY K 8644, $0.1–0.2\ \mu\mathrm{mol}\,\mathrm{l}^{-1}$. Similar findings were obtained when noradrenaline was used to increase the amplitude of i_{Ca}. These results suggest that i_{Ca} is an important factor underlying both phases of the staircase and not just the fast phase.

If it is assumed that the Ca^{2+} transient in guinea-pig papillary muscle is largely the result of Ca^{2+} release from the sarcoplasmic reticulum, the results shown in Fig. 8 are consistent with the proposal that Ca^{2+} loading of the sarcoplasmic reticulum at high rates is in part, at least, dependent on Ca^{2+} influx via the Ca^{2+} current. However, because Ca^{2+} release from the sarcoplasmic reticulum is proportional to i_{Ca}, the results do not exclude the possibility that the staircase is a result of a beat-to-beat increase in i_{Ca}. If it is assumed that the Ca^{2+} transient in guinea-pig papillary muscle is largely the result of Ca^{2+} entry from the extracellular fluid, the results in Fig. 8 suggest that the staircase is the result of a beat-to-beat increase in i_{Ca}.[8]

The role of intracellular Na$^+$ in the staircase

Purkinje fibres

Fig. 9 shows changes in the force of contraction and a^i_{Na} of a sheep Purkinje fibre on changing the rate of stimulation (left) or on commencing stimulation after a rest (centre and right). When the fibre was stimulated after a long rest, the first contraction was characteristically large (in contrast to the small first beat of guinea-pig ventricular muscle – Fig. 8), but this was followed by a dramatic decrease in force in the next beat (the result of the NIEA). The decrease in force was not related to any

---

[8] Although the results in Fig. 8 suggest that i_{Ca} does have an important role to play in the staircase, it is important to sound a word of caution. Ca^{2+} channel antagonists and agonists will affect action potential duration and it is possible that their actions on the staircase may be the result of these changes in action potential duration rather than their effects on i_{Ca}. To eliminate this possibility the experiments in Fig. 8 need to be repeated under voltage clamp control. In addition, the conclusion reached may not be valid if the Ca^{2+} channel antagonists and agonists at the concentration used either are use-dependent or have other actions.

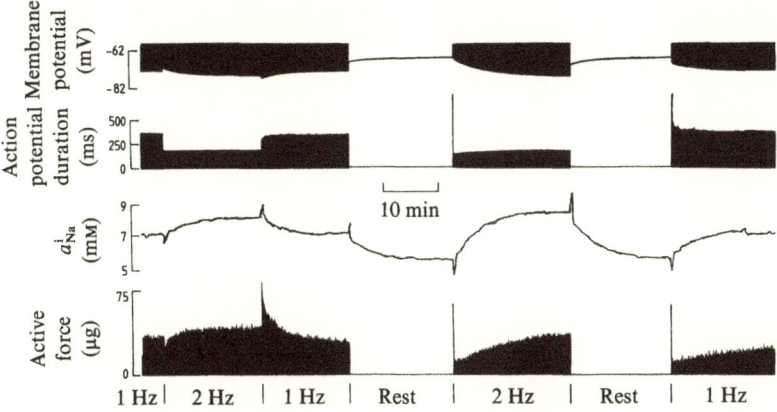

Fig. 9. Rate-dependent changes in the contraction and a^i_{Na} of a sheep Purkinje fibre. The traces show the membrane potential (upper trace; during stimulation only the bottom of the action potentials can be seen), action potential duration (measured electronically), a^i_{Na} (measured with an Na^+-sensitive microelectrode) and active force (lower trace; active force is the force developed during each contraction and was obtained by subtracting resting force from the total force). The stimulation rate is shown below the records. The transients on the a^i_{Na} signal on changing the stimulation rate or on starting or stopping stimulation are artefacts. Bathing Ca^{2+}, $2\,\text{mmol}\,l^{-1}$; temperature, $37\,°C$.

change in a^i_{Na}. The initial fall in force was followed by a positive staircase, i.e. a progressive increase in force. This increase in force was accompanied, over a similar time course, by an increase in a^i_{Na}. When the fibre was stimulated at 1 Hz after a rest (Fig. 9, right) rather than at 2 Hz (centre) the rise in a^i_{Na} was less as was the slow increase in force during the staircase. When the stimulation rate was increased from 1 to 2 Hz and then returned to 1 Hz (Fig. 9, left), there were slow changes in force, which were once again accompanied by slow changes in a^i_{Na}. Notice that a change in the stimulation rate (from 1 to 2 Hz or 2 to 1 Hz) also resulted in an immediate change in force, which was unrelated to any change in a^i_{Na}.

Boyett et al. (1987b) have examined in detail the changes in a^i_{Na} and force during the staircase in sheep Purkinje fibres. Two results from this study are shown in Figs. 10 and 11. To test whether the changes in force during the staircase are the consequence of the rise in a^i_{Na}, the rise in a^i_{Na} was reduced by the application of TTX to block the Na^+ current, i_{Na} (the rate-dependent rise in a^i_{Na} is in large part the result of Na^+ influx via i_{Na} – see below for further discussion of this point). The result of this

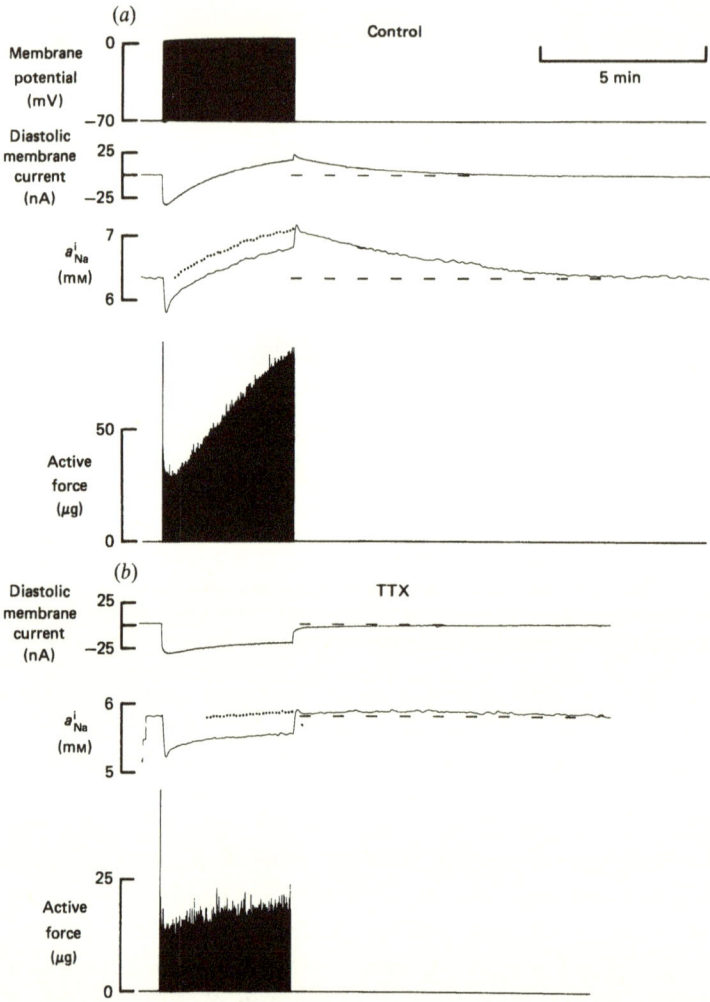

Fig. 10. The effect of block of the Na$^+$ current, i_{Na}, by tetrodotoxin (TTX) on the force staircase of a sheep Purkinje fibre. The result in (*a*) was obtained under control conditions, whereas that in (*b*) was obtained from the same fibre in the presence of TTX 2.5×10^{-5} mol l^{-1}. Each panel shows the membrane potential, diastolic membrane current, a^i_{Na} and active force before, during and after a 4 min train of voltage clamp pulses. Holding potential, -70 mV; pulse potential, $+4$ mV; pulse duration, 100 ms; pulse frequency, 2.5 Hz. During the trains the a^i_{Na} signal was offset (an artefact) and the dotted line (fitted by hand) possibly indicates a more realistic level of a^i_{Na}. The dashed lines indicate the resting level of the variable. Cs$^+$, 2 mmol l^{-1}, was present throughout. Bathing Ca^{2+}, 2 mmol l^{-1}; temperature, 37 °C. From Boyett *et al.* (1987*b*) with permission.

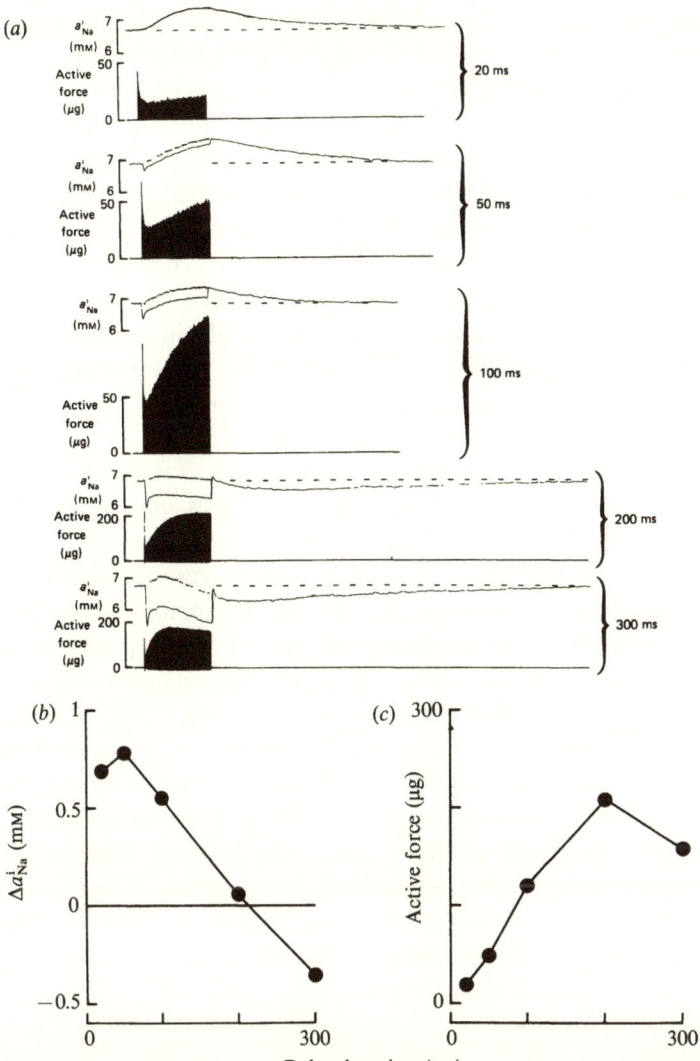

Fig. 11. The effect of pulse duration on the force staircase of a sheep Purkinje fibre during a 4 min train of voltage clamp pulses after a rest. (a) a^i_{Na} and active force during trains of voltage clamp pulses of different duration. The pulse duration is shown next to each pair of traces. Note that force is shown on a lower gain in the two lower records. See the legend to Fig. 10 for the significance of the dotted and dashed lines. (b, c) The change in a^i_{Na} during the train (b) and the active force at the end of the train (c) plotted as a function of the pulse duration. From the same experiment as panel (a). Holding potential, -70 mV; pulse potential, 0 mV; pulse frequency, 2.5 Hz. Bathing Ca^{2+}, 2 mmol 1^{-1}; temperature, 37 °C. (From Boyett et al., 1987b with permission.)

experiment is shown in Fig. 10. Under control conditions (Fig. 10(a)) a^i_{Na} rose by about 1 mmol l^{-1} during a 4 min train of 100 ms duration voltage clamp pulses at a rate of 2.5 Hz and this was accompanied by a progressive increase in the force of contraction over a similar time course. After the application of TTX, the rise of a^i_{Na} was abolished and the increase in force was also much reduced (Fig. 10(b)). This suggests that the slow increase in a^i_{Na} during the staircase is an important factor underlying the slow rise in force (see Boyett et al., 1987b, for further evidence). The result in Fig. 11, however shows, not unexpectedly, that other factors must also be involved. Fig. 11(a) shows changes in a^i_{Na} and force during 4 min trains of voltage clamp pulses of different duration (in all other respects the trains were identical). During the train of 20 ms pulses there was a substantial rise in a^i_{Na} and a small progressive rise in force. With the train of 50 ms pulses the rise of a^i_{Na} was slightly greater as was the progressive increase in force – this is consistent with the hypothesis that the rise in a^i_{Na} is an important factor underlying the positive staircase. However, with trains of longer pulses the rise of a^i_{Na} was less, whereas the progressive rise of force during the staircase was greater. This is summarised in Figs. 11(b) and (c). Note that, although during the train of 300 ms pulses there was a net *fall* of a^i_{Na}, there was still a substantial increase in force during the staircase. The results in Figs. 10 and 11 show that, although a^i_{Na} may be an important factor in the staircase, it cannot be the only one. The large increase in force during the train of 300 ms pulses could have been the result of i_{Ca}, as outlined in the previous section, or alternatively it could have been the result of the voltage-dependence of the Na–Ca exchanger (see below for further discussion). The results in Figs. 10 and 11 also confirm that the immediate decrease in force on commencing stimulation after a rest is not related to a change in a^i_{Na}.

Ventricular muscle

Purkinje tissue is a specialised conducting tissue and it is poorly contractile. Therefore, although much work has been successfully carried out on Purkinje fibres using Na$^+$-sensitive microelectrodes (*because* Purkinje fibres are poorly contractile), it is important to determine whether similar mechanisms operate in ventricular muscle. It has been shown that a^i_{Na} in ventricular muscle, like that in Purkinje fibres, increases at higher rates of stimulation (see above – p. 122). There is also evidence to show that this rise in a^i_{Na} may be an important factor in the staircase in ventricular muscle. Fig. 12 is taken from the study of Seibel (1986). The trace labelled

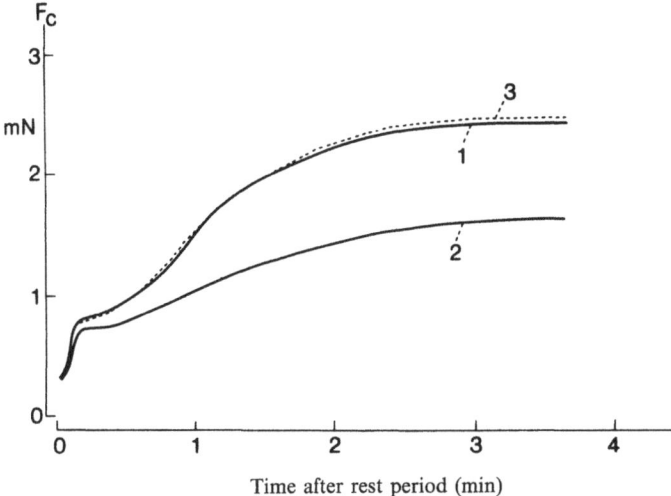

Fig. 12. Effect of block of the Na^+ current, i_{Na}, by TTX on the staircase of a guinea-pig papillary muscle after a 10 min rest. Ordinate, peak force of contraction; abscissa, time of stimulation at 1 Hz. The changes in the force of contraction during three staircases are superimposed. The numbers indicate the sequence of the stimulation periods during which the following concentrations of TTX were present: (1) and (3), 3×10^{-8} mol l^{-1}; (2) 10^{-5} mol l^{-1}. Bathing Ca^{2+}, 2 mmol l^{-1}, temperature, 35 °C. (From Seibel, 1986 with permission.)

'1' shows the envelope of the contractions when a guinea-pig papillary muscle was stimulated at a rate of 1 Hz after a rest under control conditions. Once again it shows that the increase of force during the staircase of guinea-pig ventricular muscle occurs in two phases – a fast phase and a slow phase. The trace labelled '2' in Fig. 12 shows the changes in force during a staircase in the presence of TTX – a sufficient concentration of TTX was used to approximately halve the size of i_{Na} and this presumably reduced the rise in a^i_{Na} during the staircase as in the experiment shown in Fig. 10. Fig. 12 shows that in the presence of TTX the rise in force during the slow phase of the staircase was reduced – this is similar to the result obtained from sheep Purkinje fibres (Fig. 10). Note that TTX had no effect on the fast phase of the staircase. In addition, Seibel (1986) observed that interventions expected to increase the rise of a^i_{Na} during the staircase (cardiac glycosides and veratridine) markedly increased the rise in force during the slow phase of the staircase, though they had no effect on the fast phase. These data show that a^i_{Na} may have

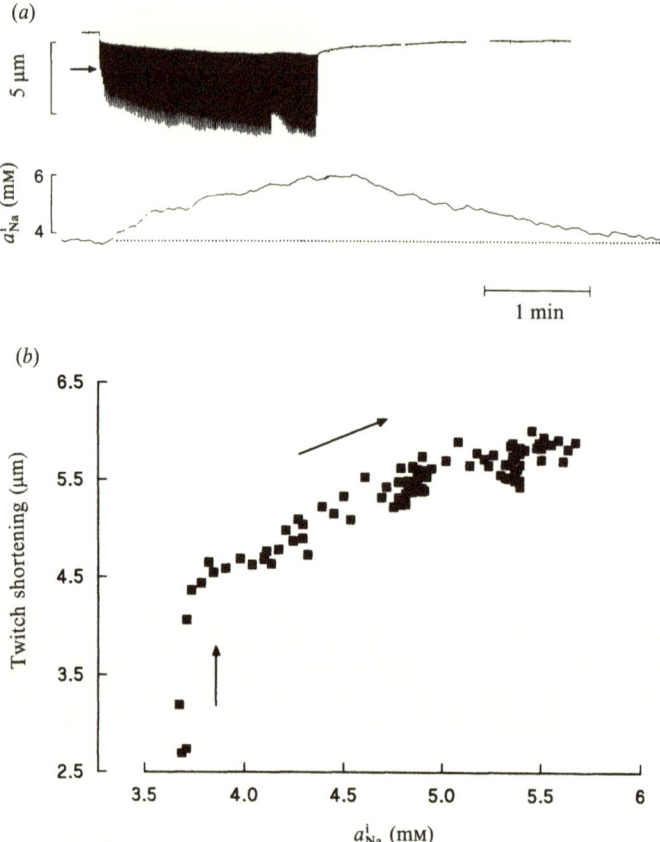

Fig. 13. Changes in the contraction and a^i_{Na} of a guinea-pig ventricular myocyte during a staircase at 1 Hz after a rest. (*a*) Cell length (measured optically; the contractions appear as downward-going deflections) and a^i_{Na} (measured with the Na^+-sensitive fluorescent dye, SBFI) before, during and after the staircase. The dotted line indicates the resting level of a^i_{Na}. The arrow highlights the first contraction after the rest. (*b*) The shortening of the cell during each twitch contraction during the staircase plotted against a^i_{Na}. The arrows indicate the time sequence of the data. Same experiment as the upper panel. Bathing Ca^{2+}, 1 mmol l⁻¹; temperature, 26 °C.

an important role to play in the slow phase (but not the fast phase) of the staircase of ventricular muscle.[9]

---

[9] Once again a word of caution should be sounded. TTX is expected to lead to changes in action potential duration and theoretically at least the effects on the staircase could be the result of these changes rather than an effect on a^i_{Na}. Seibel (1986) discounts this possibility, but ideally the experiment in Fig. 12 should be repeated under voltage clamp control.

Recently, Boyett & Harrison (1990) have recorded simultaneously a^i_{Na} and the contractions of isolated guinea-pig ventricular myocytes. Fig. 13(a) shows changes when a myocyte was stimulated at a rate of 1 Hz after a 4 min rest. Once again the strength of contraction increased in two phases during the staircase. During the fast phase of the staircase there was little change in a^i_{Na}, but during the slow phase the contraction and a^i_{Na} increased hand-in-hand. This is confirmed by Fig. 13(b) which shows that during the slow phase, but not the fast phase, there was a linear relationship between the two variables. On average twitch shortening increased by $1.8 \pm 0.3 \, \mu m$ per $mmol\,l^{-1}$ rise in a^i_{Na} (mean $\pm$ s.e.m.; $n = 16$). To test whether the increase in the twitch was the result of the rise in a^i_{Na}, in other experiments strophanthidin, a cardiac glycoside, at a concentration of $10^{-5} \, mol\,l^{-1}$, was used to elevate a^i_{Na}. This resulted in a $1.8 \pm 0.3 \, \mu m$ increase in twitch shortening per $mmol\,l^{-1}$ rise in a^i_{Na} ($n = 10$), which is not statistically different from the value obtained during the control staircase. The staircase of rat ventricular myocytes after a rest exhibits both fast and slow phases, but unlike guinea-pig ventricular myocytes twitch shortening declines rather than increases during the fast phase. Changes in the contraction and a^i_{Na} during a 1-Hz staircase from a rat ventricular myocyte after a 4 min rest are shown in Fig. 14(a). The first contraction after the rest, like that of Purkinje fibres (Fig. 9), was large, in contrast to the small first beat of guinea-pig ventricular myocytes (Fig. 8). During the next few beats the strength of contraction declined despite little change of a^i_{Na}. This was followed by a slow increase in both twitch shortening and a^i_{Na}. As in guinea-pig ventricular myocytes, there was a linear relationship between twitch shortening and a^i_{Na} during the slow phase, but not the fast phase, of the staircase (Fig. 14(b)). On average twitch shortening increased by $2.4 \pm 0.6 \, \mu m$ per $mmol\,l^{-1}$ rise in a^i_{Na} ($n = 5$). Strophanthidin, $10^{-4} \, mol\,l^{-1}$, resulted in a $1.8 \pm 0.2 \, \mu m$ increase in twitch shortening per $mmol\,l^{-1}$ rise in a^i_{Na} ($n = 5$), which is not statistically different from the value obtained during the control staircase. The data in Figs. 13 and 14 suggest that a^i_{Na} may be involved in the slow phase, but not the fast phase, of the staircase of ventricular muscle. This is consistent with the results obtained by Seibel (1986).

The results in Figs. 9, 10, 12, 13 and 14 suggest that a^i_{Na} has an important role to play in the slow phase of the staircase in both Purkinje fibres and ventricular muscle. Once again the interpretation of these findings depends on the source of Ca^{2+} for the Ca^{2+} transient. If the Ca^{2+} transient is largely the result of Ca^{2+} release from the sarcoplasmic reticulum (as in the case of sheep Purkinje fibres and rat ventricular

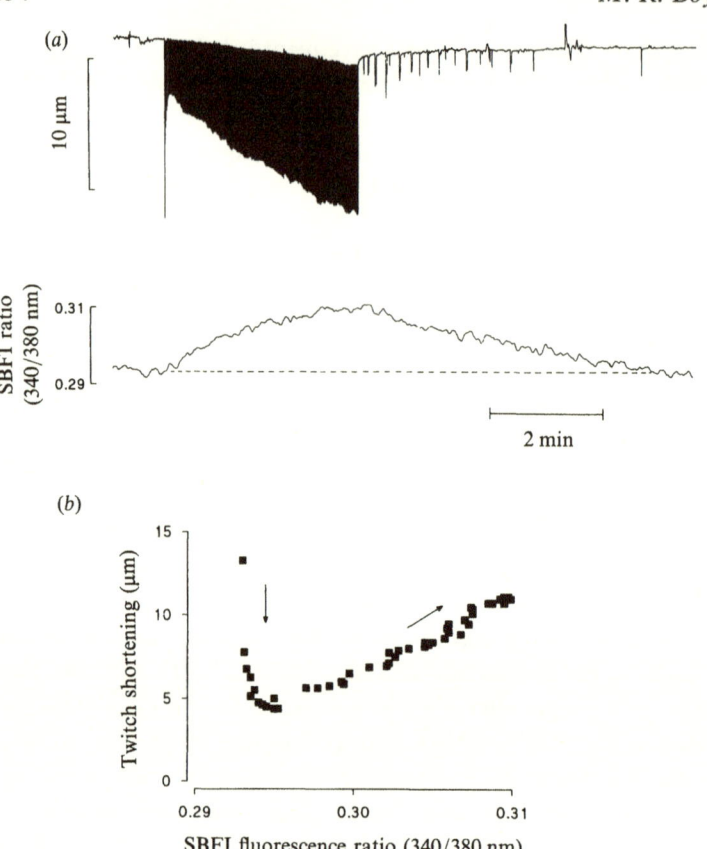

Fig. 14. Changes in the contraction and a^i_{Na} of a rat ventricular myocyte during a staircase at 2 Hz after a rest. (*a*) Cell length (measured optically; the contractions appear as downward-going deflections) and a^i_{Na} (measured with the Na^+-sensitive fluorescent dye, SBFI) before, during and after the staircase. In this experiment, the SBFI was not calibrated and the ordinate of the second trace shows the ratio of the SBFI fluorescence in response to excitation at 340 nm to the fluorescence in response to excitation at 380 nm. This ratio is a linear function of a^i_{Na}. The dashed line indicates the resting level of a^i_{Na}. (*b*) The shortening of the cell during each twitch contraction during the staircase plotted against the SBFI ratio. The arrows indicate the time sequence of the data. Same experiment as the upper panel. Bathing Ca^{2+}, 1 mmol l^{-1}; temperature, 30 °C.

muscle at least – Valdeolmillos & Eisner, 1985), the results are consistent with the mechanism proposed earlier: a rise of a^i_{Na} leading to Ca^{2+} loading of the sarcoplasmic reticulum via the Na–Ca exchanger. On the other hand, if the Ca^{2+} transient is largely the result of Ca^{2+} entry (as has been suggested for guinea-pig ventricular muscle – Bers & Hess, 1988), it suggests that the beat-to-beat increase in Ca^{2+} influx responsible for the staircase is related to the rise in a^i_{Na}. There is no evidence for such an action of a^i_{Na} on i_{Ca}, but the rise could theoretically at least lead to a beat-to-beat increase in Ca^{2+} influx via the Na–Ca exchanger during each action potential, if it is assumed that the exchanger reverses direction during the plateau of the action potential – Fig. 7 shows that a rise in a^i_{Na} increases Ca^{2+} influx via the exchanger (compare curves (c) and (d)).

Because the slow rise of a^i_{Na} at high rates may be an important determinant of the increase in the strength of contraction during the staircase, the factors responsible for the increase in a^i_{Na} will be briefly considered. In sheep Purkinje fibres, Boyett et al. (1987a) showed that the rise in a^i_{Na} during the staircase is in part the result of Na^+ influx via i_{Na} and they suggested that it is in part the result of Na^+ influx via the Na–Ca exchanger (this is considered in more detail below). The rise in a^i_{Na} occurs despite a reduction in Na^+ influx via the pacemaker current i_f and another pathway (perhaps a Na^+ leak channel or Na–Ca exchange[10]) during each action potential. If the rise of a^i_{Na} is important, the characteristic time course of the slow phase of the staircase could be the result of the slow rise of a^i_{Na}. The slow rise of a^i_{Na} is the result of the sensitivity of the Na–K pump to a^i_{Na}. On increasing the stimulation rate, Na^+ influx increases. This results in a rise in a^i_{Na} because Na^+ influx is now greater than Na^+ efflux via the Na–K pump. The activity of the Na–K pump is controlled by a^i_{Na} and this must rise by several $mmol\, l^{-1}$ until Na^+ efflux via the pump is once again equal to Na^+ influx. It takes several minutes for a^i_{Na} to rise sufficiently because the Na^+ influx associated with each action potential is only sufficient to increase a^i_{Na} by 3.5 $\mu mol\, l^{-1}$ (Bountra et al., 1988a). If the sensitivity of the Na–K pump to Na^+ was greater, the rise in a^i_{Na} would be more rapid, because a smaller rise in a^i_{Na} would be required to stimulate the pump.

---

[10] Because the Na–Ca exchanger can reverse, the exchanger, theoretically at least, can result in a net influx or efflux of Na^+. Fig. 11 (from Boyett et al., 1987b) shows that a train of short voltage clamp pulses resulted in a rise of a^i_{Na} (part of which was not dependent on i_{Na}) whereas a train of long voltage clamp pulses resulted in a fall of a^i_{Na}. It is possible that in the study of Boyett et al. (1987a) during a train of short voltage clamp pulses the exchanger resulted in net Na^+ influx – the effect of the Ca^{2+} transient on the exchanger (to stimulate Ca^{2+} efflux and Na^+ influx) would be greater than the effect of membrane depolarisation (which favours Ca^{2+} influx and Na^+ efflux). However, during a train of long voltage clamp pulses in the study of Boyett et al. (1987a) it is possible that the exchanger resulted in net Na^+ efflux because the effect of membrane depolarisation on the exchanger was greater than the effect of the Ca^{2+} transient.

Membrane potential modulation of the transmembrane Ca^{2+} flux via the Na–Ca exchanger is also important for rate and rhythm dependent changes in contractility

Involvement in the staircase

Gibbons & Fozzard (1975) studied the staircase of sheep Purkinje fibres during a train of just 10 voltage clamp pulses at a frequency of 0.5 Hz after a rest of 90 s or longer. If the voltage clamp pulses were short, e.g. 60 ms in duration, force declined during the staircase, but if the pulses were long, e.g. 1000 ms in duration, force steadily increased. The experiment shown in Fig. 11 is similar to this except that 4 min trains of voltage clamp pulses at a frequency of 2.5 Hz were applied. Once again, with the longer pulses, the increase in force during the staircase was greater. It is clear from Fig. 11 that the effect of pulse duration on the staircase is not the result of a^i_{Na}, because with long pulses a^i_{Na} fell rather than rose. The large increase in force during a train of long pulses could either be the result of the longer period during which i_{Ca} is flowing, or of the decrease in Ca^{2+} extrusion via the exchanger because of the longer time spent at the more positive potential. In this instance it is not possible to distinguish between these two possibilities. However, the experiment shown in Fig. 15(*a*) suggests that the effect of membrane potential on the exchanger is an important factor in the genesis of the staircase.

Figure 15(*a*) is taken from the study of Gibbons & Fozzard (1975) and shows changes in the force of contraction of a sheep Purkinje fibre during trains of voltage clamp pulses at 1 Hz after a rest of 90 s or longer. This time, pulse duration was held constant (300 ms) and the voltage during the pulses was varied in the different runs. During a train of pulses to a relatively negative potential, e.g. -34 mV, there was a progressive decrease in force during the staircase, but during a train of pulses to more positive potentials, e.g. $+40$ mV, there was a progressive increase in force. The effect of the pulse potential on the staircase is unlikely to be the result of any change in a^i_{Na}, because the rate-dependent rise in a^i_{Na}, theoretically at least, is expected to be smaller at pulse potentials more positive than 0 mV because of the reduction in i_{Na}. The effect of the pulse potential on the staircase was not the result of the voltage dependence of i_{Ca}, because i_{Ca} is maximal at about 0 mV and it declines at more positive potentials as the equilibrium potential for Ca^{2+}, E_{Ca}, is approached. Therefore, during the train of pulses to $+2$ mV, i_{Ca} and the associated Ca^{2+} influx will have been larger than that during the train of pulses to $+40$ mV, and yet despite this the rise in force was substantially greater during the train of pulses to +40 mV.

Another view of this experiment is provided by Fig. 15(b). The bell-shaped curve labelled 'a' in Fig. 15(b) shows the amplitude of the first beat of the trains plotted against the pulse potential. The voltage dependence of the first beat is possibly a reflection of the voltage dependence of i_{Ca}, which is also maximal at about 0 mV and less at more negative and positive potentials. Because the Ca^{2+} transient responsible for the twitch in sheep Purkinje fibres is believed to be the result of Ca^{2+}-induced Ca^{2+} release from the sarcoplasmic reticulum triggered by the Ca^{2+} current, the amplitude of the Ca^{2+} transient should be proportional to i_{Ca} (if the Ca^{2+} content of the sarcoplasmic reticulum is constant, as it should be in the case of the first beat after a rest). The curve labelled 'b' shows the amplitude of the last beat of the trains plotted against the pulse potential. The curve is no longer bell shaped. By the end of the train, the curve will not only reflect the voltage dependence of the trigger for Ca^{2+} release from the sarcoplasmic reticulum (presumably i_{Ca}), but also the voltage dependence of the mechanism responsible for increasing (or decreasing) the Ca^{2+} content of the sarcoplasmic reticulum during the staircase. The simplest interpretation of Fig. 15(b) is that this mechanism is tending to deplete the sarcoplasmic reticulum of Ca^{2+} at the more negative potentials and increase it at the more positive potentials. There is no sign that the Ca^{2+} loading of the sarcoplasmic reticulum reached a maximum at the most positive potential studied. This behaviour is not consistent with the voltage dependence of i_{Ca}, but it is consistent with the voltage dependence of the Na–Ca exchanger – Ca^{2+} influx via the exchanger which is expected to be greater the more positive the potential (Fig. 6).

The result in Fig. 15 was obtained using a Purkinje fibre, but duBell & Houser (1989) have obtained similar results using cat ventricular myocytes, and Fig. 16 shows a similar result obtained in our laboratory from a ferret ventricular myocyte. It shows changes in twitch shortening during a chain of 10 voltage clamp pulses (200 ms in duration) after a rest. During the train of pulses to −17 mV there was a gradual decline in the twitch, whereas during the train of pulses to +43 mV there was a progressive increase in the amplitude of the twitch. This behaviour suggests that the voltage dependence of the Na–Ca exchanger is also an important factor in the staircase in ventricular muscle.

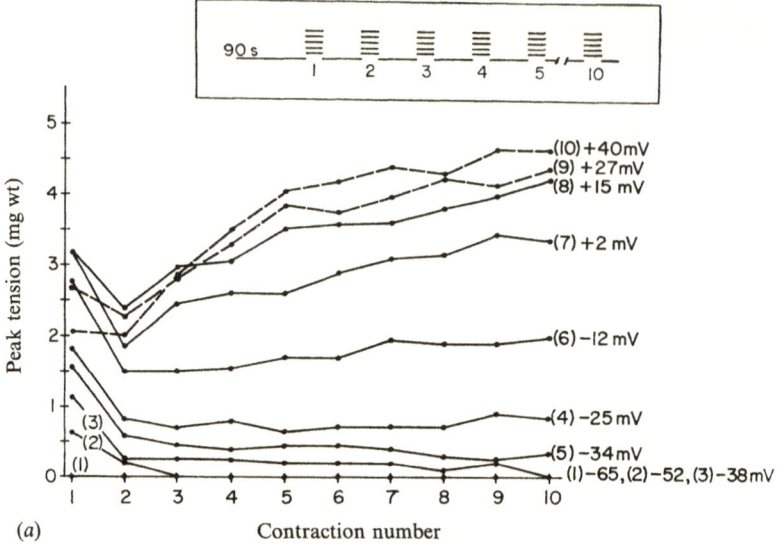

Fig. 15. The effect of the pulse potential on the changes in the force of contraction of a sheep Purkinje fibre during a train of 10 voltage clamp pulses after a 90 s rest. (a) Plot of peak tension against the number of the pulse during the train. The results from a number of trains are superimposed. The pulse potential was varied in the different runs and is shown next to each trace. (b) Plot of the peak tension of the first (curve a) and eleventh (curve b) contractions against the pulse potential during the trains. Same experiment as panel (a). The experimental protocols are shown in the insets. Holding potential, -75 mV; pulse duration, 300 ms; pulse frequency, 1 Hz. Bathing Ca^{2+}, 2.7 mmol l^{-1}; temperature, 36 °C. (From Gibbons & Fozzard (1975) with permission.)

Involvement in paired pulse stimulation

A phenomenon related to the staircase is paired pulse stimulation, and the voltage dependence of the Na–Ca exchanger may be of particular importance in this situation (Boyett, Kirby & Orchard, 1989*b*). Paired pulse stimulation is illustrated by Fig. 17. Fig. 17 shows the contractions of a ferret ventricular myocyte in response to 200 ms voltage clamp pulses. The pulses were applied at a frequency of 0.5 Hz and the cell was allowed to reach a steady state. Five pairs of voltage clamp pulses were then applied. In the different runs, the interval between the pair of pulses was varied from 0 to 800 ms. With an interval of 0 ms, the duration of the pulses was effectively doubled from 200 to 400ms, whereas the frequency of the pulses remained constant at 0.5 Hz. With an interval of 800 ms, the 200 ms pulses were regularly spaced and the frequency of regularly spaced pulses was effectively doubled from 0.5 to 1 Hz. After the five pairs of

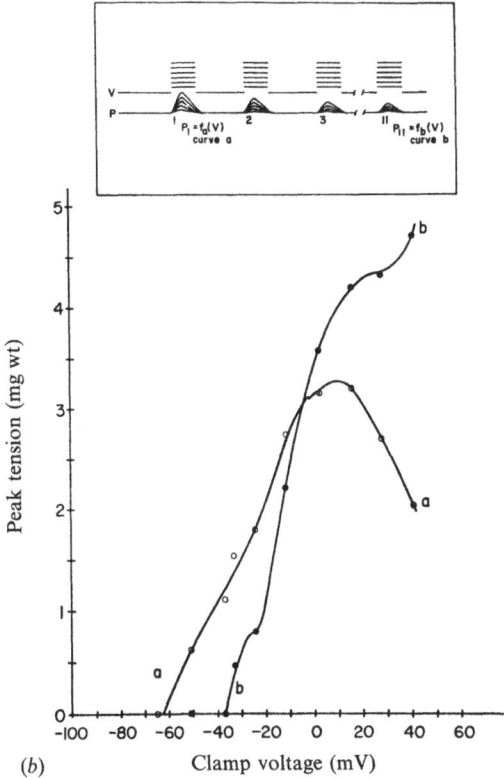

(b)

Fig. 15 (contd).

pulses, normal stimulation at 0.5 Hz was resumed. It is well known that paired pulse stimulation results in a positive inotropic effect (e.g. Hoffman, Bindler & Suckling, 1956; Brutsaert, 1966) and Fig. 17 shows that the inotropic effect is dependent upon the interval between the pair of pulses – the increase in twitch shortening was maximal with an interval of 100 ms between the pair of pulses and it was less with longer intervals. The corollary of this is that true paired pulse stimulation (with an interval of 100 ms between the pair of pulses, for example) results in a more substantial increase in the strength of contraction than doubling the stimulus frequency (i.e. with an interval of 800 ms between the pulses). This is well known (Hoffman et al., 1956; Allen, 1975). In Fig. 18(a), the amplitude of the second contraction of the pair (as a percentage of the control) is plotted against the interval between the pair of pulses. The resulting curve is a so-called 'mechanical restitution' curve. In Fig. 18(b), the amplitude of the first beat of the last pair (as a percentage of the

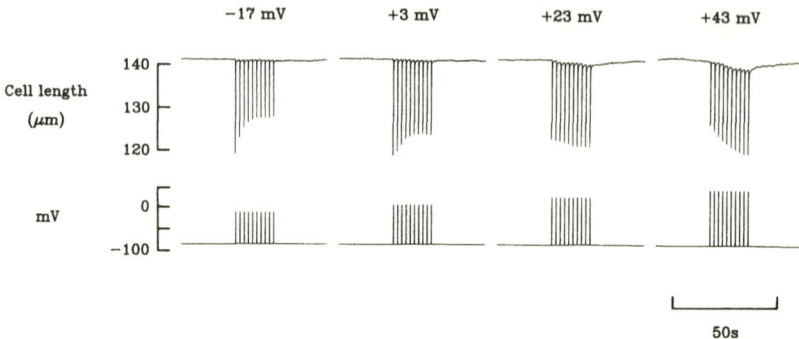

Fig. 16. The effect of the pulse potential on the changes in the contraction of a ferret ventricular myocyte during a train of 10 voltage clamp pulses after a rest. The traces show the changes in the cell length (measured optically; the contractions appear as downward-going deflections) and the membrane potential during four trains of pulses. The membrane potential during the pulses is shown above the traces. Holding potential, -85 mV; pulse duration, 200 ms; pulse frequency, 0.5 Hz. Bathing Ca^{2+}, 2 mmol l^{-1}; temperature, 34 °C.

control), an index of the inotropic effect of paired pulse stimulation, is plotted against the interval between the pair of pulses. Fig. 18(*b*) confirms that the inotropic effect of paired pulse stimulation was greatest with an interval of 100 ms. Fig. 18 shows that, as the interval between the pair of pulses was increased, the amplitude of the second contraction of each pair increased and the potentiation of the first beat of each pair declined. The possible significance of this will be considered later.

The inotropic effect of paired pulse stimulation could be the result of doubling Ca^{2+} influx via i_{Ca} (the number of Ca^{2+} currents is doubled as a result of the doubling of the number of pulses). Alternatively, the inotropic effect could be the result of doubling the time the membrane is depolarised and the effect of this on Na–Ca exchange. To distinguish between these alternatives, the voltage dependence of paired pulse potentiation was investigated and the results are shown in Fig. 19. Fig. 19(*a*) shows the results of three runs similar to those in Fig. 17 but with the interval between the pair of pulses held constant (it is not possible to separate visually the second contraction of the pair from the first) and the potential during the second pulse of each pair varied in different runs. Fig. 19(*a*) shows that the the inotropic effect of paired pulse stimulation was greater when the membrane was clamped to a more positive potential during the second pulse of the pair, and this is confirmed graphically in Fig. 19(*b*). If paired pulse potentiation is the result of an increase in Ca^{2+}

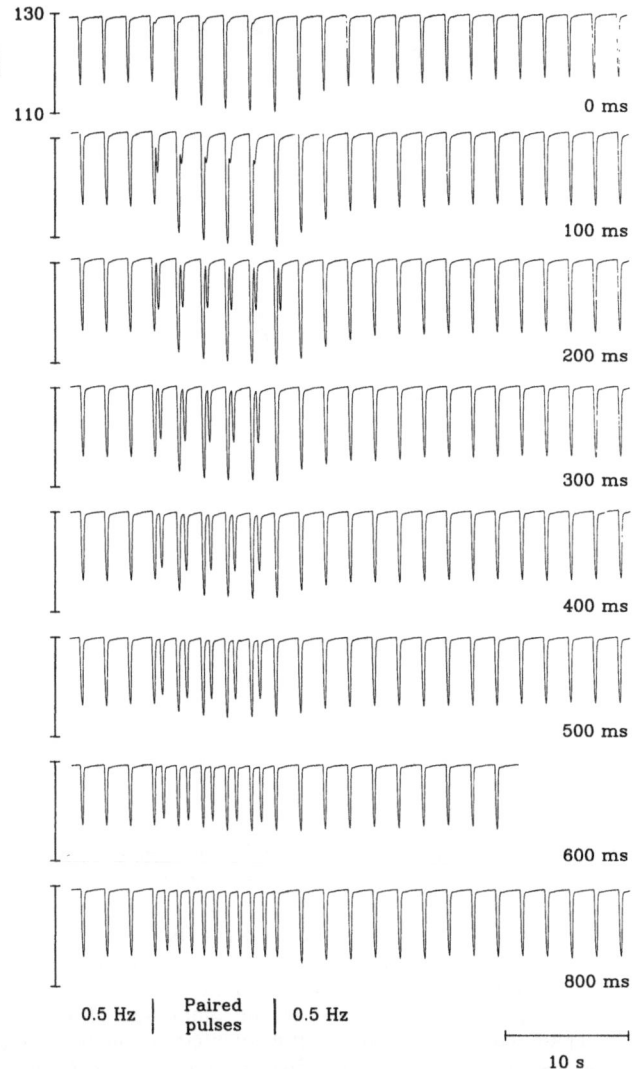

Fig. 17. The effect of the interval between the pair of pulses on paired pulse potentiation of a ferret ventricular myocyte. Single voltage clamp pulses at a frequency of 0.5 Hz were applied to a ferret ventricular myocyte. When the cell was at a steady state, five pairs of pulses were applied at the basic frequency of 0.5 Hz. After paired pulse stimulation, normal stimulation was resumed. In different runs, the interval between the pair of pulses was varied; the interval is shown next to each trace. The stimulation protocol is shown at the bottom of the figure. Holding potential, -69 mV; pulse potential, -9 mV; pulse duration 200 ms. Bathing Ca^{2+}, 2 mmol l^{-1}; temperature, 30 °C.

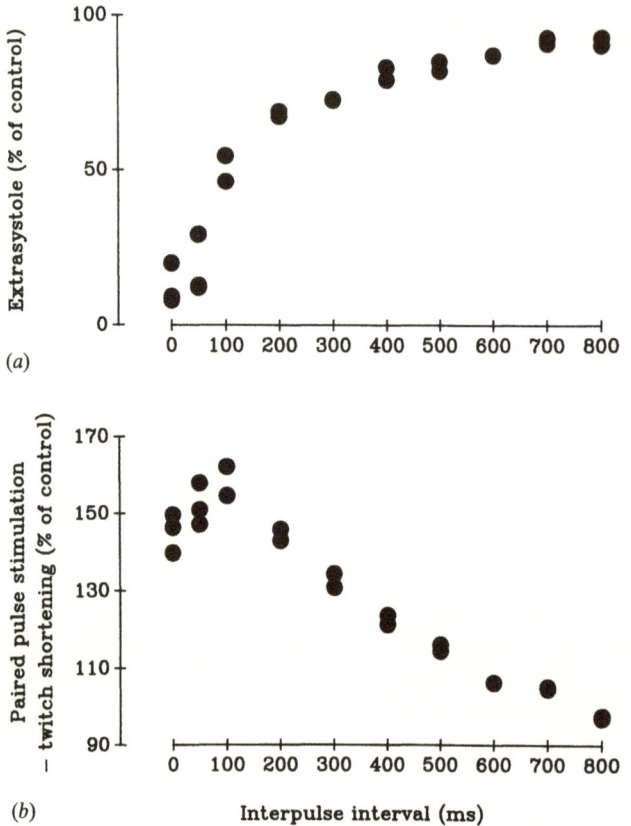

(a)

(b)

Fig. 18. The degree of potentiation of a ferret ventricular myocyte during paired pulse stimulation is inversely proportional to the amplitude of the second contraction of the pair. (a) The dependence of the amplitude of the second contraction (or extrasystole) of the first pair on the interval between the pair of pulses. The amplitude of the extrasystole is expressed as a percentage of the amplitude of a control contraction during regular stimulation at 0.5 Hz prior to paired pulse stimulation. (b) The dependence of the amplitude of the first contraction of the final pair (a measure of paired pulse potentiation) on the interval between the pair of pulses. The amplitude of the final contraction is expressed as a percentage of the amplitude of a control contraction prior to paired pulse stimulation. For intervals greater than 50 ms the potentiation of the first contraction of the pair during paired pulse potentiation is inversely proportional to the amplitude of the second contraction of the pair. Same experiment as Fig. 17.

influx via i_{Ca} the inotropic effect would be expected to decline at potentials positive to 0 mV as a result of the decrease in i_{Ca} over this potential range. This was not the case. The voltage dependence of paired pulse potentiation

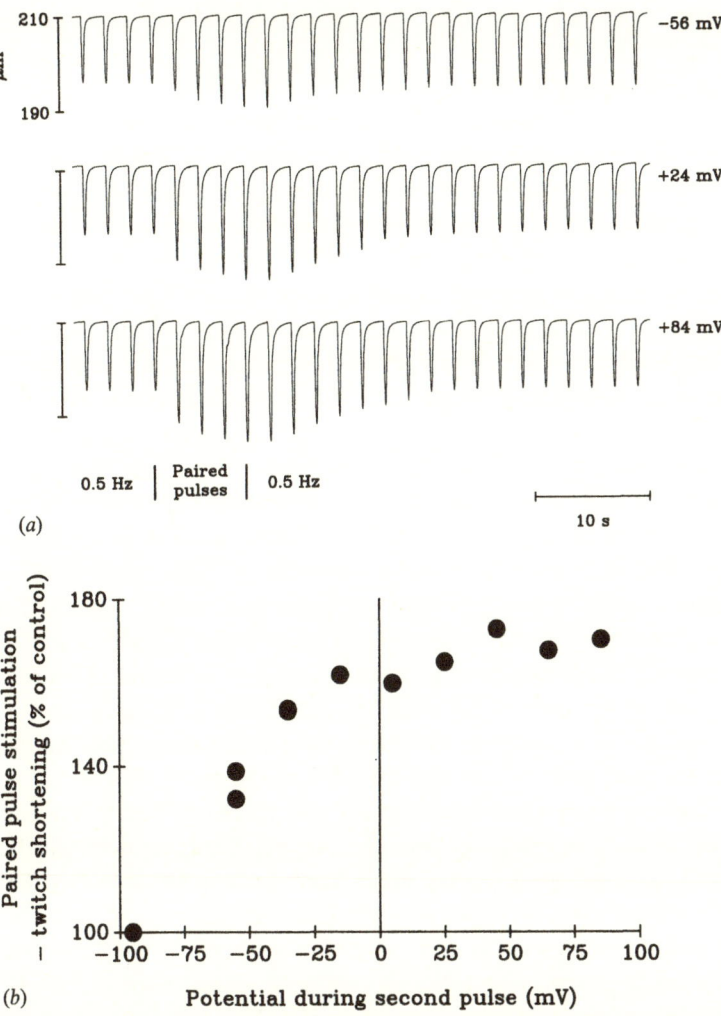

Fig. 19. The effect of the membrane potential during the second pulse of the pair on paired pulse potentiation of a ferret ventricular myocyte. 200 ms voltage clamp pulses to -34 mV were regularly applied to a ferret ventricular myocyte at a frequency of 0.5 Hz. When the cell had reached a steady state five pairs of pulses were applied to the cell, after which normal stimulation of 0.5 Hz was resumed. The interval between the pairs of pulses was 5 ms. In different runs the membrane potential during the second pulse of the pair was varied (the membrane potential during the first pulse of the pair was kept constant at -34 mV). (a) Changes in cell length (the contractions appear as downward deflections) during three runs when the membrane potential during the second pulse of the pair was clamped to -56, $+24$ and $+84$ mV. The stimulation protocol is shown beneath the traces. (b) The dependence of the amplitude of the first contraction of the final pair (a

(continued on next page)

is, however, consistent with the voltage dependence of the Na–Ca exchanger (Fig. 6) – Ca^{2+} influx via the exchanger is greater the more positive the membrane potential.

Fig. 20 illustrates a hypothesis, similar to that put forward by Hilgemann & Noble (1987), to explain paired pulse potentiation. It shows a pair of Ca^{2+} transients triggered by a pair of voltage-clamp pulses. The second Ca^{2+} transient is smaller than the first, a situation analogous to paired pulse stimulation. The driving force on the Na–Ca exchanger is the difference between the reversal potential (eqn. 1) and the membrane potential (upper panel). During the first pulse, because of the large rise in $[Ca]_i$ the reversal potential shifts in the positive direction and for part of the pulse at least the reversal potential is more positive than the membrane potential and this results in net Ca^{2+} efflux (hatched area) via the exchanger. In contrast during the second pulse of the pair, the rise in $[Ca]_i$ is less and as a consequence the reversal potential is negative to the membrane potential and this results in Ca^{2+} influx (dotted area) via the exchanger. This is expected to lead to a loading of the sarcoplasmic reticulum and a positive inotropic effect in subsequent beats.[11] This model explains the findings shown in Figs. 17 and 18 – according to this model, the inotropic effect of paired pulse stimulation is less at longer interpulse intervals because the second contraction (and hence Ca^{2+} transient) of the pair is larger as a result of more complete 'mechanical restitution'. During the second pulse of the pair the shift of the reversal potential of the exchanger to more positive potentials will therefore be greater and the driving force bringing Ca^{2+} into the cell via the exchanger will be reduced or even eliminated. On the other hand the driving force bringing Ca^{2+} into the cell via the exchanger (the difference between the reversal potential and the membrane potential) will be greater the more positive the membrane potential during the second pulse of the pair; the model can therefore explain the findings shown in Fig. 19.

The experimental findings presented in this section were obtained using

---

[11] Note that this scheme can only work if the Ca^{2+} transient is primarily dependent on Ca^{2+} release from the sarcoplasmic reticulum.

Caption for Fig. 19 (*cont.*)
measure of paired pulse potentiation) on the membrane potential during the second pulse of the pair. The amplitude of the first contraction is expressed as a percentage of a control contraction during regular stimulation at 0.5 Hz prior to paired pulse stimulation. Holding potential, -95 mV. Bathing Ca^{2+}, 2 mmol l^{-1}; temperature, $30\,^{\circ}C$.

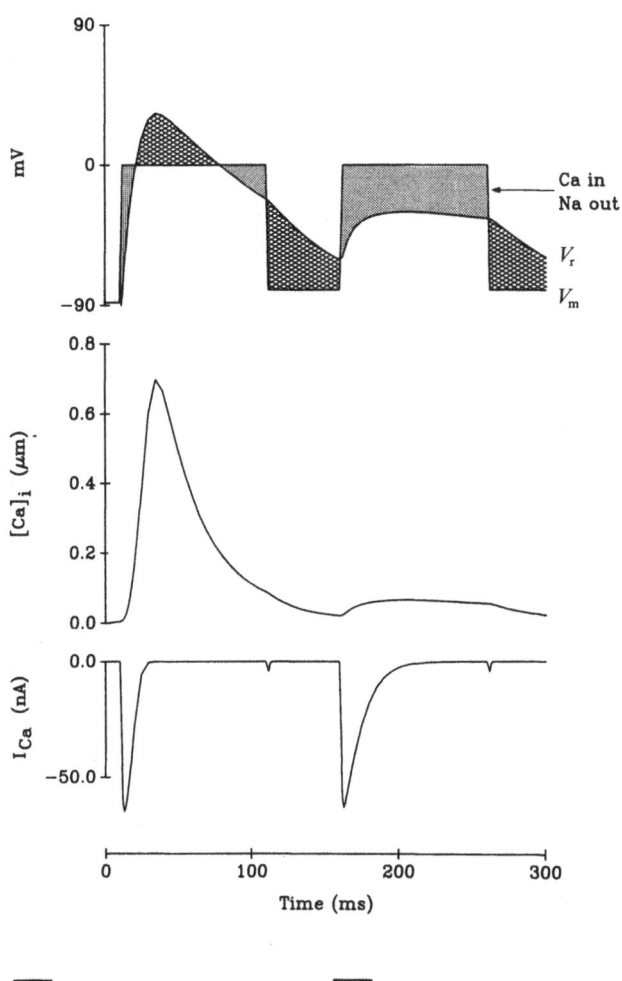

Fig. 20. Calculated changes in the reversal potential of the Na–Ca exchanger, V_r (top), the intracellular Ca^{2+} concentration, $[Ca]_i$ (middle), and the Ca^{2+} current, I_{Ca} (bottom), during a pair of voltage clamp pulses (top). In the upper panel the dotted areas indicate when the membrane potential (V_m) is more positive than the reversal potential of the exchanger and there is net Ca^{2+} influx and Na^+ efflux via the exchanger, and the hatched areas indicate when the membrane potential is more negative than the reversal potential of the exchanger and there is net Ca^{2+} efflux and Na^+ influx via the exchanger. The changes were calculated using the Hilgemann & Noble (1987) version of the 'Heart' program written by D. Noble. Holding potential, -80 mV; pulse potential, 0 mV; pulse duration, 100 ms; interval between the pair of pulses, 50 ms.

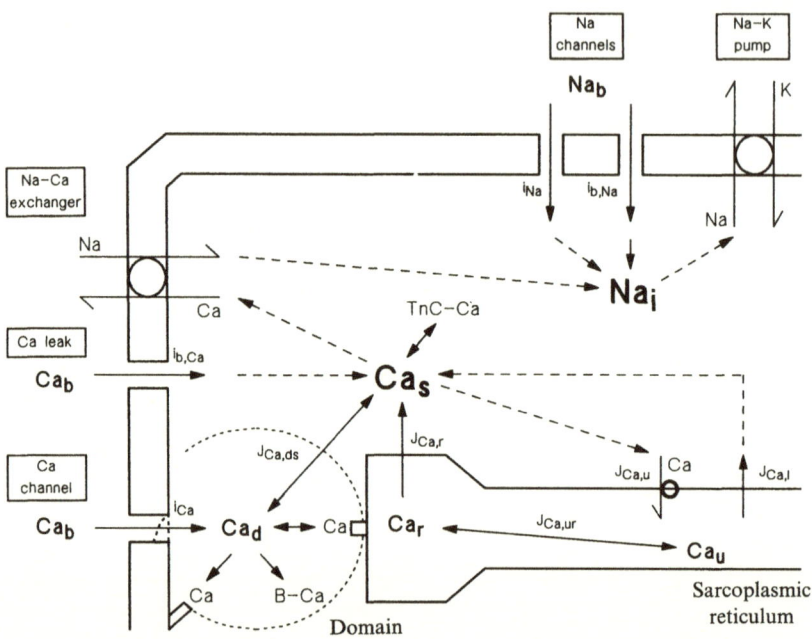

Fig. 21. A schematic diagram of the model of excitation–contraction coupling. See text for explanation and Table 1 for the meaning of the abbreviations.

sheep Purkinje fibres and ferret ventricular myocytes – in both of these tissues the Ca^{2+} transient depends primarily on Ca^{2+} release from the sarcoplasmic reticulum. The results are consistent with the mechanism presented earlier and the membrane potential dependence of the Na–Ca exchanger can lead to an increase in the Ca^{2+} content of the sarcoplasmic reticulum both during the staircase (Fig. 15) and during paired pulse stimulation (e.g. Fig. 19). In tissues in which the Ca^{2+} transient is primarily dependent on Ca^{2+} influx, the membrane potential dependence of the Na–Ca exchanger will be of importance if Ca^{2+} influx via the exchanger, as well as i_{Ca}, contributes to the Ca^{2+} transient.

A computer model of the staircase

The experiments described above suggest that i_{Ca} and the Na–Ca exchanger are important factors in the generation of the staircase. To test in a quantitative manner if these mechanisms can account for the staircase a mathematical model of a single cardiac cell has been constructed. The

Table 1. *Model variables and constants*

Symbol	Variable or constant	Value	Unit
t	time	–	s
F	Faraday's constant	96 500	C mol^{-1}
R	Universal gas constant	8.31	joules mol^{-1} K^{-1}
T	Temperature	303	K
E_m	Membrane potential	–	V
V_c	Cell volume	35×10^{-12}	l
V_d, V_r, V_u, V_s	Volume of domains, release and uptake sites and sarcoplasm	–	l
$[Na]_b$	Bathing Na$^+$ concentration	140×10^{-3}	mol l^{-1}
$[Na]_i$	Intracellular Na$^+$ concentration	–	mol l^{-1}
$[K]_b$	Bathing K$^+$ concentration	5.4×10^{-3}	mol l^{-1}
$[K]_i$	Intracellular K$^+$ concentration	140×10^{-3}	mol l^{-1}
$[Ca]_b$	Bathing Ca^{2+} concentration	2×10^{-3}	mol l^{-1}
$[Ca]_s$	Sarcoplasmic Ca^{2+} concentration	–	mol l^{-1}
$[Ca]_d$	Ca^{2+} concentration in the domains	–	mol l^{-1}
$[Ca]_r$	Ca^{2+} concentration in the release site	–	mol l^{-1}
$[Ca]_u$	Ca^{2+} concentration in the uptake site	–	mol l^{-1}
$[B]_d$	Concentration of Ca^{2+} buffer in the domains	400×10^{-6}	mol l^{-1}
$[B]_s$	Concentration of Ca^{2+} buffer in the sarcoplasm	200×10^{-6}	mol l^{-1}
E_{Na}	Na$^+$ equilibrium potential	–	V
E_{Ca}	Ca^{2+} equilibrium potential	–	V
i_{Na}	Main Na$^+$ current	–	A
g_{Na}	Main Na$^+$ conductance	4×10^{-6}	S
E_{mh}	Reversal potential of i_{Na}	–	V
m, h	i_{Na} gating variables	–	–
$\alpha_m, \beta_m, \alpha_h, \beta_h$	i_{Na} rate constants	–	s^{-1}
$i_{b,Na}$	Background Na$^+$ current	–	A
$g_{b,Na}$	Background Na$^+$ conductance	0.0002×10^{-6}	S
i_p	Na–K pump current	–	A
$i_{p,max}$	Maximum i_p	0.6×10^{-9}	A
$K_{m,K}$	$[K]_b$ at which i_p is half-maximally activated	1×10^{-3}	mol l^{-1}
$K_{m,Na}$	$[Na]_i$ at which i_p is half-maximally activated	15×10^{-3}	mol l^{-1}
n	Hill coefficient for the activation of i_p by Na$^+$	1.5	–
i_{Ca}	Main Ca^{2+} current	–	A
$i_{Ca,max}$	Maximum i_{Ca}	–	A
P_{Ca}	Main Ca^{2+} permeability	150	–
d, f_1, f_2, f_3	i_{Ca} gating variables	–	–
$\alpha_d, \beta_d, \alpha_{f1}, \beta_{f1}, \alpha_{f2}, \beta_{f2}$	i_{Ca} rate constants	–	s^{-1}
$K_{m,i}$	$[Ca]_d$ at which i_{Ca} is half-maximally inactivated	1×10^{-6}	mol l^{-1}
$i_{b,Ca}$	Background Ca^{2+} current	–	A

Table 1 (cont.)

$g_{b,Ca}$	Background Ca^{2+} conductance	0.0006×10^{-6}	S
$J_{Ca,r}$	Ca^{2+} flux from release site into sarcoplasm	–	mol s^{-1}
α_r	Rate constant for $J_{Ca,r}$	66.7	s^{-1}
$K_{m,r}$	$[Ca]_d$ at which $J_{Ca,r}$ is half-maximally activated	1×10^{-6}	mol l^{-1}
R	Available fraction of Ca^{2+} release sites	–	–
α_i	Rate constant of inactivation of Ca^{2+} release channels	10^7	s^{-1}
β_i	Rate constant of recovery from inactivation of Ca^{2+} release channels	1.0	s^{-1}
$J_{Ca,u}$	Ca^{2+} flux from sarcoplasm into uptake site	–	mol l^{-1}
$J_{Ca,u,max}$	Maximum $J_{Ca,u}$	0.06×10^{-12}	mol l^{-1}
$K_{m,u}$	$[Ca]_s$ at which $J_{Ca,u}$ is half-maximally activated	150×10^{-9}	mol l^{-1}
$J_{Ca,1}$	Ca^{2+} leak from uptake site into sarcoplasm	–	mol s^{-1}
a_1	Rate constant of Ca^{2+} leak from uptake site into sarcoplasm	1.72	s^{-1}
$J_{Ca,ur}$	Ca^{2+} flux from uptake to release site	–	mol s^{-1}
a_{ur}	Rate constant of Ca^{2+} flux from uptake to release site	2.857×10^{12}	s^{-1}
i_{NaCa}	Na–Ca exchange current	–	A
k_{NaCa}	Scaling factor for i_{NaCa}	0.48	A (mol l)$^{-4}$
r	Partition coefficient for i_{NaCa}	1.0	–
$J_{Ca,ds}$	Ca^{2+} flux from domains into sarcoplasm	–	mol s^{-1}
α_{ds}	Rate constant of Ca^{2+} flux from domains to sarcoplasm	3.3×10^3	s^{-1}
U_d	Fraction of Ca^{2+} free (unbound) in the domains	–	–
U_s	Fraction of Ca^{2+} free (unbound) in the sarcoplasm	–	–
$K_{m,b}$	[Ca] at which the Ca^{2+} buffer is half-maximally saturated	2×10^{-6}	mol l^{-1}

model is based on the model published by DiFrancesco and Noble (1985) and Hilgemann and Noble (1987). The Ca^{2+} movements envisaged in the model are similar to those proposed by others (e.g. Kaufmann et al., 1974; Allen, Jewell & Wood, 1976). In the model the Ca^{2+} transient is primarily dependent on Ca^{2+} release from the sarcoplasmic reticulum. A schematic diagram of the model is shown in Fig. 21. Na$^+$ enters the cell via voltage-dependent Na$^+$ channels, background Na$^+$ channels and the Na–Ca exchanger. It is pumped out of the cell via the Na–K pump. Ca^{2+}

enters the cell via voltage-dependent Ca^{2+} channels (the main Ca^{2+} channels) and background Ca^{2+} channels. Inactivation of the main Ca^{2+} channels is, in part, the result of voltage-dependent inactivation and in part Ca^{2+}-dependent inactivation. Ca^{2+} flows through the main Ca^{2+} channels and accumulates in miniature 'domains' centred on the openings of Ca^{2+} channels on the inner face of the membrane. Within the domains Ca^{2+} can bind to (i) a Ca^{2+} buffer, (ii) a receptor and bring about Ca^{2+}-dependent inactivation of the Ca^{2+} channel, and (iii) one of the subsarcolemmal cisternae (which are thought to be the site of Ca^{2+} storage and may be in close juxtaposition to the Ca^{2+} channels – Cohen & Lederer, 1988) and bring about Ca^{2+} release from the cisternae. In the model this Ca^{2+} is not released into the domains next to the Ca^{2+} channels; instead it is released into the general sarcoplasm. The Ca^{2+} within the domains is also able to diffuse into the sarcoplasm. The Ca^{2+} within the sarcoplasm can bind to a buffer (such as troponin-C), leave the cell via the Na–Ca exchanger, or be taken back up into the sarcoplasmic reticulum via a Ca^{2+} pump. In common with many models of excitation–contraction coupling in the heart, Ca^{2+} is taken up by a separate uptake site. The Ca^{2+} can then diffuse from the uptake site to the release site of the sarcoplasmic reticulum. In the model there is also a leak of Ca^{2+} out of the uptake site of the sarcoplasmic reticulum into the sarcoplasm.

Description of the equations

The variables and constants used in the model are listed in Table 1.

The principal route for Na^+ influx is via the voltage-dependent Na^+ current, i_{Na}. This current is calculated from a set of equations taken from DiFrancesco & Noble (1985) with g_{Na} scaled down for a single cell:

$$i_N{}^a = m^3 h g_N{}^a (E_M - E_{MM}) \tag{2}$$

$$E_{mh} = \frac{RT}{F} \log_e \frac{[Na]_b + 0.12[K]_b}{[Na]_i + 0.12[K]_i} \tag{3}$$

$$\frac{dm}{dt} = \alpha_m(1 - m) - \beta_m m \tag{4}$$

$$\frac{dh}{dt} = \alpha_h(1 - h) - \beta_h h \tag{5}$$

$$\alpha_m = \frac{200(1000E_m + 41)}{1 - \exp(-0.1(1000E_m + 41))} \tag{6}$$

$$\beta_m = 8000 \exp(-0.056(1000E_m + 66)) \tag{7}$$

$$\alpha_h = 20 \exp(-0.125(1000E_m + 75)) \tag{8}$$

$$\beta_h = \frac{2000}{320 \exp(-0.1(1000E_m + 75)) + 1} \tag{9}$$

Na^+ also flows into the cell via a background Na^+ current, $i_{b,Na}$ (from DiFrancesco & Noble, 1985):

$$i_{b,Na} = g_{b,Na}(E_m - E_{Na}) \tag{10}$$

where

$$E_{Na} = \frac{RT}{F} \log_e \frac{[Na]_b}{[Na]_i} \tag{11}$$

Na^+ is primarily removed from the cell via the Na–K pump. The Na–K pump current, i_p, is given by the following equation (after Boyett & Fedida, 1988):

$$i_p = i_{p,max} \cdot \frac{[K]_b}{K_{m,K} + [K]_b} \cdot \frac{[Na]_i^n}{K_{m,Na}^n + [Na]_i^n} \tag{12}$$

A change in the $[Na]_i$ will depend on the balance of Na^+ influx and efflux:

$$\frac{d[Na]_i}{dt} = \frac{-i_{Na} + i_{b,Na} + 3i_{NaCa} + 3i_p}{FV_c} \tag{13}$$

The intracellular Na^+ activity, a^i_{Na}, was calculated by multiplying $[Na]_i$ by an activity coefficient of 0.76.

The principal means of Ca^{2+} influx is via the voltage dependent Ca^{2+} current, i_{Ca}:

$$i_{Ca} = df_1 f_2 f_3 i_{Ca,max} \tag{14}$$

where d is the voltage-dependent activation variable which is given by the following equations taken from DiFrancesco & Noble (1985):

$$\frac{\mathrm{d}d}{\mathrm{d}t} = \alpha_d(1 - d) - \beta_d d \tag{15}$$

$$\alpha_d = \frac{30(1000E_m + 24)}{1 - \exp(-(1000E_m + 24)/4)} \tag{16}$$

$$\beta_d = \frac{12(1000E_m + 24)}{\exp((1000E_m + 24)/10) - 1} \tag{17}$$

i_{Ca} has fast and slow phases of voltage-dependent inactivation (Boyett & Kirby, 1988) and these are governed by the inactivation variables f_1 and f_2 in eqn. 14. The fast and slow phases of inactivation have not been fully characterised and in the model the rate constants for these processes are only crudely described. The following equations have been used for f_1 and f_2:

$$\frac{\mathrm{d}f_1}{\mathrm{d}t} = \alpha_{f1}(1 - f_1) - \beta_{f1} f_1 \tag{18}$$

$$\frac{\mathrm{d}f_2}{\mathrm{d}t} = \alpha_{f2}(1 - f_2) - \beta_{f2} f_2 \tag{19}$$

At $-80\,\mathrm{mV}$: $\alpha_{f1} = 2.5$, $\beta_{f1} = 0$

At $> -80\,\mathrm{mV}$: $\alpha_{f1} = 5$, $\beta_{f1} = 5$

At $-80\,\mathrm{mV}$: $\alpha_{f2} = 0.1$, $\beta_{f2} = 0$

At $> -80\,\mathrm{mV}$: $\alpha_{f2} = 0.01$, $\beta_{f2} = 0.09$

A substantial component of inactivation of i_{Ca} is known to be Ca^{2+} dependent inactivation (for review, see Eckert & Chad, 1984). In the model Ca^{2+}-dependent inactivation is described using a scheme put forward by Eckert & Chad (1984; see also Standen & Stanfield, 1982). The Ca^{2+} flows through the Ca^{2+} channels and accumulates in small domains on the inner surface of the membrane. The domains may be the result of the slow diffusion away from the Ca^{2+} channels rather than true anatomical structures. Within the domains it is suggested that Ca^{2+} can bind to a site (with a binding constant, $K_{m,i}$) and bring about inactivation of the channel. f_3 in eqn. 14 is the inactivation variable for Ca^{2+}-dependent inactivation – it is the proportion of Ca^{2+} channels not inactivated by

Ca^{2+}. It is given by

$$f_3 = 1 - \frac{[Ca]_d}{K_{m,i} + [Ca]_d} \tag{20}$$

The maximum Ca^{2+} current, $i_{Ca,max}$, in eqn. 14 is given by the following equation from DiFrancesco and Noble (1985):

$$i_{Ca,max} = \frac{4P_{Ca}(E_m - 0.05)F/(RT)}{1 - \exp(-(E_m - 0.05)2F/(RT))}$$

$$\times \left\{ [Ca]_d \exp\left(\frac{F}{10RT}\right) - [Ca]_b \exp\left(\frac{-(E_m - 0.05)2F}{RT}\right) \right\} \tag{21}$$

Ca^{2+} also flows into the cell via a background Ca^{2+} current, $i_{b,Ca}$ (from DiFrancesco & Noble, 1985):

$$i_{b,Ca} = g_{b,Ca}(E_m - E_{Ca}) \tag{22}$$

where

$$E_{Ca} = \frac{RT}{2F} \log_e \frac{[Ca]_b}{[Ca]_s} \tag{23}$$

Ca^{2+} efflux from the cell is via the Na–Ca exchanger, which is assumed to have a stoichiometry of $3Na^+ : 1Ca^{2+}$. The Na–Ca exchanger current, i_{NaCa}, is given by the following equation from Noble (1986) and Kimura, Miyamae and Noma (1987):

$$i_{NaCa} = k_{NaCa} \left\{ [Na]_i^3 [Ca]_b \exp\left(\frac{rE_m F}{RT}\right) \right.$$

$$\left. - [Na]_b^3 [Ca]_s \exp\left(-\frac{(1 - r)E_m F}{RT}\right) \right\} \tag{24}$$

A change in the sarcoplasmic Ca^{2+} concentration, $[Ca]_s$, will depend on the balance of entry and exit of Ca^{2+} into and out of the sarcoplasm:

$$\frac{d[Ca]_s}{dt} = \frac{U_s}{V_s} \left(J_{Ca,ds} - \frac{i_{b,Ca}}{2F} + \frac{i_{NaCa}}{F} + J_{Ca,r} - J_{Ca,u} + J_{Ca,l} \right) \tag{25}$$

Equation 25 shows that $[Ca]_s$ is the result of Ca^{2+} movements within the cell as well as across the cell membrane.

In the model the Ca^{2+} transient is predominantly the result of release of Ca^{2+} from the release site of the sarcoplasmic reticulum by Ca^{2+}-

dependent Ca^{2+} release: Ca^{2+} within the domains is able to bind to a
site (with a binding constant $K_{m,r}$) on the sarcoplasmic reticulum to bring
about release. The Ca^{2+} flux from the release site into the sarcoplasm,
$J_{Ca,r}$ in eqn. 25, is given by an equation adapted from the work of
DiFrancesco and Noble (1985):

$$J_{Ca,r} = \alpha_r R \frac{[Ca]_d^2}{K_{m,r}^2 + [Ca]_d^2} V_r [Ca]_r \tag{26}$$

Fabiato (1985) demonstrated that Ca^{2+} inactivates as well as activates
Ca^{2+} release. R in eqn. 26 is an inactivation variable and it is the
proportion of Ca^{2+} release channels not inactivated by Ca^{2+}. It has been
assumed that Ca^{2+}-dependent inactivation occurs via a first-order binding reaction to the channel:

$$\frac{dR}{dt} = -\alpha_i [Ca]_d R + \beta_i (1 - R) \tag{27}$$

In the model, relaxation is the result of Ca^{2+} uptake into the uptake
site of the sarcoplasmic reticulum. It has been assumed that the Ca^{2+} flux
into the uptake site, $J_{Ca,u}$ in eqn. 25, is the result of a fourth-order binding
of Ca^{2+} to the Ca^{2+}-pump of the sarcoplasmic reticulum:

$$J_{Ca,u} = J_{Ca,u,max} \cdot \frac{[Ca]_s^4}{K_{m,u}^4 + [Ca]_s^4} \tag{28}$$

Ca^{2+} is also able to leak from the uptake site back into the sarcoplasm –
this Ca^{2+} flux, $J_{Ca,l}$ in eqn. 25, is given by

$$J_{Ca,l} = \alpha_l V_u [Ca]_u \tag{29}$$

Once Ca^{2+} has been taken up into the uptake site it diffuses to the
release site:

$$J_{Ca,ur} = \alpha_{ur} V_u ([Ca]_u - [Ca]_r) \tag{30}$$

where $J_{Ca,ur}$ is the flux of Ca^{2+} from the uptake to the release site.

Ca^{2+} entering the cell as i_{Ca} flows into the sarcoplasm via the domains.
The flux of Ca^{2+} from the domains to the sarcoplasm, $J_{Ca,ds}$ in eqn. 25, is
given by

$$J_{Ca,ds} = \alpha_{ds} V_d ([Ca]_d - [Ca]_s) \tag{31}$$

In both the sarcoplasm and the domains, Ca^{2+} is able to bind to a
buffer with a binding constant, $K_{m,b}$, of 2 μmol l^{-1} (Hilgemann & Noble,
1987). The concentration of buffer in the sarcoplasm, $[B]_s$ – 200 μmol l^{-1},

is approximately the same as that assumed by Hilgemann and Noble (1987) and the major part of it is thought to be troponin-C. The concentration of Ca^{2+} buffer in the domains, $[B]_d$, is assumed to be double $[B]_s$. In the sarcoplasm and domains the fractions of unbound Ca^{2+}, U_s (in eqn. 25) and U_d (in eqn. 36) respectively, are given by

$$U_s = 1 - \frac{[B]_s}{K_{m,b} + [Ca]_s + [B]_s} \tag{32}$$

$$U_d = 1 - \frac{[B]_d}{K_{m,b} + [Ca]_d + [B]_d} \tag{33}$$

The concentration of Ca^{2+} in the release and uptake sites and domains is given by equations analogous to eqn. 25:

$$\frac{d[Ca]_r}{dt} = \frac{J_{Ca,ur} - J_{Ca,r}}{V_r} \tag{34}$$

$$\frac{d[Ca]_u}{dt} = \frac{J_{Ca,u} - J_{Ca,1} - J_{Ca,ur}}{V_u} \tag{35}$$

$$\frac{d[Ca]_d}{dt} = \frac{U_d}{V_d}\left(J_{Ca,ds} - \frac{i_{Ca}}{2F}\right) \tag{36}$$

The volume of the cell, V_c, is assumed to be 35 pl (cf. Boyett, Frampton & Kirby, 1990). The volumes of the compartments within the cell are calculated according to the following formulae:

$$V_u = 0.05V_c \tag{37}$$

$$V_r = 6V_u \tag{38}$$

$$V_d = 0.01V_c \tag{39}$$

$$V_s = V_c - V_u - V_d \tag{40}$$

The fractional volumes of the release and uptake sites are similar to those used by DiFrancesco and Noble (1985) and Hilgemann and Noble (1987). The release site is assumed to have a negligible anatomical volume, but a large effective volume ($6 \times V_c$), because of the presence of Ca^{2+} buffering by calsequestrin within the release site (Hilgemann & Noble, 1987).

Not all of the membrane currents known to exist in cardiac cells have been included in the model. In order to reduce computation time, only those which have a direct role in excitation–contraction coupling have

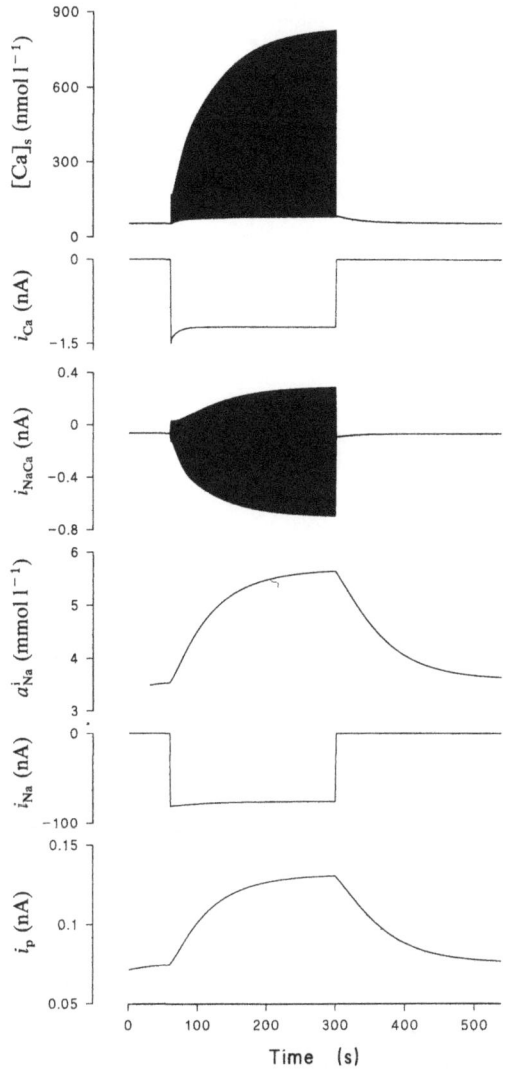

Fig. 22. Computer simulation of the staircase. Calculated changes in $[Ca]_s$ (top), i_{Ca}, i_{NaCa}, a^i_{Na}, i_{Na} and i_p (bottom) during a 4 min train of voltage clamp pulses at 1 Hz after a rest. Because of the slow time base used it is not possible to see the individual Ca^{2+} transients or the changes in i_{NaCa} during each beat. Peak i_{Ca} and peak i_{Na} only have been plotted for simplicity. Holding potential, -80 mV; pulse potential, 0 mV; pulse duration, 200 ms.

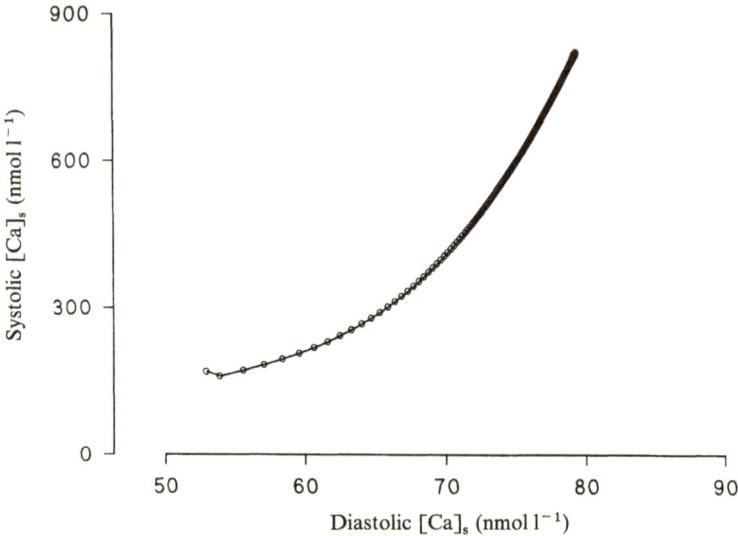

Fig. 23. The relationship between systolic Ca^{2+} (the sarcoplasmic Ca^{2+} concentration at the peak of the Ca^{2+} transient) and diastolic Ca^{2+} (the sarcoplasmic Ca^{2+} concentration prior to the Ca^{2+} transient) during the simulated 1 Hz staircase. From the simulation shown in Fig. 22.

been incorporated. Because of the lack of some membrane currents, voltage clamp control was used in the model. Also note that the model only computes the Ca^{2+} transient – it does not compute the mechanical event of muscle contraction. The program was written in Turbo Pascal (version 4) and ran on IBM compatible computers. A simulation could take up to five days to compute.

Fig. 22 shows that this model of the cardiac cell can indeed reproduce the staircase. At rest, the sarcoplasmic Ca^{2+} concentration, $[Ca]_s$, was 53 nmol l^{-1} and a^i_{Na} was 3.6 mmol l^{-1}. During stimulation a^i_{Na} gradually rose to 5.6 mmol l^{-1} over about 4 min (cf. Fig. 9). Each voltage clamp pulse resulted in a transient rise in $[Ca]_s$. During the train of pulses there were rises in both the Ca^{2+} concentration at the peak of the Ca^{2+} transient and the diastolic Ca^{2+} concentration between Ca^{2+} transients. At the end of the train of pulses both $[Ca]_s$ and a^i_{Na} slowly returned to their original values. In the model the increase in the Ca^{2+} transient is the result of a gradual increase in the Ca^{2+} content of the uptake site. This, in turn, is the result of greater uptake of Ca^{2+} into the sarcoplasmic reticulum as a result of the increase in $[Ca]_s$ between pulses. In Fig. 23 the sarcoplasmic Ca^{2+} concentration at the peak of the Ca^{2+} transient

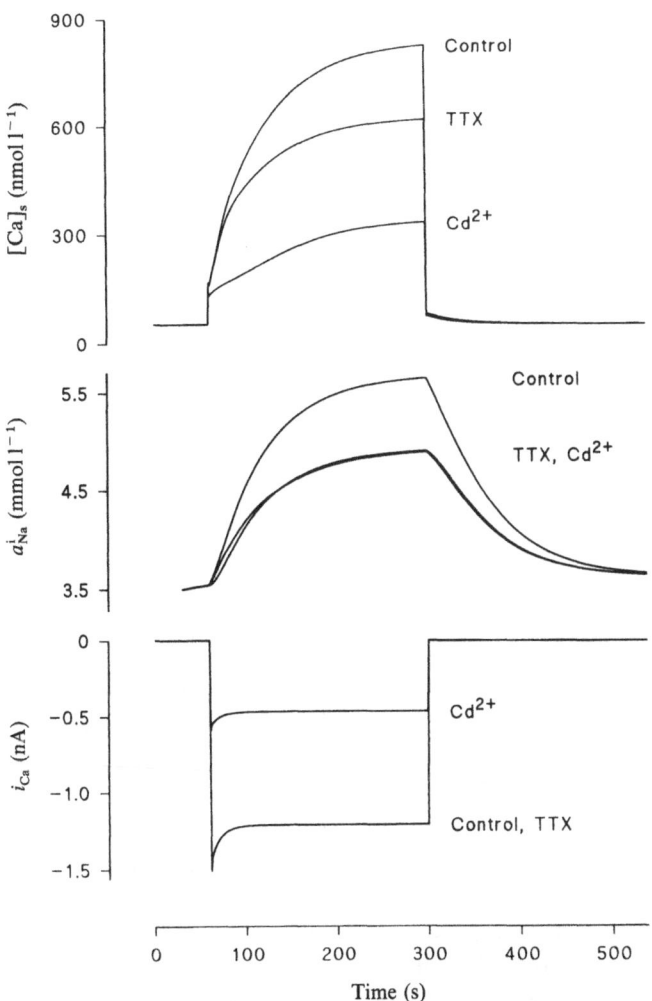

Fig. 24. Computer simulation of the effect of TTX and Cd²⁺ on the staircase. The action of TTX was simulated by setting g_{Na} (eqn. 2) to zero (control value 4×10^{-6} S) and Cd²⁺ was simulated by setting P_{Ca} (eqn. 21) to 50 (control value 150). The effects of TTX and Cd²⁺ on the changes in $[Ca]_s$ (top), a^i_{Na} and i_{Ca} (bottom) during a train of voltage clamp pulses after a rest are shown. Results obtained under control conditions and in the presence of 'TTX' and 'Cd²⁺' are superimposed. Peak $[Ca]_s$ and peak i_{Ca} are shown only for simplicity. Holding potential, -80 mV; pulse potential, 0 mV; pulse duration, 200 ms; pulse frequency, 1 Hz; duration of train, 4 min.

during the staircase has been plotted against the sarcoplasmic Ca^{2+} concentration during diastole between Ca^{2+} transients. This plot is therefore equivalent to the plot of experimental data shown in Fig. 3(b). Although there is not a linear relationship between systolic and diastolic Ca^{2+} in the model, it is clear that a rise in diastolic Ca^{2+} is accompanied by a rise in systolic Ca^{2+}. During the staircase diastolic Ca^{2+} rose from 53 to 79 nmol l^{-1}, whereas systolic Ca^{2+} rose from 169 to 827 nmol l^{-1}. This corresponds to a slope (ratio of the change in systolic Ca^{2+} to the change in diastolic Ca^{2+}) of 25, which although higher is comparable to the values of 4 to 9 observed experimentally. Fig. 24 shows the effect of blocking i_{Na} and i_{Ca} on the simulated staircase. Complete block of i_{Na} reduced the rise in a^i_{Na} during the train and reduced the increase in the Ca^{2+} transient during the later phase of the staircase; it had no effect on the early phase of the staircase. The effects of block of i_{Na} in the model are similar to the effects of TTX shown in Figs. 10 and 12. The effect of partial block of i_{Ca} on the simulated staircase is also similar to the result observed experimentally (Fig. 8). 67% block of i_{Ca} markedly reduced the increase in the Ca^{2+} transient during the early phase of the staircase, but in addition it reduced the increase in the Ca^{2+} transient during the later phase. The early phase of the staircase in the model is almost exclusively the result of the sudden increase in Ca^{2+} influx (via i_{Ca}) on commencing stimulation after the rest. After partial block of i_{Ca}, the decrease of the later phase of the staircase is, in part, the result of the decrease in the rise of a^i_{Na}.[12] The decrease in the rise in a^i_{Na} in the presence of Cd^{2+} may be a surprise, although theoretically at least it is to be expected. The total extra Na^+ influx per beat (presumably via i_{Na} as well as the Na–Ca exchanger) has been estimated to be 10 pmol l^{-1} cm^{-2} in the dog heart (Conn & Wood, 1959; calculated using a surface area:volume ratio of 4000 cm^{-1}), 16.5 pmol l^{-1} cm^{-2} in dog papillary muscle (Langer, 1967; calculated using a surface area:volume ratio of 4000 cm^{-1}) and 1.7 pmol l^{-1} cm^{-2} and 1.2 pmol l^{-1} cm^{-2} in sheep Purkinje fibres (Ellis, 1985; Bountra et al., 1988a). The extra Ca^{2+} influx per beat has been estimated to be 0.13 pmol l^{-1} cm^{-2} in the frog heart (Niedergerke et al., 1969) and 10 pmol l^{-1} cm^{-2} in guinea-pig ventricular muscle (Isenberg, 1982 – see footnote 4). If this Ca^{2+} is extruded from the cell via the Na–Ca exchanger alone, it will result in a Na^+ influx of either 0.39 or 30

---

[12] It is clear that the effect of Cd^{2+} on the staircase is not entirely attributable to the reduction in the rise of a^i_{Na}, because the rise in a^i_{Na} was roughly the same in the presence of either TTX or Cd^{2+} and yet the rise in the Ca^{2+} transient in the presence of Cd^{2+} was much less than that in the presence of TTX.

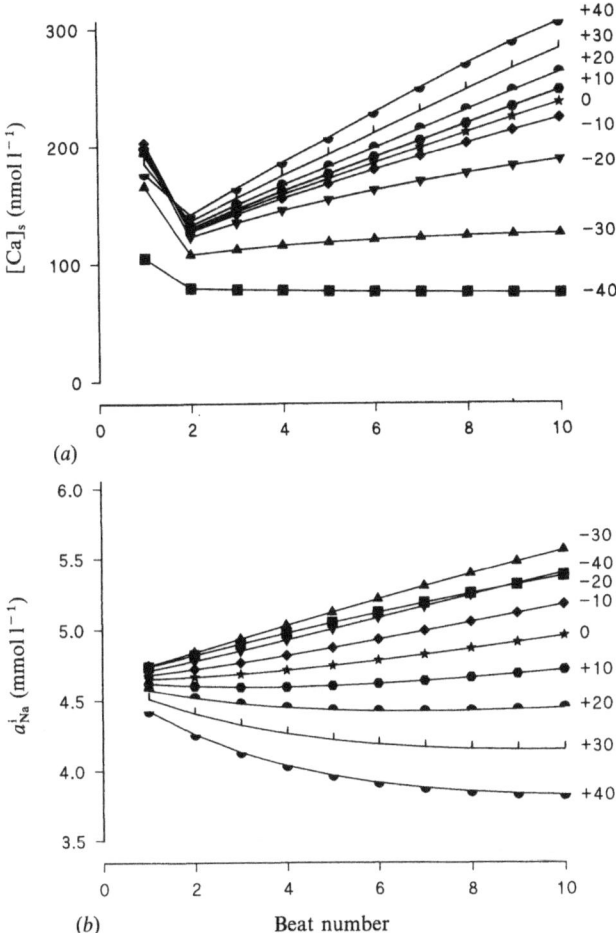

Fig. 25. The effect of the pulse potential on the simulated staircase. Calculated changes in [Ca]$_s$ (top) and a^i_{Na} (bottom) during trains of 10 voltage clamp pulses after a rest. Peak [Ca]$_s$ is shown only for simplicity. In the different runs, the membrane potential during the pulses (shown to the right of each trace) was varied. Holding potential, -80 mV; pulse duration, 800 ms; pulse frequency, 1 Hz.

pmol l^{-1} cm^{-2} (based on the assumption that the stoichiometry of the exchanger is 3Na⁺:1Ca²⁺). This is comparable to the total extra Na⁺ influx per beat. Therefore, theoretically at least, block of i_{Ca} is expected to reduce the rise a^i_{Na} during stimulation. There is some experimental evidence to support this conjecture. Both Boyett $et\ al.$ (1987a) and Bountra $et\ al.$ (1988b) (see also Falk & Cohen, 1984) have shown that the application of a Ca²⁺ channel antagonist reduces the rate-dependent

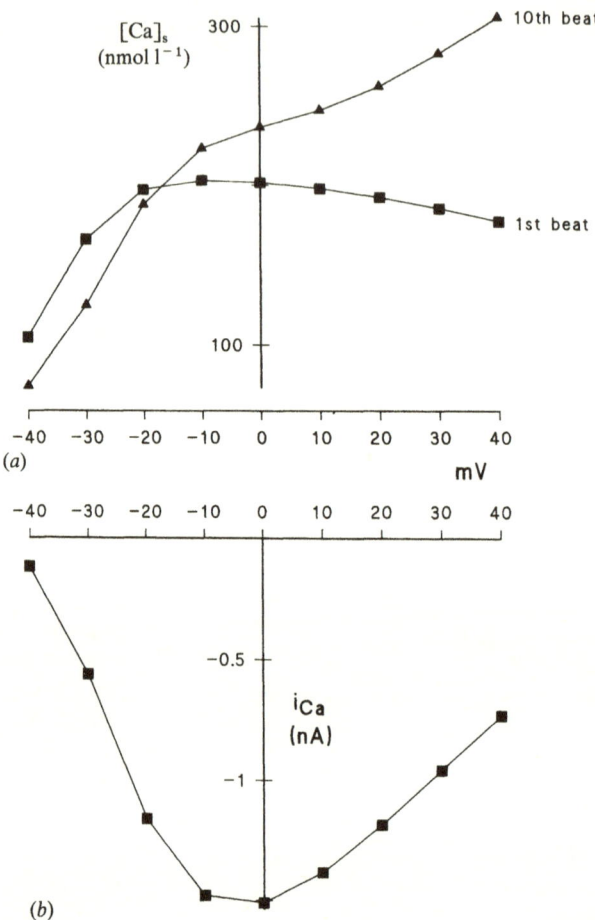

Fig. 26. The effect of the pulse potential on the simulated staircase. The peak [Ca]$_s$ during the first and tenth beats of the train (*a*) and the peak i_{Ca} during the first beat of the train (*b*) are plotted against the membrane potential during the pulses. Same experiment as Fig. 25.

rise in a^i_{Na} in sheep Purkinje fibres (although it should be borne in mind that the Ca^{2+} channel antagonist used, D600, has a direct inhibitory action on i_{Na}). Furthermore, Boyett *et al.* (1987*a*) reported that, after complete block of i_{Na} by TTX, there could still be a small increase in a^i_{Na} during repetitive stimulation in sheep Purkinje fibres.

The simulation in Fig. 25 shows that, in the model, the modulation of the Na–Ca exchanger by the membrane potential is an important influence on the staircase. Fig. 25 shows the changes in the peak of the

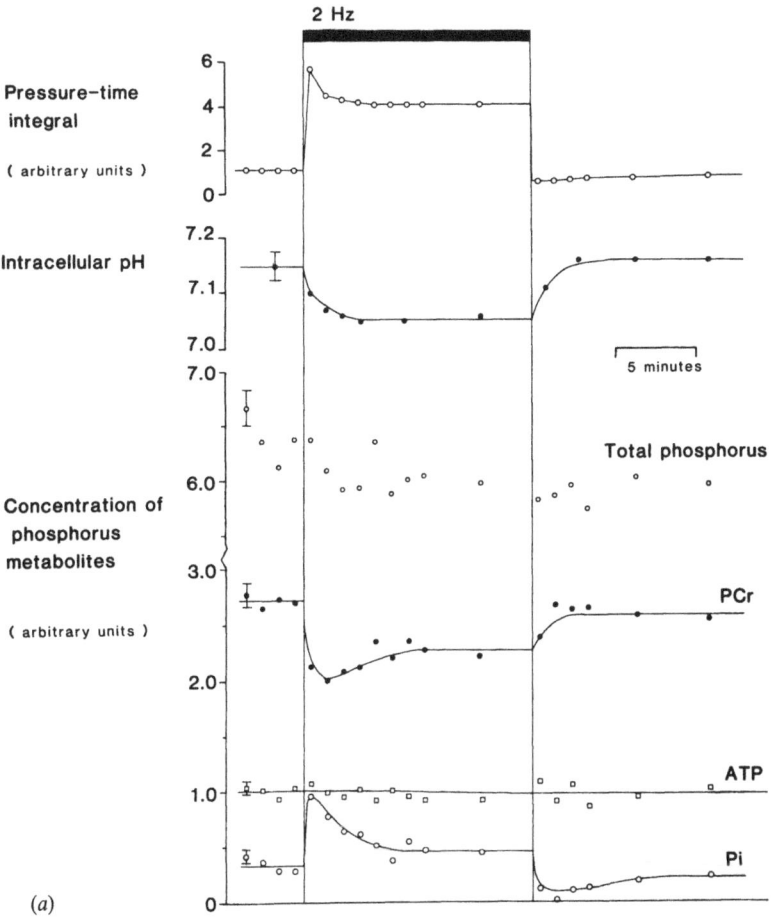

Fig. 27. The metabolic effects of an increase in the stimulation rate in isolated ferret hearts. (*a*) The effect of an increase in the stimulation rate from 0.1–0.7 Hz to 2 Hz on the time integral of the left ventricular developed pressure (a measure of the work output of the heart; top), intracellular pH, total phosphorus, phosphocreatine (PCr), ATP and inorganic phosphate (P$_i$; bottom). Apart from the left ventricular developed pressure, all measurements were made using ^{31}P nuclear magnetic resonance; intracellular pH was determined from P$_i$ chemical shift. Concentrations have been normalised to the start of each experiment. Data from six Langendorff perfused ferret hearts. Bars show ±1 s.e.m. Lines drawn

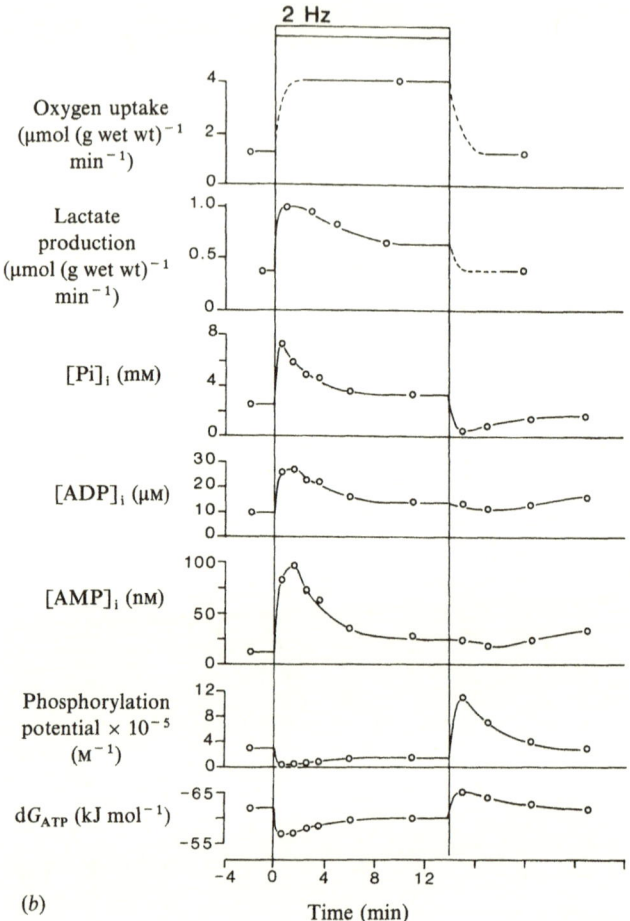

(b)

Time (min)

by hand (*b*) The effect of an increase in the stimulation rate to 2 Hz on oxygen uptake (top), lactate production, intracellular concentrations of P_i, ADP and AMP, phosphorylation potential and dG_{ATP}. The oxygen uptake of four hearts was calculated from the oxygen tension of the effluent. Lactate in the effluent was measured using a diagnostic kit from Sigma in five hearts. Measurement of P_i are taken from the data in panel (*a*). ADP and AMP were calculated assuming that the creatine kinase and myokinase reactions are at equilibrium. Lines drawn by hand. Bathing Ca^{2+}, 2 mmol l^{-1}; temperature, 30 °C. For further details of the methods see Elliott (1987). From Elliott (1987) with permission.

Ca^{2+} transient as well as a^i_{Na} during a train of 10 voltage clamp pulses applied after a rest. The pulse frequency was 1 Hz and the pulse duration was 800 ms (there was, therefore, just 200 ms between pulses). During the train of pulses to -20 mV, for example, there was a small progressive increase (after an initial decrease) in the Ca^{2+} transient during the train and a rise in a^i_{Na}. During the train of pulses to $+40$ mV there was a large increase in the Ca^{2+} transient and this was despite the fact that i_{Ca} was smaller than at -20 mV (Fig. 26(b)) and a^i_{Na} fell rather than rose. The results in Fig. 25(a) are summarised in Fig. 26(a) – the peak value of the Ca^{2+} transients during the first and tenth beats of the trains has been plotted against the pulse potential. For comparison, the amplitude of i_{Ca} during the first beat of the train has been plotted against the pulse potential in Fig. 26(b). In the first beat of the train the size of the Ca^{2+} transient (Fig. 26(a)) is a reflection of the size of i_{Ca} (Fig. 26(b)), but by the tenth beat of the train this is not the case. These results are very similar to the experimental results obtained by Gibbons and Fozzard (1975) shown in Fig. 15. In the model the large increase in the Ca^{2+} transient during the train of pulses to $+40$ mV, for example, was the result of Ca^{2+} influx via the Na–Ca exchanger during the pulses to $+40$ mV.[13] The reversal of the exchanger was also the cause of the fall of a^i_{Na} during the train of pulses to $+40$ mV (Fig. 25(b)). The computed result in Fig. 25 is also similar to the experimental result in Fig. 11, which shows that, in sheep Purkinje fibres during a train of long voltage clamp pulses, there is a large increase in the twitch and a fall in a^i_{Na} – this could be equivalent to the simulated changes during the train of 800 ms pulses to $+40$ mV in Fig. 25.

In summary, the model shows that (i) the increase in Ca^{2+} influx via i_{Ca}, (ii) the rise of a^i_{Na} and (iii) the modulation of the Na–Ca exchanger by the membrane potential can theoretically at least account for the increase in the strength of contraction during the staircase.

Changes in inorganic phosphate and intracellular pH during the staircase

So far in this chapter discussion has centred on changes in intracellular Ca^{2+} and a^i_{Na} during the staircase. However, there may also be changes

[13] To simulate the experimental result from a sheep Purkinje fibre in Fig. 15, the partition coefficient r in eqn. 24 for the Na–Ca exchanger, was set to 1.0. r determines the voltage-dependence of the Ca^{2+} flux via the exchanger. By setting r to 1.0, Ca^{2+} influx via the exchanger increases steeply at potentials positive to E_{NaCa}. Kimura *et al.* (1987) have reported r to be 0.34 in guinea-pig ventricular myocytes. It is possible that the value of r is greater in sheep Purkinje fibres. Note that the behaviour shown in Figs. 22, 23 and 24 is not dependent on the precise value of r.

in intracellular levels of inorganic phosphate (P_i) and phosphorus metabolites and intracellular pH (pH_i) and this final section is concerned with
the possible impact of these changes on the contraction during the
staircase.

Elliott (1987) has studied heart rate dependent changes in P_i, phosphorus-
metabolites and pH_i in isolated perfused ferret hearts using ^{31}P nuclear
magnetic resonance and results from his study are shown in Fig.
27. After an increase in the stimulation rate from 0.1–0.7 Hz to 2 Hz there
was no change in ATP, but a transient fall in phosphocreatine (PCr) and a
transient increase in P_i. The changes in PCr and P_i reached their greatest
extent in the first two minutes of stimulation at 2 Hz. In addition to the
transient changes in PCr and P_i, during maintained stimulation at 2 Hz
PCr remained lower and P_i remained higher than their levels at the lower
frequency. Note that there was also a transient increase in lactate
production after the increase in rate. A possible explanation of these
changes will now be considered. After the increase in rate, ATP hydrolysis
will increase leading to a rise in P_i. Immediately after the increase in
stimulation rate aerobic glycolysis may not keep pace with the demand
for ATP. Regeneration of ATP may therefore be the result of the
breakdown of PCr (which would explain the fall in PCr) as well as
anaerobic glycolysis (which would explain the rise in lactate production).
With time, aerobic glycolysis may increase (as indicated by the increase
in oxygen consumption – Fig. 27) – this is thought to be the result of the
rise of the intramitochondrial Ca^{2+} concentration (which in turn is the
result of the rise in $[Ca]_s$ discussed at length above) and the consequent
activation of Ca^{2+}-sensitive intramitochondrial dehydrogenases (see, for
example, McCormack et al., 1990; Unitt et al., 1989). As aerobic glycolysis
increases, the increase in ATP production leads to the fall in P_i, and Cr
is rephosphorylated to replenish the pool of PCr. What effects if any will
these changes have on the contraction during the staircase? Kentish (1986)
has studied the effects of P_i, PCr and creatine on tension development by
skinned cardiac muscle fibres. Although PCr has a small effect on tension
production, the relatively small rate-dependent change in PCr is unlikely
to have a substantial effect on the contraction. P_i affects both the Ca^{2+}
sensitivity of the myofilaments and the maximum tension developed by
the myofilaments. Elliott (1987) using the data of Kentish (1986) estimates
that the transient increase in P_i from about 3 to 7 mmol$\,l^{-1}$ in Fig. 27 is
expected to result in a transient decrease in tension development by about
40%. Changes in P_i are therefore expected to affect the staircase. It should
be pointed out that Katz, Koretsky and Balaban (1988) and Katz et al.

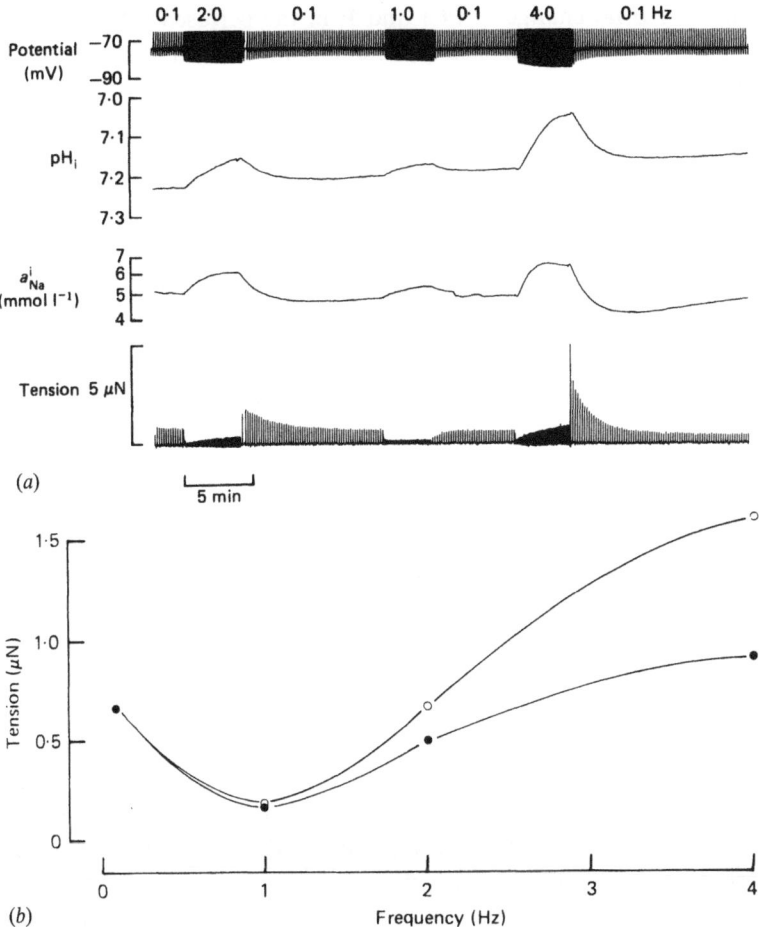

Fig. 28. Rate-dependent changes in intracellular pH in a sheep Purkinje fibre. (a) The effect of the stimulation rate on the membrane potential (upper trace; the bottoms only of the action potentials can be seen), pH_i and a^i_{Na} (measured with pH and Na⁺ sensitive microelectrodes) and tension (lower trace; bandpass filtered at 0.1–10 Hz). The fibre was stimulated at a basic rate of 0.1 Hz and for short periods at 2, 1 and 4 Hz, as indicated above the traces. (b) Influence of the rate-dependent acidosis upon the force–frequency relationship. Closed circles show steady-state twitch tension plotted as a function of the stimulation rate. Same experiment as panel (a). Open circles show the predicted relationship if the rate-dependent acidosis observed in panel (a) had not occurred (see Bountra *et al.*, 1988a, for details of the calculations). Bathing Ca^{2+}, 2.5 mmol l⁻¹; temperature, 37 °C. From Bountra *et al.* 1988a with permission.

(1989) measured no change in PCr and P_i in the perfused rat heart and the dog heart *in vivo* under steady-state conditions after the heart rate had been roughly doubled. However, these authors did not look for possible transient changes on changing the heart rate.

Fig. 27 shows that in the perfused ferret hearts an intracellular acidosis of about 0.1 pH units developed over about 5 min on roughly doubling the stimulation rate. Bountra *et al.* (1988a,b) have observed a similar rate-dependent acidosis in isolated sheep Purkinje fibres. An example of the changes in pH_i in a sheep Purkinje fibre is shown in Fig. 28(a) – changes in membrane potential, a^i_{Na} and tension are also shown. Note that the change in pH_i was greater at higher stimulation rates – in general the change in pH_i in sheep Purkinje fibres showed a linear dependence on stimulation rate with a mean slope of 0.023 pH units Hz^{-1}. Fig. 28(a) shows that the changes in pH_i occurred slowly – a new steady state was generally reached 3–30 min after an increase in the stimulation rate. Vanheel and de Hemptinne (1985) have also observed rate-dependent changes in pH_i in isolated sheep Purkinje fibres and Heinemeyer and Bay (1987) have observed a rate-dependent acidosis in guinea-pig and cat ventricular muscle. Both Elliott (1987) and Bountra *et al.* (1988b) suggest that part of the rate-dependent intracellular acidosis is the result of anaerobic metabolism and the resultant build-up of lactic acid (Fig. 27). A fall in pH_i is well known to depress the strength of contraction of cardiac muscle, on which it has a number of effects (for a recent review see Orchard & Kentish, 1990). For example, it inhibits the Na–Ca exchanger and the sarcoplasmic reticulum and reduces i_{Ca}, all of which are involved in the staircase. In addition a fall in pH_i decreases the Ca^{2+} sensitivity of the myofilaments as well as the maximum force generated by the myofilaments (e.g. Fabiato & Fabiato, 1978). Elliott (1987) estimated that the fall in pH_i in the ferret hearts (Fig. 27) would depress developed pressure by about 20%. In sheep Purkinje fibres Vaughan-Jones, Eisner and Lederer (1987) measured the effect of pH_i on sheep Purkinje fibres and Bountra *et al.* (1988a) used this to estimate the effect of the rate-dependent acidosis on the tension developed by a sheep Purkinje fibre at different stimulation rates. The filled circles in Fig. 28(b) show the steady-state tension at each rate, whereas the open circles show the estimated tension if pH_i had remained constant. At 4 Hz, for example, tension would have been 100% greater. It should be pointed out that Katz *et al.* (1989) observed no change in pH_i in the dog heart *in vivo* on roughly doubling the stimulation rate.

Summary and conclusions

The increase in the strength of contraction after an increase in the stimulation rate or on commencing stimulation after a rest is the result of an increase in the Ca^{2+} transient. In species in which the Ca^{2+} transient is thought to be primarily dependent on Ca^{2+} release from the sarcoplasmic reticulum, the increase in the Ca^{2+} transient during the staircase is thought to be the result of an increase in the Ca^{2+} content of the sarcoplasmic reticulum. It has been suggested that this, in turn, is the result of an increase in the sarcoplasmic Ca^{2+} concentration between beats. The increase of the sarcoplasmic Ca^{2+} concentration between beats and hence the Ca^{2+} content of the sarcoplasmic reticulum is the result of (i) an increase in Ca^{2+} influx via the Ca^{2+} current, i_{Ca}, and (ii) a decrease in Ca^{2+} efflux via the Na–Ca exchanger as a result of an increase in the intracellular Na^+ activity, a^i_{Na}. The membrane potential will also modulate the Na–Ca exchanger and thus the changes in the strength of contraction during the staircase. In species in which the Ca^{2+} transient is primarily dependent on Ca^{2+} influx in that beat, the increase in the Ca^{2+} transient during the staircase is presumably the result of a beat-to-beat increase in the Ca^{2+} influx via either i_{Ca} or the Na–Ca exchanger. A beat-to-beat increase in i_{Ca} may be an intrinsic property of this current and Ca^{2+} influx via the exchanger may increase as a result of the rise in a^i_{Na}. Finally, the changes in the strength of contraction during the staircase may be modulated by metabolic-induced changes in inorganic phosphate and intracellular pH.

Acknowledgements

This work was supported by the British Heart Foundation, the Medical Research Council and the Wellcome Trust.

References

Allen D. G. (1975). The variations in contractility of cardiac muscle. PhD thesis, University of London.

Allen, D. G. & Blinks, J. R. (1978). Calcium transients in aequorin-injected frog cardiac muscle. *Nature*, **273**, 509–13.

Allen, D. G., Jewell, B. R. & Wood, E. H. (1976). Studies of the contractility of mammalian myocardium at low rates of stimulation. *Journal of Physiology*, **254**, 1–17.

Allen, D. G. & Kurihara, S. (1980). Calcium transients in mammalian ventricular muscle. *European Heart Journal*, **1** (Suppl A), 5–15.

Bers, D. M. (1983). Early transient depletion of extracellular Ca during individual cardiac muscle contractions. *American Journal of Physiology*, **244**, H462–8.

Bers, D. M. (1985). Ca influx and sarcoplasmic reticulum Ca release in cardiac muscle activation during postrest recovery. *American Journal of Physiology*, **248**, H366–81.

Bers, D. M., Bridge, J. H. B. & MacLeod, K. T. (1987). The mechanism of ryanodine action in rabbit ventricular muscle evaluated with Ca-selective microelectrodes and rapid cooling contractures. *Canadian Journal of Physiology and Pharmacology*, **65**, 610–18.

Bers, D. M. & Hess, P. (1988). The influence of rest periods on calcium currents and contractions in isolated ventricular myocytes from guinea-pig and rabbit hearts. In *Biology of Isolated Adult Cardiac Myocytes*, ed. W. A. Clark, R. S. Decker and T. K. Borg, pp. 410–13. Elsevier Science Publishing Co., Inc.

Bountra, C., Kaila, K. & Vaughan-Jones, R. D. (1988*a*). Effect of repetitive activity upon intracellular pH, sodium and contraction in sheep cardiac Purkinje fibres. *Journal of Physiology*, **398**, 341–60.

Bountra, C., Kaila, K. & Vaughan-Jones, R. D. (1988*b*). Mechanism of rate-dependent pH changes in the sheep cardiac Purkinje fibre. *Journal of Physiology*, **406**, 483–501.

Bowditch, H. P. (1871). Über die Eigenthümlichkeiten der Reizbarkeit, welche die Muskelfasern des Herzens zeigen. *Berichte der Königlich–Sächsischen Gesellschaft der Wissenschaften*, **23**, 652–89.

Boyett, M. R., Capogrossi, M. C., duBell, W. H., Lakatta, E. G. & Spurgeon, H. A. (1989*a*). Cytosolic Ca^{2+} modulation of the action potential in rat ventricular myocytes. *Journal of Physiology*, **415**, 109P.

Boyett, M. R. & Fedida, D. (1984). The effect of heart rate on the membrane currents of isolated sheep Purkinje fibres. *Journal of Physiology*, **399**, 467–91.

Boyett, M. R. & Fedida, D. (1988). A computer simulation of the effect of heart rate on ion concentrations in the heart. *Journal of Theoretical Biology*, **132**, 15–27.

Boyett, M. R., Frampton, J. E. & Kirby, M. S. (1990). The length, width and volume of isolated rat and ferret ventricular myocytes during twitch contractions and changes in osmotic strength. *Experimental Physiology*, **76**, 259–70.

Boyett, M. R. & Harrison, S. M. (1990). The relationship between the intracellular sodium activity (a^i_{Na}), measured with SBFI, and the strength of contraction of ventricular myocytes isolated from the guinea-pig. *Journal of Physiology*, **423**, 60P.

Boyett, M. R., Hart, G. & Levi, A. J. (1987*a*). Factors affecting intracellular sodium during repetitive activity in isolated sheep Purkinje fibres. *Journal of Physiology*, **384**, 405–29.

Boyett, M. R., Hart, G., Levi, A. J. & Roberts, A. (1987*b*). Effects of repetitive activity on developed force and intracellular sodium in isolated sheep and dog Purkinje fibres. *Journal of Physiology*, **388**, 295–322.

Boyett, M. R. & Kirby, M. S. (1988). Use-dependent changes and ultra-slow inactivation of the Ca^{2+} current in ferret ventricular myocytes. *Journal of Molecular and Cellular Cardiology*, **20**, Supp. IV, S37.

Boyett, M. R., Kirby, M. S. & Orchard, C. H. (1989*b*). Paired pulse potentiation in isolated ferret ventricular muscle. *Journal of Physiology*, **410**, 66P.

Brutsaert, D. L. (1966). Studies on the potentiation of contractility of heart papillary muscle by paired stimulation. *Archives Internationales de Physiologie et de Biochimie*, **74**, 642–64.

Bryerly, L., Chase, P. B. & Stimers, J. R. (1985). Permeation and interaction of divalent cations in calcium channels of snail neurones. *Journal of General Physiology*, **85**, 491–518.

Capogrossi, M. C., Kort, A. A., Spurgeon, H. A. & Lakatta, E. G. (1986). Single adult rabbit and rat cardiac myocytes retain the Ca^{2+}- and species-dependent systolic and diastolic contractile properties of intact muscle. *Journal of General Physiology*, **88**, 589–613.

Cohen, C. J., Fozzard, H. A. & Sheu, S.-S. (1982). Increase in intracellular sodium ion activity during stimulation in mammalian cardiac muscle. *Circulation Research*, **50**, 651–62.

Cohen, N. M. & Lederer, W. J. (1988). Changes in the calcium current of rat heart ventricular myocytes during development. *Journal of Physiology*, **406**, 115–46.

Conn, H. L., Jr. & Wood, J. C. (1959). Sodium exchange and distribution in the isolated heart of the normal dog. *American Journal of Physiology*, **197**, 631–6.

DiFrancesco, D. & Noble, D. (1985). A model of cardiac electrical activity incorporating ionic pumps and concentration changes. *Philosophical Transactions of the Royal Society (Series B)*, **307**, 353–98.

duBell, W. H. & Houser, S. R. (1989). Voltage and beat dependence of Ca^{2+} transient in feline ventricular myocytes. *American Journal of Physiology*, **257**, H746–59.

Eckert, R. & Chad, J. E. (1984). Inactivation of Ca channels. *Progress in Biophysics and Molecular Biology*, **44**, 215–67.

Edman, K. A. P. & Jóhannsson, M. (1976). The contractile state of rabbit papillary muscle in relation to stimulation frequency. *Journal of Physiology*, **254**, 565–81.

Ehara, T., Matsuoka, S. & Noma, A. (1989). Measurements of reversal potential of Na^+–Ca^{2+} exchange current in single guinea-pig ventricular cells. *Journal of Physiology*, **410**, 227–49.

Eisner, D. A. (1990). Intracellular sodium in cardiac muscle: effects on contraction. *Experimental Physiology*, **75**, 437–57.

Eisner, D. A., Lederer, W. J. & Vaughan-Jones, R. D. (1981). The dependence of sodium pumping and tension on intracellular sodium activity in voltage-clamped sheep Purkinje fibres. *Journal of Physiology*, **317**, 163–87.

Elliott, A. C. (1987). Phosphorus nuclear magnetic resonance studies on metabolite levels and intracellular pH in muscle. PhD thesis, University of London.

Ellis, D. (1985). Effects of stimulation and diphenylhydantoin on the intracellular sodium activity in Purkinje fibres of the sheep heart. *Journal of Physiology*, **359**, 81–105.

Fabiato, A. (1985). Time and calcium dependence of activation and inactivation of calcium-induced release of calcium from the sarcoplasmic reticulum of a skinned canine cardiac Purkinje cell. *Journal of General Physiology*, **85**, 247–89.

Fabiato, A. & Fabiato, F. (1978). Effects of pH on the myofilaments and the sarcoplasmic reticulum of skinned cells from cardiac and skeletal muscles. *Journal of Physiology*, **276**, 233–55.

Falk, R. T. & Cohen, I. S. (1984). Membrane current following activity in canine cardiac Purkinje fibers. *Journal of General Physiology*, **83**, 771–99.

Frampton, J. E., Orchard, C. H. & Boyett, M. R. (1990*a*). The relationship between diastolic and systolic intracellular [Ca^{2+}] ([Ca^{2+}]$_i$) in ventricular myocytes isolated from rat hearts. *Journal of Physiology*, **425**, 53P.

Frampton, J. E., Orchard, C. H. & Boyett, M. R. (1990*b*). Caffeine-induced calcium release in myocytes isolated from the ventricles of rat hearts changes during inotropic interventions. *Journal of Physiology*, **429**, 19P.

Gibbons, W. R. & Fozzard, H. A. (1975). Relationships between voltage and tension in sheep cardiac Purkinje fibres. *Journal of General Physiology*, **65**, 345–65.

Henry, P. D. (1975). Positive staircase effect in the rat heart. *American Journal of Physiology*, **228**, 360–4.

Heinemeyer, D. & Bay, W. (1987). Intracellular pH in quiescent and stimulated ventricular myocardium. Effect of extracellular chloride concentration. *Pflügers Archiv*, **409**, 142–4.

Hilgemann, D. W. & Noble, D. (1987). Excitation–contraction coupling and extracellular calcium transients in rabbit atrium: reconstruction of basic cellular mechanisms. *Proceedings of the Royal Society (Series B)*, **230**, 163–205.

Hoffman, B. F., Bindler, E. & Suckling, E. E. (1956). Postextrasystolic potentiation of contraction in cardiac muscle. *American Journal of Physiology*, **185**, 95–102.

Hotokebuchi, N., Yano, T., Nishizono, Y. & Nishi, K. (1987). Changes in intra- and extracellular potassium and intracellular sodium activities induced by repetitive stimulation and their relation to membrane potential in guinea-pig papillary muscle. *Japanese Journal of Physiology*, **37**, 797–819.

Isenberg, G. (1982). Ca entry and contraction as studied in isolated bovine ventricular myocytes. *Zeitschrift für Naturforschung*, **37c**, 502–12.

Isenberg, G. & Wendt-Gallitelli, M. F. (1987). X-ray microprobe analysis of the elemental distribution applied to isolated guinea-pig ventricular myocytes shock-frozen under voltage clamp conditions. *Journal of Physiology*, **390**, 54P.

Katz, L. A., Koretsky, A. P. & Balaban, R. S. (1988). Activation of dehydrogenase activity and cardiac respiration: a ^{31}P-NMR study. *American Journal of Physiology*, **255**, H185–8.

Katz, L. A., Swain, J. A., Portman, M. A. & Balaban, R. S. (1989). Relation between phosphate metabolites and oxygen consumption of heart *in vivo*. *American Journal of Physiology*, **256**, H265–74.

Kaufmann, R., Bayer, R., Furniss, T., Krause, H. & Tritthart, H. (1974). Calcium-movement controlling cardiac contractility II. Analog computation of cardiac excitation–contraction coupling on the basis of calcium kinetics in a multi-compartment model. *Journal of Molecular and Cellular Cardiology*, **6**, 543–59.

Kentish, J. C. (1986). The effects of inorganic phosphate and creatine phosphate on force production in skinned muscles from rat ventricle. *Journal of Physiology*, **370**, 585–604.

Kimura, J., Miyamae, S. & Noma, A. (1987). Identification of sodium-calcium exchange current in single ventricular cells of guinea-pig. *Journal of Physiology*, **384**, 199–222.

Koch-Weser, J. & Blinks, J. R. (1963). The influence of the interval between beats on myocardial contractility. *Pharmacological Reviews*, **15**, 601–52.

Lado, M. G., Sheu, S.-S. & Fozzard, H. A. (1982). Changes in intracellular Ca^{2+} activity with stimulation in sheep cardiac Purkinje strands. *American Journal of Physiology*, **243**, H133–7.

Lakatta, E. G. & Spurgeon, H. A. (1980). Force staircase kinetics in mammalian cardiac muscle: modulation by muscle length. *Journal of Physiology*, **299**, 337–52.

Langer, G. A. (1965). Calcium exchange in dog ventricular muscle: relation to frequency of contraction and maintenance of contractility. *Circulation Research*, **17**, 78–90.

Langer, G. A. (1967). Sodium exchange in dog ventricular muscle. Relation to frequency of contraction and its possible role in the control of myocardial contractility. *Journal of General Physiology*, **50**, 1221–39.

Langer, G. A. (1968). Ion fluxes in cardiac excitation and contraction and their relation to myocardal contractility. *Physiological Reviews*, **48**, 708–57.

Langer, G. A. (1983). The 'sodium pump lag' revisited. *Journal of Molecular and Cellular Cardiology*, **15**, 647–51.

Langer, G. A. & Brady, A. J. (1963). Calcium flux in the mammalian ventricular myocardium. *Journal of General Physiology*, **46**, 703–20.

Lederer, W. J. & Sheu, S.-S. (1983). Heart rate-dependent changes in intracellular sodium activity and twitch tension in sheep cardiac Purkinje fibres. *Journal of Physiology*, **345**, 44P.

Lee, K. S. (1987). Potentiation of the calcium-channel currents of internally perfused mammalian heart cells by repetitive depolarization. *Proceedings of the National Academy of Sciences, USA*, **84**, 3941–5.

Lee, C. O., Im, W. B. & Sonn, J. K. (1987). Intracellular sodium ion activity: reliable measurement and stimulation-induced change in cardiac Purkinje fibers. *Canadian Journal of Physiology and Pharmacology*, **65**, 954–62.

Lewartowski, B. & Pytkowski, B. (1987). Cellular mechanism of the relationship between myocardial force and frequency of contractions. *Progress in Biophysics and Molecular Biology*, **50**, 97–120.

McCormack, J. G., Halestrap, A. P. & Denton, R. M. (1990). Role of calcium ions in regulation of mammalian intramitochondrial metabolism. *Physiological Reviews*, **70**, 391–425.

Narahashi, T., Tsunoo, A. & Yoshi, M. (1987). Characterisation of two types of calcium channels in mouse neuroblastoma cells. *Journal of Physiology*, **383**, 231–49.

Niedergerke, R., Page, S. & Talbot, M. S. (1969). Calcium fluxes in frog heart ventricles. *Pflügers Archiv*, **306**, 357–60.

Noble, D. (1986). Sodium-calcium exchange and its role in generating electric current. In *Cardiac Muscle: Excitation and Regulation of Contraction*, ed. R. D. Nathan. London: Academic Press.

Noble, S. & Shimoni, Y. (1981). The calcium and frequency dependence of the slow inward current 'staircase' in frog atrium. *Journal of Physiology*, **310**, 57–75.

Orchard, C. H. & Kentish, J. C. (1990). Effects of changes of pH on the contractile function of cardiac muscle. *American Journal of Physiology*, **258**, C967–81.

Orchard, C. H. & Lakatta, E. G. (1985). Intracellular calcium transients and developed tension in rat heart muscle. *Journal of General Physiology*, **86**, 637–51.

Payett, M. D., Schanne, O. F. & Ruiz-Ceretti, E. (1981). Frequency dependence of the ionic currents determining the action potential repolarization in rat ventricular muscle. *Journal of Molecular and Cellular Cardiology*, **13**, 207–15.

Ruch, S., Kennedy, R. H. & Seifen, E. (1988). Effect of stimulation frequency on intracellular Na^+ activity in rat atrial muscle. *Canadian Journal of Physiology and Pharmacology*, **66**, 1565–9.

Sands, S. D. & Winegrad, S. (1970). Treppe and total calcium content of the frog ventricle. *American Journal of Physiology*, **218**, 908–10.

Schouten, V. J. A. & ter Keurs, H. E. D. J. (1986). The force–frequency relationship in rat myocardium. The influence of muscle dimensions. *Pflügers Archiv*, **407**, 14–17.

Schramm, M., Thomas, G., Towart, R. & Franckowiak, G. (1983). Novel dihydropyridines with positive inotropic action through activation of calcium channels. *Nature*, **303**, 535–7.

Seibel, K. (1986). The slow phase of the staircase in guinea-pig papillary muscle, influence of agents acting on transmembrane sodium flux. *Naunyn-Schmiedeberg's Archives of Pharmacology*, **334**, 92–9.

Seibel, K., Karema, L. Takeya, K. & Reiter, M. (1978). Effect of noradrenaline on an early and a late component of the myocardial contraction. *Naunyn-Schmiedeberg's Archives of Pharmacology*, **305**, 65–74.

Smith, G. L., Valdeolmillos, M., Eisner, D. A. & Allen, D. G. (1988). Effects of rapid applications of caffeine on intracellular calcium concentration in ferret papillary muscles. *Journal of General Physiology*, **92**, 351–68.

Standen, N. B. & Stanfield, P. R. (1982). A binding-site model for calcium channel inactivation that depends on calcium entry. *Proceedings of the Royal Society (Series B)*, **217**, 101–10.

Unitt, J. F., McCormack, J. G., Reid, D., MacLachlan, L. K. & England, P. J. (1989). Direct evidence for a role of intramitochondrial Ca^{2+} in the regulation of oxidative phosphorylation in the stimulated rat heart. Studies using ^{31}P n.m.r. and ruthenium red. *Biochemical Journal*, **262**, 293–301.

Valdeolmillos, M. & Eisner, D. A. (1985). The effects of ryanodine on calcium-overloaded sheep cardiac Purkinje fibres. *Circulation Research*, **56**, 452–6.

Vanheel, B. & de Hemptinne, A. (1985). Intracellular pH in depolarized cardiac Purkinje strands. *Pflügers Archiv*, **405**, 118–26.

Vaughan-Jones, R. D., Eisner, D. A. & Lederer, W. J. (1987). Effects of changes of intracellular pH on contraction in sheep cardiac Purkinje fibres. *Journal of General Physiology*, **89**, 1015–32.

Wang, D. Y., Chae, S. W., Gong, Q. Y. & Lee, C. O. (1988). Role of a^i_{Na} in positive force–frequency staircase in guinea-pig papillary muscle. *American Journal of Physiology*, **255**, C798–807.

Wendt-Gallitelli, M. F. (1985). Presystolic calcium loading of the sarcoplasmic reticulum influences time to peak force of contraction. X-ray microanalysis on rapidly frozen guinea-pig ventricular muscle preparations. *Basic Research in Cardiology*, **80**, 617–25.

Wendt-Gallitelli, M. F. & Jacob, R. (1982). Rhythm-dependent role of different calcium stores in cardiac muscle: X-ray microanalysis. *Journal of Molecular and Cellular Cardiology*, **14**, 487–92.

Wier, W. G. & Yue, D. (1986). Intracellular calcium transients underlying the short-term force–interval relations in ferret ventricular myocardium. *Journal of Physiology*, **376**, 507–30.

Quantitative aspects of cellular calcium regulation during post-rest stimulation in cardiac muscle: implications for steady-state conditions

BOHDAN LEWARTOWSKI

Stimulation- and rest-dependent changes in cellular Ca^{2+} content

Long periods of rest in the ventricular myocardium of most mammalian species result in a decrease of contractility. If the rest is long enough, its further prolongation does not result in any further decrease in contractile force. A contraction initiated after such a long rest is called a 'rested state contraction' (Allen, Jewell & Wood, 1976; Edman & Jóhannsson, 1976; Koch-Weser & Blinks, 1963). The characteristic feature of a rested state contraction is a prolonged time to peak tension and abrupt transition to the relaxation phase. This time course is typical for contractions initiated in mammalian myocardium, the internal calcium store of which has been deprived of Ca^{2+}. Indeed, it has been shown by several experimental approaches that there is a net loss of Ca^{2+} from the resting myocardium, whereas stimulation after the prolonged rest, resulting in the recovery of contractile force (Bowditch effect), is associated with net Ca^{2+} gain (for a recent review, see Lewartowski & Pytkowski, 1987).

Although rest decay and post-rest recovery of contraction are not physiological phenomena, they are extreme forms of physiological force–frequency relation. During rest decay and post-rest recovery, it is possible to carry out quantitative analysis of Ca^{2+} fluxes and this may help us to understand the Ca^{2+} fluxes under steady-state conditions.

The total cellular Ca^{2+} content measured with atomic absorption spectrophotometry amounts in the stimulated guinea-pig ventricular muscle to 2.2 mmol/kg wet weight of the tissue (Lewartowski, Pytkowski & Janczewski, 1984). Complete equilibrium of the stimulated muscle with a perfusate containing the isotope $^{45}Ca^{2+}$ results in labelling of about 75% of the total Ca^{2+} (1.6 mmol). After a rest sufficiently long for subsequent beats to have a low contractility which is constant regardless of the amount of further time rest is prolonged (the rested state contraction), about 70% of exchangeable Ca^{2+} is lost from guinea-pig ventricular muscle and 46% is lost in rabbit (Lewartowski et al., 1984; Lewartowski & Pytkowski, 1987; Pytkowski, 1989). The rat differs from other species in that there is no loss of Ca^{2+} from the resting myocardium, which shows sustained post-rest potentiation irrespective of the duration of rest (Janczewski & Lewartowski, 1986). In guinea-pig and rabbit ventricular muscle, post-rest stimulation results in re-uptake of the exchangeable Ca^{2+} parallel to recovery of contractile force. The content of exchangeable Ca^{2+} correlates linearly with contractile force during rest-decay, post-rest recovery and steady-state stimulation of the muscle at the various rates (Lewartowski et al., 1984).

The rest- and stimulation-dependent fraction of cellular Ca^{2+} is of considerable interest as it reflects all the Ca^{2+} fluxes related to activity of cardiac muscle. The following section reviews the evidence concerning the components of this fraction, their subcellular localisation and the shifts related to the functional state of the muscle. It is convenient to begin the analysis with the sarcoplasmic reticulum as its Ca^{2+} content reflects the net sarcolemmal calcium flux (see below).

Sources and sinks of the rest- and stimulation-dependent cellular Ca^{2+}: quantitative aspects

Sarcoplasmic reticulum (SR)

The SR is one of the best known subcellular Ca^{2+} stores. It is composed of two main parts: the net of longitudinal tubules wrapping the sarcomeres and the terminal cisternae placed in apposition to the outer sarcolemma or to the walls of the T tubules (if present). The longitudinal tubules of the SR contain the Ca-ATPase which transports Ca^{2+} into their lumen. The membranes of the terminal cisternae form the 'feet' traversing the narrow space between them and sarcolemma or T tubules. The feet have been proved to be identical with the ryanodine receptor, i.e. they are built of the proteins of the SR Ca^{2+} release channels (Rardon et al., 1989). The Ca^{2+} trapped by the tubular part of the SR is transported to the terminal cisternae. Their release channels are activated by rapid increase in the sarcoplasmic Ca^{2+} concentration and inhibited by higher and sustained Ca^{2+} concentration. These results, which were obtained by Fabiato (1983, 1985) in skinned myocytes have been recently confirmed in experiments on isolated fragments of the SR (Meissner & Henderson, 1987; Meissner, Darling & Eveleth, 1986). The SR is postulated to provide a source of most of the Ca^{2+} activating contraction.

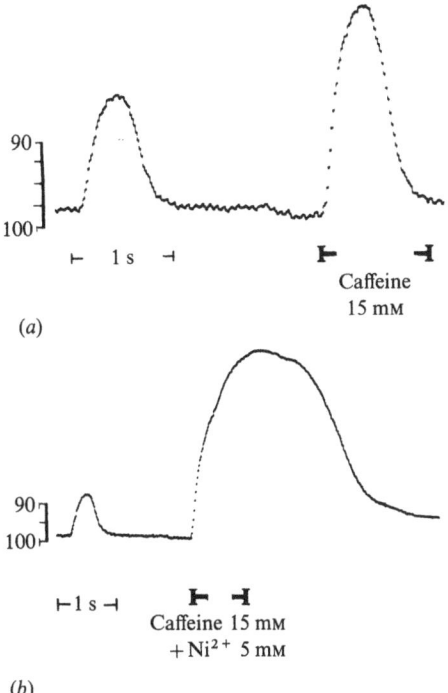

(a)

(b)

Fig. 1. (a) Electrically stimulated contraction of a single myocyte of guinea-pig heart (left) and contractures initiated by caffeine applied for 1 s by means of a rapid superfusion system (right, between bars). (b) Effect of adding nickel ions with caffeine. Horizontal axis: time. Vertical axis: cell shortening as a percentage of resting length. Note differences in both axes between (a) and (b).

Recently it became possible to investigate the SR Ca^{2+} content by exposing isolated cardiac myocytes to high concentrations of caffeine (10–15 mM) injected from a micropipette (du Bell & Houser, 1990; Lewartowski *et al.*, 1990; Stern *et al.*, 1988) or applied by means of a rapid perfusion system (Lewartowski *et al.*, 1990). This results in rapid release of Ca^{2+} from the SR, as does rapid cooling below $+5\,°C$ (Bers, Bridge & Spitzer, 1989; Hryshko, Stiffel & Bers, 1989; Lewartowski *et al.*, 1990). The resulting transient increase in sarcoplasmic $[Ca^{2+}]$ and/or transient contracture (Fig. 1) may be used as an index of the SR Ca^{2+} content. In guinea-pig (Bers *et al.*, 1989; Lewartowski *et al.*, 1990), rabbit (Hryshko *et al.*, 1989) and feline myocytes (du Bell & Houser, 1990) it has been shown by both methods that the SR Ca^{2+} content decreases during prolonged rest more or less in parallel to the decrease in contractility.

No, or only negligible, responses to caffeine or cooling are observed when the rested state contraction is attained.

The Ca^{2+} released from the SR by rapid cooling is partly extruded from the cell and partly taken back by the SR (Bers *et al.*, 1989). The Ca^{2+} released by caffeine is completely extruded from the cell. No SR re-uptake of Ca^{2+} occurs under these experimental conditions, as shown by the lack of any contractile response to the next application of caffeine unless the cell is stimulated (Lewartowski & Zdanowski, 1990). As suggested by the effect of nickel ions (Ni^{2+}) in Fig. 1, the outward transport occurs by the Na/Ca exchange system. It operates from the very beginning of release of Ca^{2+} by caffeine, since the rate of rise of the contracture is accelerated when the cell is superfused with a solution deprived of Na^+ and Ca^{2+} or containing 5.0 mM of Ni^{2+}. Ni^{2+} has been proved to inhibit the Na/Ca exchange current (Callewaert, Cleeman & Morad, 1989; Kimura, Miyamae & Noma, 1987). Thus the Ca^{2+} transient or contracture initiated by caffeine is a resultant of Ca^{2+} release from the SR and Ca^{2+} extrusion from the cell. The difference between the effects of cooling and caffeine probably depend on the following: cooling activates the SR Ca^{2+} release channels but it inhibits the Ca^{2+} transport systems. Thus Ca^{2+} released from the SR largely remains in the cell (Bers *et al.*, 1989). Upon re-warming, this Ca^{2+} is taken up by SR. Caffeine activates the SR Ca^{2+} release channels (Rousseau & Meissner, 1989) which renders the SR unable to retain Ca^{2+} if taken up by the SR Ca^{2+}-ATPase. Thus all the released Ca^{2+} is extruded from the cell. No recovery of the contractile response to the second application of caffeine was found in guinea-pig myocytes irrespective of the duration of the delay between the applications (Lewartowski & Zdanowski, 1990). Thus the only source of Ca^{2+} activating post-caffeine contractions seems to be the sarcolemma. The initial post-caffeine contractions are very weak (mean about 18% of the pre-caffeine control). In many cells they are hardly visible in the records. Subsequent stimulation results in recovery of the pre-caffeine contractile amplitude within a few beats (Fig. 2). Thus the effect of caffeine resembles the effect of prolonged rest, as under both conditions the SR Ca^{2+} is depleted and contractility is strongly inhibited. However, there is an important difference: the post-caffeine recovery of the contractile amplitude is completed during a few subsequent beats, whereas post-rest recovery of contractility requires steady-state stimulation of the cells for about 1 min. Even when the rested state contraction has been attained, further prolongation of rest results in delay of recovery (Lewartowski, unpublished observations). The most likely explanation is that caffeine

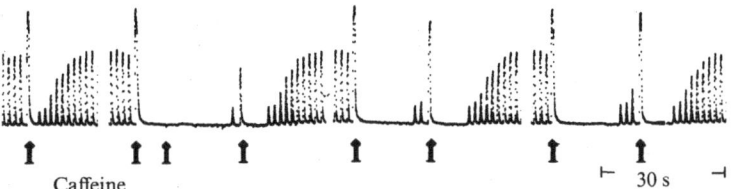

Fig. 2. Electrically stimulated contractions and caffeine contractures (arrows) initiated in an isolated single myocyte of guinea-pig heart. Vertical deflections (uncalibrated) indicate cell shortening. Restoration of contractile response to the second application of caffeine by electrically stimulated contractions.

releases Ca^{2+} selectively from the SR whereas the other cellular Ca^{2+} stores remain untouched. The long rest results in the loss of Ca^{2+} from all cellular stores due to long-lasting extrusion of Ca^{2+} from the cell. The longer the rest period, the more complete is the depletion. During post-rest stimulation the SR, the other Ca^{2+} stores and the contractile proteins compete for Ca^{2+} diffusing into the sarcoplasm. Saturation of those sinks is a time-consuming process. During post-caffeine stimulation, however the only competitor for the contractile proteins is the SR; the other sinks are still saturated with Ca^{2+}. Hence, a cell exposed previously to caffeine is a very attractive model, as it seems to be selectively deprived of the SR Ca^{2+}. The post-caffeine recovery of contractility would reflect in such a cell the kinetics of a selective repletion of the SR Ca^{2+}.

A single electrically stimulated contraction immediately restores a contractile response to the second application of caffeine (Fig. 2). Thus the amplitude of this restored caffeine contracture may be regarded as an index of the amount of Ca^{2+} which diffused to the sarcoplasm during a single excitation and was taken up by the SR. This contracture has a mean amplitude of 58% of that of the control caffeine contracture initiated after steady-state electrically stimulated contractions, although it may be nearly as high as that of a steady-state contraction. An estimate of the content of Ca^{2+} in the SR after a single excitation is difficult for at least three reasons:

1. Caffeine has been shown to increase the sensitivity of the contractile system to Ca^{2+} (Fabiato, 1981; Wendt & Stephenson, 1983).
2. Calcium transients initiated by caffeine develop more slowly and last longer than the Ca^{2+} transients during electrical stimulation (du Bell & Houser, 1990). Therefore, the lower amount of released Ca^{2+} may initiate a stronger contractile response (Yue, 1987).

3. The relationship between the activation of the contractile proteins and Ca^{2+} is sigmoid (Harrison, Lamont & Miller, 1988) and it is not known at which part of the curve to place the signals.

However, another approach to the semi-quantitative estimation of the amount of Ca^{2+} at a single post-caffeine excitation is possible. As shown in Fig. 2, full amplitude of the caffeine contracture may be attained after three post-caffeine electrically driven contractions. Bers et al. (1989) showed that rapid cooling of a single stimulated guinea-pig cardiomyocyte results in an increase in sarcoplasmic $[Ca^{2+}]$ from about 150 nM to 13–32 μM. Allowing for the buffering of Ca^{2+} by the intracellular binding sites, 140–235 (Pierce, Rich & Langer, 1985) or 85–115 μM/kg wet weight (Fabiato, 1983) would be required to bring free $[Ca^{2+}]$ to 13–32 μM. This amount of Ca^{2+} is apparently released from the SR by cooling, i.e., at least this amount of Ca^{2+} is contained in the SR during the steady-state stimulation of a cell. This value fits well to the estimates of the SR Ca^{2+} content based on the other experimental approaches (Dani, Cittadim & Inesi, 1979; Levitsky et al., 1981; Solaro & Briggs, 1974). It also fits with the result of Pytkowski (1989) who found that short exposure to 12.5 mM caffeine resulted in a decrease in the exchangeable Ca^{2+} content in the stimulated rabbit ventricular myocardium by 170 μmol/kg wet weight.

Thus it may be expected that the SR Ca^{2+} content in our experiments was about 150–200 μmol/kg wet weight. This amount of Ca^{2+} could be accumulated during three electrically driven beats (Bowditch effect) by an SR previously completely depleted of Ca^{2+} by caffeine. If the Ca^{2+} influx at each beat were equal, this would give about 50–70 μM Ca^{2+}/kg wet weight per beat. This increase in cellular Ca^{2+} content roughly corresponds to that calculated by Wendt-Gallitelli and Isenberg (1989) from the post-rest calcium currents measured in isolated guinea-pig myocytes (73–90 μmol/kg wet weight/post-rest excitation). However, the influx at the first beat is probably the largest and it decreases during the subsequent contractions (Lewartowski et al., 1984; Pytkowski et al., 1983). Therefore it may be expected that Ca^{2+} uptake by the SR during the first post-caffeine contraction is (in the guinea-pig cardiomyocyte) about 100 μmol/kg wet weight. This estimate would fit with the data of Lewartowski et al. (1984), who found that, during the first post-rest beat, exchangeable Ca^{2+} content in the isolated perfused guinea-pig ventricle may increase by as much as 200 μM/kg wet weight. The corresponding Ca^{2+} influx into the rabbit ventricular myocardium seems to be much less: 73 μM (Pytkowski, 1989) and 13.6 μM (Pierce et al., 1987).

There is some other evidence suggesting that the SR may take up, during the first post-caffeine contraction, the amount of Ca^{2+} which might otherwise have directly activated a strong twitch. This evidence has been provided by experiments in which SR function was selectively impaired by ryanodine or menadione. A plant alkaloid, ryanodine, has been shown to lock the SR Ca^{2+} release channel in the semi-opened state. When applied to multicellular myocardial preparations or to single cardiac myocytes, it dramatically accelerates the leak of Ca^{2+} from the SR. The leak becomes so rapid, that it is possible to initiate the caffeine contracture only during the relaxation phase of the preceding contraction (Lewartowski *et al.*, 1990). By the time relaxation is complete, no contractile response to caffeine may be initiated. Thus the SR Ca^{2+} is already depleted when the next electrical stimulus is initiated. The 2-methyl-1,4-naphthoquinone (menadione) has been shown by Floreani & Carpenedo (1989) and by Floreani, Santi Soncin & Carpenedo (1989) to inhibit, relatively selectively, the SR Ca^{2+}-ATPase. Both compounds inhibit the contractile response to the first application of caffeine and the restoration by a single excitation of the contractile response to the second caffeine application. The first post-caffeine contraction increases as the caffeine contractures decrease (Fig. 3(*a*)). Eventually, the amplitude of the post-caffeine contraction becomes as high as that of the steady state contractions (Lewartowski *et al.*, 1990, 1991). When the first electrical stimulus after caffeine was applied, the SR had been deprived of Ca^{2+} by ryanodine or menadione application. Thus the only change imposed by these compounds was that the SR was no longer able to retain or to trap Ca^{2+}, respectively. A manyfold increase in Ca^{2+} influx under the effect of ryanodine is unlikely (Mitchell *et al.*, 1984). The effect of menadione on i_{Ca} has never been investigated. It is conceivable that the initial post-caffeine electrically stimulated contraction is so small not because there is no Ca^{2+} to be released from the SR to activate contractile proteins, but because Ca^{2+} diffusing to the sarcoplasm from sources other than the SR is trapped by this organelle before it can reach the contractile system. After the ability of the SR to trap or to retain Ca^{2+} is abolished by menadione or ryanodine, respectively, Ca^{2+} diffusing to the sarcoplasm may bypass the SR and reach the contractile system. The amount of this Ca^{2+} is apparently sufficient to activate a contraction of amplitude equal to that of the steady-state contractions. A similar explanation may apply to the rested state contraction. It is hardly decreased with respect to the steady-state contractions in guinea-pig cells treated with menadione (Lewartowski *et al.*, 1990*b*). (See note at end of chapter.)

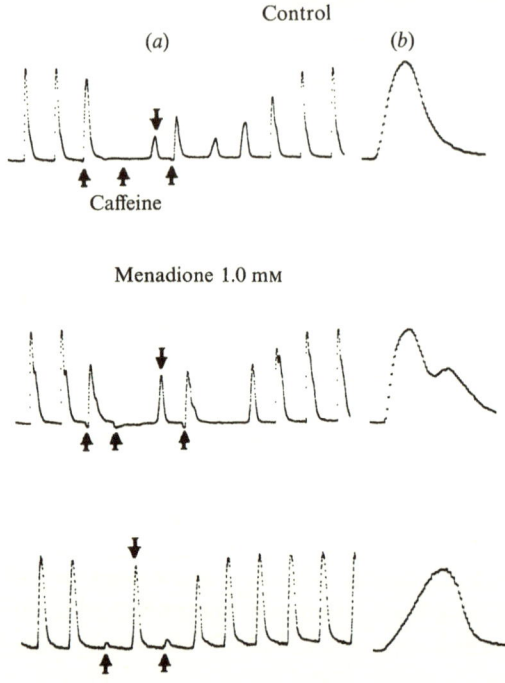

Fig. 3. (a) The effect of menadione (water soluble) on the electrically stimulated contractions and caffeine contractures (arrows pointing upwards) in an isolated myocyte of guinea-pig heart. The first electrically stimulated post-caffeine contraction is indicated by the arrows directed downwards. (b) Electrically stimulated contractions registered at higher paper speed.

The amplitude of steady-state contractions decreased slightly or not at all after menadione or ryanodine treatment despite depletion of the SR Ca^{2+} (Lewartowski et al., 1990, 1991). The time to peak amplitude of these contractions increased significantly (Fig. 3(b)) in the cells treated with menadione. Initially a slow late phase of contraction appeared, super-imposed on the relaxation phase. After the full effect of menadione had developed, the first rapid phase disappeared completely whereas the amplitude of the slow phase reached the value of the original amplitude of the rapid phase. Thus it seems clear that the first phase resulted from release of Ca^{2+} from the SR whereas the second phase resulted from release of Ca^{2+} into sarcoplasm from sources other than the SR. The amount of this Ca^{2+} was sufficient for activation of a strong contraction. It appears that, after menadione, the amplitude of the steady-state contractions, of post-caffeine contractions and of post-rest contractions is equal and that all these contractions are activated by Ca^{2+} derived from sources other than the SR. This does not mean necessarily that Ca^{2+} influx in the normal cells is sufficient for direct activation of the steady state contractions. As described in the paragraph on the effect of rate of stimulation on Ca^{2+} influx (below), it may be enhanced in cells in which the SR has been deprived of Ca^{2+}. Moreover, although the amplitude of the Ca^{2+} transient is decreased in cells treated with ryanodine, its duration is increased (du Bell & Houser, 1990; Wier, Yue & Marban, 1985; Yue, 1987). This may result in more complete activation of contractile proteins despite decrease in maximal $[Ca^{2+}]_i$ (Yue, 1987).

The above evidence and estimates suggest that the Ca^{2+} influx into, and the SR uptake from, the sarcoplasm in a single post-caffeine excitation is of the order of 100 μmol/kg wet weight. Similar influx may occur during the initial post-rest contraction and in cells treated with ryanodine or menadione. Two sources of this Ca^{2+} may be considered: mitochondria and the sarcolemma.

Mitochondria

As shown by Hansford *et al.* (1990) and by Wolska & Lewartowski (1991), the mitochondrial Ca^{2+} content is 1.5–2.5 nmol/mg of mitochondrial protein higher in the stimulated than in the rested guinea-pig ventricular myocardium. Taking the mitochondrial protein content as 40 g/kg wet weight (Hansford, 1985), this would make 60–100 μmol of mitochondrial stimulation-dependent Ca^{2+}/kg wet weight of the muscle. It is not known how many beats are required in order to accumulate this amount of mitochondrial Ca^{2+}. These results show that a considerable fraction of the rest- and stimulation-dependent Ca^{2+} described by Lewartowski *et al.* (1984) is contained in mitochondria. This Ca^{2+} could be released from the mitochondria in the cells allowed to rest after caffeine application and could be taken up by the SR. However, if this were the case, mitochondrial Ca^{2+} would be taken up by the SR irrespective of stimulation or quiescence of the cells. As pointed out above, stimulation is an indispensable condition of recovery of the contractile response to the second application of caffeine. Thus a mitochondrial source seems unlikely.

Sarcolemma

Three routes of sarcolemmal Ca^{2+} influx into the sarcoplasm may be considered.

Calcium channels

Calculations of the influx of extracellular Ca^{2+} based on measurements of the second inward current yielded a very broad range of values from a fraction of a μmol to several tens of μmoles. In multicellular preparations, a net gain in intracellular Ca^{2+} of between 1.0 and 50 μmol/kg wet weight has been calculated by Beeler & Reuter (1970a,b) and between 0.5 and 5.0 μmol by New & Trautwein (1972). The value obtained by Vassort & Rougier (1972) in frog atrial muscle was 10.0 μmol/kg wet weight per beat. Beeler & Reuter (1970b) did not explain in their paper on which experimental conditions this broad range of magnitude of i_{Ca}-mediated calcium influx depended. Reuter, referring to this paper in his review article (1974) wrote that, with an extracellular Ca^{2+} concentration of 2.0 mM, the gain in intracellular Ca^{2+} ions during an action potential is (in the dog myocardium) of the order of 1–5.0 μmoles per litre cell volume.

Results of calculations of Ca^{2+} influx in isolated bovine and guinea-pig ventricular myocytes have been reported over the last decade by Isenberg and his co-workers. The calculations are based on the assumption that the calcium current is carried exclusively by calcium ions. An early estimate in bovine myocytes amounted to an increase of 25 μmol in total $[Ca^{2+}]_i$ per excitation with a physiological Ca^{2+} concentration in the superfusing solution (Isenberg, 1982). The influx increased in the presence of adrenaline. A similar influx was estimated in guinea-pig ventricular myocytes by London & Kreuger (1986). Higher values of net cellular Ca^{2+} gain were proposed in two later publications. In guinea-pig isolated myocytes, i_{Ca} was found to reach a peak, at 0 mV, of 85 μA/cm^2 of the cell surface. This i_{Ca} was supposed to load the cell within 320 ms with 75 μmoles Ca^{2+} (Isenberg et al., 1987). A net Ca^{2+} gain of 473 μmoles/kg wet weight per five post-rest calcium currents was reported by Wendt-Gallitelli & Isenberg (1989) in single guinea-pig ventricular myocytes. If the Ca^{2+} influx at each post-rest excitation were equal, this would give about 90 μmol/kg wet weight per beat. However, in the last paper of this group (Shepherd, Vornanen & Isenberg, 1990) a net Ca^{2+} gain in guinea-pig cells of ~17 μmol was reported. Although it is not quite clear in the paper, it seems that this influx was calculated from i_{Ca} measured under conditions of steady state stimulation. Moreover, the cells worked under isometric conditions which has been shown in this paper to decrease the magnitude of i_{Ca}.

Allowing for the buffering of Ca^{2+} by the cellular components (Fabiato, 1983), a net cellular Ca^{2+} gain of up to 25.0 μmol/kg wet weight of the cells would directly activate not more than 10% of the maximal tension. Even higher capacity of the cellular Ca^{2+} buffers was proposed by Pierce, Philipson & Langer (1985), i.e. greater Ca^{2+} influx would be needed to activate a given percentage of maximal tension. These considerations lead to the conclusion that only the highest Ca^{2+} influx calibrated from i_{Ca} could account for significant direct activation of contractile proteins. The respective currents were recorded in isolated cells and apparently after prolonged rest (at least in the paper by Wendt-Gallitelli & Isenberg, 1989). It is conceivable that the magnitude of i_{Ca} is greater in isolated cells than in multicellular preparations. This could result from destruction of the extracellular structures associated with the sarcolemma, like the glycocalyx (Isenberg & Klockner, 1980), and of the net of protein fibres. Also the difference in the geometry, and in Ca^{2+} buffering of the extracellular space, between the isolated cells and multicellular preparations could account for the increase in the i_{Ca} in the cells (Fabiato, 1983). The magnitude of i_{Ca} is largest after rest and decreases during post-rest stimulation (see below).

Sodium/calcium exchange

Calcium may be transported into the cells by means of Na/Ca exchange working in the 'in mode' during the initial phase of the plateau of the action potential (Wier & Beuckelmann, 1989). The amount of this Ca^{2+} is difficult to estimate. However, it does not seem to exceed the amount of Ca^{2+} carried by the i_{Ca} (Powell & Noble, 1989). According to the calculations of Kimura *et al.* (1987), the magnitude of the inward Na/Ca exchange current flowing during the plateau of the action potential is 0.5 μA/μF. This current magnitude corresponds to a Ca^{2+} efflux of 50 μmol/l/s assuming a volume of a guinea-pig ventricular myocyte of 20 pl. Sodium–calcium exchange may operate in the 'in mode' over about the initial 50 ms of an action potential (Wier & Beuckelmann, 1989). If the mean magnitude of the initial Ca^{2+} influx were equal to the magnitude of Ca^{2+} efflux over the later phases of the action potential, the influx would be 2–3 μmol/l.

These estimates of *trans*-sarcolemmal Ca^{2+} fluxes based on the measurements of i_{Ca} and $i_{Na, Ca}$ or on changes in the intracellular Ca^{2+} content, can be compared with measurements of extracellular Ca^{2+} transients by means of extracellular Ca^{2+}-sensitive dyes or extracellular Ca^{2+}-sensitive microelectrodes.

Extracellular calcium transients

The changes in extracellular calcium ion concentration $[Ca^{2+}]_o$ related to the functional states of the myocytes have been investigated by means of extracellular Ca^{2+}-sensitive dyes and extracellular Ca^{2+}-sensitive microelectrodes in the amphibian and mammalian myocardium. These experiments have confirmed that there is a depletion of $[Ca^{2+}]_o$ (net cellular gain) during post-rest stimulation, a repletion of $[Ca^{2+}]_o$ (net cellular loss) at rest and an increase in $[Ca^{2+}]_o$ associated with potentiated contractions.

Repetitive post-rest stimulation at a rate of 2 Hz for 15 s resulted in depletion of 20 µM Ca^{2+} from the extracellular space of isolated rabbit papillary muscle as measured with Ca^{2+}-sensitive microelectrodes (Bers & MacLeod, 1986). The $[Ca^{2+}]_o$ in the superfusing solution was 0.2 mM. Assuming that the volume of extracellular space is 0.3 l/kg wet weight, the cellular Ca^{2+} uptake would be 6.6 µmol/kg wet weight. An increase in $[Ca^{2+}]_o$ to 2.0 mM resulted in an increase in depletion to 80 µM, i.e. an increase in the cellular uptake to 26.4 µmol/kg wet weight. The phasic depletions associated with single steady-state beats, measured with the same technique in the same preparation, amounted to 45 µM with $[Ca^{2+}]_o = 2.0$ mM. This would correspond to a cellular uptake of 11–16 µmol Ca^{2+}/kg wet weight, assuming that the volume of the extracellular space is 24–35% (Bers, 1983). Thus the cumulative uptake would not be larger than 2–3 times the phasic influx.

The cumulative cellular Ca^{2+} uptake estimated from the depletion of $[Ca^{2+}]_o$ measured with Ca^{2+}-sensitive dyes in rabbit left atrium amounted to ~ 8 µmol/kg wet weight with 1 mM Ca^{2+} in the superfusing solution (Hilgemann, Delay & Langer, 1983), or ~ 6.0 µmol/kg wet weight with 250.0 µM Ca^{2+} in the superfusate (Hilgemann, 1986a). Using the uptake/ $[Ca^{2+}]_o$ relationship of roughly 0.5 estimated by Bers (1983), cellular uptake with 2.0 mM Ca^{2+} in the superfusate would be ~ 10 µmol/kg wet weight. The maximal phasic Ca^{2+} depletion measured with tetramethyl-murexide due to a steady-state contraction of the guinea-pig atrium, with free $[Ca^{2+}]_o$ of 135 µM, was 0.4 µM and the cellular uptake was 0.08 µmol/kg wet weight (Hilgemann, 1986b). Thus with 2.0 mM external Ca^{2+}, uptake of up to 2.4 µmol/kg wet weight might be expected (Hilgemann & Noble, 1987).

These Ca^{2+} depletions per single post-rest beat or per steady state contraction are even lower than the Ca^{2+} influxes calculated from i_{Ca}. However, techniques of measurement of the extracellular Ca^{2+} transients seem to underestimate *trans*-sarcolemmal Ca^{2+} fluxes. Changes in $[Ca^{2+}]_o$ resulting from these fluxes may be damped by two mechanisms:

1. They may be compensated by Ca^{2+} exchange between the superfusing solution and the interstitial space.
2. They may be damped by extracellular Ca^{2+} buffers such as the outer surface of the sarcolemma and related structures. The possible effect of extracellular buffering has been clearly shown by Hilgemann (1986a): addition of citrate to the superfusing solution abolished the extracellular Ca^{2+} transients without affecting contractions.

Sarcolemmal calcium pool

If the influx into the sarcoplasm from the two former sources is regarded to be too small to account for activation of contraction in the cells after the SR has been deprived of Ca^{2+} (after caffeine, menadione, ryanodine or prolonged rest), the sarcolemmal rapidly exchanging pool seems to be an attractive alternative. This compartment, defined by Langer, Rich & Orner (1990), is apparently localised in the sarcolemma or at a cellular site in very rapid equilibration with sarcolemmal sites (see chapter by Langer in this volume). This compartment is postulated to contain most of the cellular exchangeable Ca^{2+} (Langer et al., 1990). Increase in its capacity results in a positive inotropic effect (Langer & Rich, 1986; Rich, Langer & Klassen, 1988). However, as this pool remains in rapid equilibrium with extracellular Ca^{2+} (Langer et al., 1990; Rich et al., 1988), influx of Ca^{2+} into the sarcoplasm from this pool should be reflected in extracellular Ca^{2+} depletion. As reviewed above, the extracellular Ca^{2+} depletion is too small to account for the large post-caffeine or post-rest Ca^{2+} uptake. If these transients really reflect quantitatively the Ca^{2+} influx, a source of Ca^{2+} other than both the SR and the extracellular space should be postulated. The possible solution may be provided by Lüllmann's hypothesis proposing the existence of a Ca^{2+} pool bound to the inner surface of the sarcolemma (Lüllmann, Peters & Preuner, 1983). The binding sites would be provided by phosphatidylserine. Their affinity would depend on the local, intrasarcolemmal pH, which would decrease during depolarisation due to increase in the outward driving force for protons. This would result in release of the sarcolemmal-bound Ca^{2+}.

The Ca^{2+} would be rebound upon repolarisation and the consequent increase in pH. Thus the sarcolemmal-bound Ca^{2+} would function as a kind of shuttle. It should remain in a kind of equilibrium with extracellular Ca^{2+}, but equilibration could be slow enough for the extracellular Ca^{2+} transients to be compensated effectively by the Ca^{2+} shifts between interstitium and superfusing solution or capillaries. Involvement of this fraction in the activation of the post-rest or post-caffeine contractions would require that it is not depleted after rest or caffeine application.

It is very important if and how prolonged rest may affect the *trans*-sarcolemmal Ca^{2+} influx. In other words, it is interesting to examine whether the steady state Ca^{2+} influx is as large as that after caffeine or prolonged rest.

The effect of rate of stimulation on calcium influx

The *trans*-sarcolemmal i_{Ca} is inhibited by the $[Ca^{2+}]_i$ and its inactivation is accelerated (Kirby, Orchard & Boyett, 1989; Boyett, Kirby & Orchard, 1988; Tseng, 1988). The decrease of the i_{Ca} may occur as a consequence of elevation of the resting $[Ca^{2+}]_i$ or due to the transient increase in $[Ca^{2+}]_i$ following stimulation. The rate of increase and maximal $[Ca^{2+}]_i$ is decreased during post-rest contractions compared to steady-state contractions (Bers, Bridge & Spitzer, 1989; DuBell & Houser, 1990), apparently due to depletion of the SR Ca^{2+}. Similar changes in the Ca^{2+} transient have been seen with ryanodine (Wier et al., 1985; Yue, 1987). This may result in an increase in maximal amplitude and in delay in inactivation of i_{Ca} (Mitchell et al., 1984). i_{Ca} is largest during the initial post-rest beats (Beeler & Reuter, 1970a; Gibbons & Fozzard, 1975; Simurda et al., 1981; Shepherd et al., 1990) and decreases to the steady state level during subsequent post-rest stimulation (Bowditch effect).

Slowing down of the upstroke and decrease in magnitude of the Ca^{2+} transient during the initial post-rest beats may also enhance the Ca^{2+} influx by means of Na/Ca exchange (Kirby et al., 1989; Powell & Noble, 1989; Wier & Beuckelmann, 1989). No evidence is available concerning the effect of rate of stimulation on Ca^{2+} release from the rapidly exchangeable sarcolemmal pool. What happens during changes in the rate of steady state stimulation is probably a continuum of the states between post-rest contraction (when the SR is deprived of Ca^{2+} and the rate of rise and amplitude of the Ca^{2+} transient is decreased) and the steady-state contraction at the optimal rate of stimulation (when the SR is loaded with Ca^{2+} and the Ca^{2+} transient is of high amplitude).

Summary and conclusions

The large diversity of estimates of the *trans*-sarcolemmal Ca^{2+} fluxes makes any firm conclusion concerning the physiological significance of influx of Ca^{2+} from the extracellular space very difficult. It is, however, possible to try to create an image of the probable course of events during changes in the rate of stimulation or during and after rest. This image will be based on principles similar to those accepted by Hilgemann & Noble (1987) for their computations of the Ca^{2+} movements during the excitation of the cardiac myocyte.

Experiments in which the SR has been deprived of Ca^{2+} by ryanodine or menadione suggest that the sarcolemmal Ca^{2+} influx (i_{Ca}, $i_{Na,Ca}$ and rapidly exchangeable Ca^{2+} pool), if not inhibited, is potentially sufficient for activation of a contraction of an amplitude equal to the amplitude of a steady state contraction of the normal cell. When sarcolemma is the only source of activator Ca^{2+} (after ryanodine, caffeine, menadione or prolonged rest) its effectiveness in activation of contraction is increased due to increased duration of the Ca^{2+} transient, although the maximal $[Ca^{2+}]_i$ may be decreased. At least two components of the Ca^{2+} influx (i_{Ca} and $i_{Na,Ca}$) are inhibited by $[Ca^{2+}]_i$. Thus negative feed-back between Ca influx and $[Ca^{2+}]_i$ is established. The $[Ca^{2+}]_i$ during cell excitation depends on the resting calcium concentration plus the Ca^{2+} transient. The rate of rise and maximal sarcoplasmic concentration of free Ca^{2+} during an action potential depends on the amount and rate of Ca^{2+} release from the SR. This is related to the SR Ca^{2+} content (Fabiato, 1983, 1985). Hence the greater the SR Ca^{2+} content, the lower the *trans*-sarcolemmal Ca^{2+} influx. The SR Ca^{2+} content increases with increase in the rate of stimulation. On the other hand, the higher rate of rise and higher amplitude of the Ca^{2+} transient at high rates of stimulation would enhance Ca^{2+} extrusion via Na/Ca exchange. Together with the decreased Ca^{2+} influx this would lead to a decrease in the SR Ca^{2+} content. Under steady-state conditions these opposite tendencies should be balanced. Under non steady-state conditions, one of them prevails. This was clearly shown by Hilgemann (1986a,b); potentiated beats initiated when the SR Ca^{2+} content was large were associated with net Ca^{2+} loss whereas post-rest beats (i.e. with the SR deprived of Ca^{2+}) were associated with net Ca^{2+} gain. The amplitude and time course of the rapid component of contraction depends on the rate and amplitude of the Ca^{2+} transient related to the SR Ca^{2+} release. Hence, lower Ca^{2+} influx, shorter time to peak tension or time to peak amplitude of contraction and larger tension or amplitude of contraction may be expected when the rate of stimulation is increased. Contraction would then consist almost exclusively of the first, rapid phase. When the rate of stimulation is low, increase in Ca^{2+} influx, increase in the time to peak tension and decrease in tension or amplitude of contraction should occur. The second, slow phase of contraction activated by the increased Ca^{2+} influx may then be visible. The post-rest or post-caffeine contractions correspond to the extremes of the decrease in the rate of stimulation. The Ca^{2+} influx is large but the post-caffeine or post-rest contractions are small because Ca^{2+} is trapped by the SR (after caffeine) or by the SR and other binding sites (after rest) on its way to the contractile system. When the ability of the SR to take up or to store Ca^{2+} is abolished (menadione, ryanodine) sarcolemma-derived Ca^{2+} may reach the contractile system and activate a strong contraction. In this case, contraction consists exclusively of the second, slow component.

Note added in proof

The effects of menadione appeared poorly reproducible in the series of experiments performed after the manuscript had been sent to publisher. Apparently they did not depend on menadione itself but on some uncontrollable factor formed in its presence. Recently we obtained identical results using tapsigargin which was shown (Thustrup *et al.*, *Proc. Natl. Acad. Sci. USA*, **87**, 2466–70, 1990) to block the SR Ca^{2+}-ATPase.

References

Allen, D. G., Jewell, B. R. & Wood, E. H. (1976). Studies of the contractility of mammalian myocardium at low rates of stimulation. *Journal of Physiology*, **254**, 1–17.

Beeler, G. W. & Reuter, H. (1970a). Membrane calcium current in ventricular myocardial fibres. *Journal of Physiology*, **207**, 191–209.

Beeler, G. W. & Reuter, H. (1970b). The relation between membrane potential, membrane currents and activation of contraction in ventricular myocardial fibres. *Journal of Physiology*, **207**, 211–19.

Bers, D. M. (1983). Early transient depletion of extracellular Ca during individual cardiac muscle contractions. *American Journal of Physiology*, **244**, H462–8.

Bers, D. M. & MacLeod, K. T. (1986). Cumulative depletions of cellular calcium in rabbit ventricular muscle monitored with calcium-sensitive microelectrodes. *Circulation Research*, **58**, 769–82.

Bers, D. M., Bridge, J. H. B. & Spitzer, K. (1989). Intracellular Ca^{2+} transients during rapid cooling contractures in guinea-pig ventricular myocytes. *Journal of Physiology*, **417**, 537–53.

Boyett, M. R., Kirby, M. S. & Orchard, C. H. (1988). Rapid regulation of the 'second inward current' by intracellular calcium in isolated rat and ferret ventricular myocytes. *Journal of Physiology*, **407**, 77–102.

Callewaert, G., Cleeman, L. & Morad, M. (1989). Caffeine-induced Ca^{2+} release activates Ca^{2+} extrusion via Na–Ca exchanger in cardiac myocytes. *American Journal of Physiology*, **257**, C147–52.

Dani, A. M., Cittadim, A. & Inesi, G. (1979). Calcium transport and contractile activity in dissociated mammalian heart cells. *American Journal of Physiology*, **237**, C147–55.

du Bell, W. H. & Houser, S. R. (1990). Rest decay of Ca^{2+} transients and contractility in feline ventricular myocytes. *American Journal of Physiology*, **259**, H395–402.

Edman, K. A. P. & Jóhannsson, M. (1976). The contractile state of rabbit papillary muscle in relation to stimulation frequency. *Journal of Physiology*, **254**, 565–81.

Fabiato, A. (1981). Effect of cyclic AMP and phosphodiesterase inhibitors on the contraction and the Ca transient detected with aequorin in skinned cardiac cells from rat and rabbit ventricles. *Journal of General Physiology*, **78**, 15a–16a.

Fabiato, A. (1983). Calcium-induced release of calcium from the cardiac sarcoplasmic reticulum. *American Journal of Physiology*, **245**, C1–14.

Fabiato, A. (1985). Time and calcium dependence of activation and inactivation of calcium-induced release of calcium from endoplasmic reticulum of a skinned canine cardiac Purkinje cell. *Journal of General Physiology*, **85**, 247–89.

Floreani, M. & Carpenedo, F. (1989) Inhibition of cardiac sarcoplasmic reticulum Ca-ATPase activity by menadione. *Archives of Biochemistry and Biophysics*, **270**, 33–41.

Floreani, M., Santi Soncin, E. & Carpenedo, F. (1989). Effects of 2-methyl-1,4-naphthoquinone (menadione) on myocardial contractility and cardiac sarcoplasmic reticulum Ca-ATPase. *Naunyn-Schmiedeberg's Archives of Pharmacology*, **399**, 448–55.

Gibbons, W. R. & Fozzard, H. A. (1975). Slow inward current and contraction of sheep cardiac Purkinje fibres. *Journal of General Physiology*, **65**, 367–84.

Hansford, R. G. (1985). Relation between mitochondrial calcium transport and control of energy metabolism. *Review of Physiology, Biochemistry and Pharmacology*, **102**, 1–72.

Hansford, R. G., Hogue, B., Wasilewska-Dziubinska, E., Prokopczuk, A. & Lewartowski, B. (1990). Activation of pyruvate dehydrogenase by electrical stimulation and low-Na^+ perfusion of guinea-pig heart. *Biochemica et Biophysica Acta*, **1018**, 282–6.

Harrison, S. M., Lamont, C. & Miller, D. J. (1988). Hysteresis and the length dependence of calcium sensitivity in chemically skinned rat cardiac muscle. *Journal of Physiology*, **401**, 115–43.

Hilgemann, D. W. (1986a). Extracellular calcium transients and action potential configuration changes related to post-stimulatory potentiation in rabbit atrium. *Journal of General Physiology*, **87**, 675–706.

Hilgemann, D. W. (1986b). Extracellular calcium transients at single excitations in rabbit atrium measured with tetramethylmurexide. *Journal of General Physiology*, **87**, 707–35.

Hilgemann, D. W., Delay, M. J. & Langer, G. A. (1983). Activation-dependent cumulative depletions of extracellular free calcium in guinea-pig atrium measured with Antipyrylazo III and tetramethylmurexide. *Circulation Research*, **53**, 779–93.

Hilgemann, D. W. & Noble, D. (1987). Excitation–contraction coupling and extracellular calcium transients in rabbit atrium: reconstruction of basic cellular mechanisms. *Proceedings of the Royal Society (Series B)*, **230**, 163–205.

Hryshko, L. V., Stiffel, V. & Bers, D. M. (1989). Rapid cooling contractures as an index of sarcoplasmic reticulum calcium content in rabbit ventricular myocytes. *American Journal of Physiology*, **257**, H1369–77.

Isenberg, G. (1982). Ca entry and contraction as studied in isolated bovine ventricular myocytes. *Zeitschrift für Naturforschung* **37**, 502–12.

Isenberg, G. & Klockner, K. (1980). Glycocalyx is not required for slow calcium current in isolated rat heart myocytes. *Nature*, **284**, 358–60.

Isenberg, G., Klockner, K., Mascher, D. & Ravens, U. (1987). Changes in contractility and membrane currents as studied with a single patch-electrode whole cell clamp technique. In *Electrophysiology of Single Cardiac Cells*. ed. D. Noble & T. Powell, pp. 25–66, Orlando Fl: Academic Press.

Janczewski, A. & Lewartowski, B. (1986). The effect of prolonged rest on calcium exchange and contractions in rat and guinea-pig ventricular myocardium. *Journal of Molecular and Cellular Cardiology*, **18**, 1233–42.

Kimura, J., Miyamae, S. & Noma, A. (1987). Identification of sodium-calcium current in single ventricular cells of guinea-pig. *Journal of Physiology*, **384**, 199–222.

Kirby, M. S., Orchard, C. H. & Boyett, M. R. (1989). The control of calcium influx by cytoplasmic calcium in mammalian heart muscle. *Molecular and Cellular Biochemistry*, **89**, 109–19.

Koch-Weser, J. & Blinks, J. R. (1963). The influence of the interval between beats on myocardial contractility. *Pharmacological Reviews*, **15**, 601–52.

Langer, G. A. & Rich, T. L. (1986). Augmentation of sarcolemmal Ca by anionic amphiphile: contractile response of three ventricular tissues. *American Journal of Physiology*, **250**, H247–54.

Langer, G. A., Rich, T. L. & Orner, F. B. (1990). Calcium exchange under non-perfusion limited conditions in rat ventricular cells. Identification of subcelluler compartments. *American Journal of Physiology*, **259**, H592–602.

Levitsky, D. O., Benevolenski, D. S., Levchenko, T. S., Smirnov, V. N. & Chazov, E. I. (1981). Calcium-binding rate and capacity of cardiac sarcoplasmic reticulum. *Journal of Molecular and Cellular Cardiology*, **13**, 785–96.

Lewartowski, B., Pytkowski, B. & Janczewski, A. (1984). Calcium fraction correlating with contractile force of ventricular muscle of guinea-pig heart. *Pflügers Archiv*, **401**, 198–203.

Lewartowski, B. & Pytkowski, B. (1987). Cellular mechanism of the relationship between myocardial force and frequency of contractions. *Progress in Biophysics and Molecular Biology*, **50**, 97–120.

Lewartowski, B., Hansford, R. G., Langer, G. A. & Lakatta, E. G. (1990). Contraction and SR Ca^{2+} content in single myocytes of guinea-pig hearts: the effect of ryanodine. *American Journal of Physiology*, **259**, H1222–9.

Lewartowski, B. & Zdanowski, K. (1990). Net Ca^{2+} influx and sarcoplasmic reticulum Ca^{2+} uptake in resting single myocytes of the rat heart: comparison with guinea-pig. *Journal of Molecular and Cellular Cardiology*, **22**, 1221–9.

Lewartowski, B., Zdanowski, K. & Wolska, B. (1991). The effect of menadione on sarcoplasmic reticulum Ca^{2+} and contractions of single guinea-pig cardiomyocytes. *Journal of Physiology and Pharmacology*, **42**, 223–36.

London, B. & Krueger, J. W. (1986). Contraction in voltage-clamped, internally perfused single heart cells. *Journal of General Physiology*, **88**, 475–505.

Lüllmann, H., Peters, T. & Preuner, J. (1983). Role of the plasmalemma for calcium homeostasis and for excitation–contraction coupling in cardiac muscle. in *Cardiac Metabolism*, ed. A. J. Drake-Holland & M. I. M. Noble, pp. 1–18, Chichester, John Wiley & Sons Ltd.

Meissner, G., Darling, E. & Eveleth, J. (1986). Kinetics of rapid Ca^{2+} release by sarcoplasmic reticulum. Effects of Ca^{2+}, Mg^{2+}, and adenosine nucleotides. *Biochemistry*, **25**, 236–44.

Meissner, G. & Henderson, J. S. (1987). Rapid calcium release from cardiac sarcoplasmic reticulum vesicles is dependent on Ca^{2+} and is modulated by Mg^{2+}, adenine nucleotides and calmodulin. *Journal of Biological Chemistry*, **262**, 3065–73.

Mitchell, M. R., Powell, T., Terrar, D. A. & Twist, V. M. (1984). Ryanodine prolongs Ca-currents while suppressing contraction in rat ventricular muscle cells. *British Journal of Pharmacology*, **81**, 13–15.

New, W. & Trautwein, W. (1972). The ionic nature of slow inward current and its relation to contraction. *Pflügers Archiv*, **334**, 24–38.

Pierce, G. N., Philipson, K. D. & Langer, G. A. (1985). Passive calcium-buffering capacity of a rabbit ventricular homogenate preparation. *American Journal of Physiology*, **249**, C248–55.

Pierce, G. N., Rich, T. L. & Langer, G. A. (1987). *Trans*-sarcolemmal Ca^{2+} movements associated with contraction of rabbit ventricular wall. *Circulation Research*, **61**, 805–14.

Powell, T. & Noble, D. (1989). Calcium movements during each heart beat. *Molecular and Cellular Biochemistry*, **89**, 103–8.

Pytkowski, B. (1989). Rest- and stimulation-dependent changes in exchangeable calcium content in rabbit ventricular myocardium. *Basic Research in Cardiology*, **84**, 22–9.

Pytkowski, B., Lewartowski, B., Prokopczuk, A., Zdanowski, K. & Lewandowska, K. (1983). Excitation- and rest-dependent shifts of Ca in the guinea-pig ventricular myocardium. *Pflügers Archiv*, **398**, 103–13.

Rardon, D. P., Cefuli, D. C., Mitchell, R. D., Seiler, S. M. & Jones, L. R. (1989). High molecular weight proteins purified from cardiac junctional sarcoplasmic reticulum vesicles are ryanodine-sensitive calcium channels. *Circulation Research*, **64**, 779–89.

Reuter, H. (1974). Exchange of calcium ions in the mammalian myocardium. Mechanism and physiological significance. *Circulation Research*, **34**, 599–605.

Rich, T. L., Langer, G. A. & Klassen, M. G. (1988). Two components of coupling calcium in single ventricular cells of rabbits and rats. *American Journal of Physiology*, **254**, H937–46.

Rousseau, E. & Meissner, G. (1989). Single cardiac sarcoplasmic reticulum Ca^{2+} release channel: activation by caffeine. *American Journal of Physiology*, **256**, H328–33.

Shepherd, N., Vornanen, M. & Isenberg, G. (1990). Force measurements from voltage-clamped guinea-pig ventricular myocytes. *American Journal of Physiology*, **258**, H452–9.

Simurda, J., Simurdova, M., Braveny, P. & Sumbera, J. (1981).

Activity-dependent changes of slow inward current in ventricular heart muscle. *Pflügers Archiv*, **362**, 209–18.

Solaro, A. & Briggs, A. M. (1974). Estimation of the functional capabilities of sarcoplasmic reticulum in cardiac muscle. *Circulation Research*, **34**, 531–40.

Stern, M. D., Silverman, H. S., Houser, S. R., Josephson, R. A., Capogrossi, M. C., Nichols, C. G., Lederer, W. J. & Lakatta, E. G. (1988). Anoxic contractile failure in rat heart myocytes is caused by failure in intracellular calcium release due to alteration of action potential. *Proceedings of the National Academy of Sciences of USA*, **85**, 6954–8.

Tseng, G.-N. (1988). Calcium current restitution in mammalian ventricular myocytes is modulated by intracellular calcium. *Circulation Research*, **63**, 468–82.

Vassort, G. & Rougier, O. (1972). Membrane potential and slow inward current dependence of frog cardiac mechanical activity. *Pflügers Archiv*, **331**, 191–203.

Wendt, I. R. & Stephenson, D. G (1983). Effects of caffeine on skinned cardiac and skeletal muscles fibres of the rat. *Pflügers Archiv*, **398**, 210–16.

Wendt-Gallitelli, M. F. & Isenberg, G. (1989). X-ray microanalysis of single cardiac myocytes frozen under voltage-clamp conditions. *American Journal of Physiology*, **256**, H574–83.

Wier, W. G., Yue, D. Y. & Marban, E. (1985). Effects of ryanodine on intracellular Ca^{2+} transients in mammalian cardiac muscle. *Federation Proceedings*, **44**, 2989–93.

Wier, W. G. & Beuckelmann, D. J. (1989). Sodium-calcium exchange in mammalian heart: current–voltage relation and intracellular calcium concentration. *Molecular and Cellular Biochemistry*, **89**, 97–102.

Wolska, B. & Lewartowski, B. (1991). Calcium in the *in situ* mitochondria of rested and stimulated myocardium. *Journal of Molecular and Cellular Cardiology*, **23**, 217–26.

Yue, D. T. (1987). Intracellular $[Ca^{2+}]$ related to rate of force development in twitch contraction of heart. *American Journal of Physiology*, **252**, H760–70.

Calcium compartmentation and contractile function of the heart

G. A. LANGER

It has been the goal over many years to define calcium (Ca) compartments within the cardiac cell in terms of their organelles of origin and their relation to contractile function (Shine, Serena & Langer, 1971; Philipson & Langer, 1979; Hunter, Haworth & Berkoff, 1981; Lewartowski, Pytkowski & Janczewski, 1984). This definition was hampered in the whole tissue (arterially or bath-perfused papillary muscle or arterially perfused heart) by the complexity of the preparations. There was always uncertainty in the definition of exchange rates and compartment sizes because the orientation of the compartments with respect to each other (series, parallel or a combination) and the magnitude of isotopic reflux were essentially unknown. The recent development of viable single cardiac cell preparations (Powell, Terrar & Twist, 1980; Piper et al., 1982) has, to a large extent, obviated these problems. The use of single cells in combination with rapid superfusion techniques (Rich, Langer & Klassen, 1988) and specific probes is now permitting further realistic definition of excitation–contraction processes in the intact, functional myocardium. The purpose of this chapter is to review these recent results and provide an update for Ca control of cardiac contraction.

Contractile function studies

The contractile response of single rat and rabbit ventricular cells to rapid changes in the perfusion medium disclosed two functional pools of Ca (Rich et al., 1988). A 'fast exchanging' pool could be totally depleted or repleted, by removal and replacement of perfusate Ca respectively, within a single diastolic period in both the rat and rabbit. The Ca within this pool was mandatory for maintenance of contraction. At 1 mM $[Ca]_o$ the 'fast' pool is nearly functionally saturated in the rat but not nearly saturated in the rabbit. A more slowly exchanging pool, also an important contributor to contraction, is demonstrated by repletion of Ca after 10 min perfusion with Ca-free perfusate. After 10 min depletion, more than 60 s of Ca repletion are required to restore contraction to control level.

The response of the rabbit cell to removal of Na from the perfusate indicated that the origin of the 'fast' pool was not simply extracellular Ca. Reduction of $[Na]_o$ produces a positive inotropic response that is fully developed within two beats and returns to control within a single beat upon return to standard $[Na]_o$. Since reduction of $[Na]_o$ does not change extracellular Ca but will only produce changes in cellular Ca the response indicates that the 'fast' pool has a cellular component.

The 'slow' pool contributes much more to contractile support in the rat than in the rabbit. After 10 min Ca depletion the first beat after return to 1 mM $[Ca]_o$ measures 60% of control in the rabbit but less than 10% in the rat. The return to 100% of control level then requires 60 s or more in both species. The studies of Bers (1985) and Fabiato (1983) have indicated that rat ventricle is among the tissues most dependent upon Ca-induced Ca release from the sarcoplasmic reticulum (SR). The responses of the rat and rabbit to Ca depletion and repletion are, then, consistent with placement of the functionally defined 'slow' pool Ca in the SR. The contractile response of the cells from the two species to ryanodine confirms this contention. It is generally accepted that ryanodine removes the contribution of the SR Ca pool to contraction. Ryanodine decreased contraction by 84% in rat cells as compared to only 18% in rabbit cells.

These results are consistent with the generally accepted model for excitation–contraction (E–C) coupling in mammalian heart muscle: there are two components of Ca which are important. One component enters through the sarcolemmal 'slow' Ca channel to serve primarily as a 'trigger' to induce Ca release from the SR. This mechanism is most developed in the rat. In contrast to the rat, in the rabbit this component seems to contribute directly to myofilament activation in addition to serving as a 'trigger' for SR Ca release. The second component of Ca resides in the SR and is dependent upon Ca from the first component to induce its release (Fabiato, 1983). Recent studies using rapid cooling and caffeine to specifically release Ca from the SR support this model (Bers, Bridge & Spitzer, 1989; Hryshko, Stiffel & Bers, 1989).

The above model describes the subcellular distribution of Ca in very general terms as inferred from contractile function studies. In order to define Ca loci and movements in greater detail the chapter will now focus on the pertinent cellular organelles with respect to their role in Ca exchange. Then, an attempt will be made to place these subcellular elements within the context of the whole cell and whole tissue.

Sarcolemma

This is made up of the lipid bilayer and its covering layer of glycoproteins, glycolipids and polysaccharides called the glycocalyx (Langer, Frank & Philipson, 1982). The latter has two components – the surface coat and external lamina which separate when the cell is exposed to zero $[Ca]_o$ for short periods. Therefore it appears that Ca plays a role in the maintenance of glycocalyx integrity and some Ca is localised within this surface structure. The glycocalyx contains significant amounts of the acidic sugar, sialic acid. It had been demonstrated (Langer *et al.*, 1976) that removal of sialic acid with neuraminidase specifically increased Ca uptake by myocardial cells and a recent study indicated that this was mediated, at least in part, by a large increase in current through the transient (T) Ca channel (Yee, Weiss & Langer, 1989). These results suggest that glycosylation of the sarcolemma plays an important role in the regulation of myocardial Ca influx.

The lipid bilayer is composed largely of phospholipid and cholesterol. Its interior contains well-ordered hydrophobic fatty acid chains and the surfaces project the hydrophilic head groups, generally choline, ethanolamine, serine or inositol. Embedded in the bilayer are the membrane proteins which constitute the three sarcolemmal systems important in Ca exchange.

Ca channels

A low threshold channel (L) carries most of the Ca current after it opens at approximately $-35\,\mathrm{mV}$ during excitation. It remains open for the duration of the action potential plateau. A higher threshold channel is the transient (T) channel which carries much less current and may be particularly important in pacemaking. (For a comprehensive presentation of cardiac calcium currents see Campbell & Giles, 1990.)

The Na–Ca exchanger

A very rapid transport system which couples the movement of $3Na^+$ to $1\,Ca^{2+}$. It is capable, within the course of a contraction cycle, of removing all of the Ca which previously entered the cell across the sarcolemma. It operates in the net Ca efflux mode throughout most of the cardiac cycle in most species under normal conditions. If intracellular Na increases for any reason net Ca influx via the exchanger is increasingly favoured, e.g. at high contraction frequency or after digitalis administration (see Philipson, 1990).

The calcium pump

This has a high affinity ($K_d \sim 1$ μM) for Ca in the presence of calmodulin. It pumps 1 Ca ion for 1 molecule of ATP hydrolysed; thus it operates at half the efficiency of the SR Ca pump. The bulk of Ca efflux from the cell occurs via the Na–Ca exchanger with the pump acting as a 'fine-tuner' of cell Ca along with the SR (see Carafoli, 1990).

The organisation of the sarcolemmal lipids has been recently defined (Post *et al.*, 1988) for rat myocardial cells in culture. The cholesterol: phospholipid ratio is 0.5. The phospholipid classes are asymmetrically distributed: (1) the negatively charged, phosphatidylserine and phosphatidylinositol are located exclusively in the inner or cytoplasmic leaflet; (2) 75% of zwitterionic phosphatidylethanolamine is in the inner leaflet; (3) 93% of sphingomyelin is in the outer leaflet; (4) 43% of phosphatidylcholine is in the outer leaflet.

The presence of all the anionic lipids at the inner monolayer may be significant in the light of their effects on the Na–Ca exchanger (Philipson, 1990) and the sarcolemmal Ca pump (Carafoli, 1990). Exchanger activity is markedly augmented by anionic amphiphiles due to an increase in Ca affinity of the exchanger. This suggests an interaction between the anionic charge and the exchanger Ca-binding site. The Ca pump is also activated by acidic phospholipids. These findings direct attention to the inner sarcolemmal leaflet as the possible site for important Ca interactions with the two important systems responsible for Ca removal from the cell. This will be discussed further below.

It is also likely that the lipid environment of the sarcolemmal Ca channel has a major influence on the channel's activity. Post *et al.* (1991) have recently shown in rabbit ventricular cells that insertion of an anionic amphiphile significantly enhances L-type Ca current and greatly augments contractile force; insertion of a cationic amphiphile produces opposite effects on current and force. The current–voltage relation of the channel is also shifted in a predictable direction by the amphiphiles. The results indicate that fixed charges on the outer leaflet play a significant role in modulating the properties of voltage-gated Ca currents.

In summary, the sarcolemma harbours three systems important in cellular Ca exchange: the Ca channel(s), the Na–Ca exchanger and the Ca pump. The first controls influx, the second operates to produce net Ca efflux unless intracellular Na rises and the third is an efflux system. The first is significantly affected by change of sialic acid content within the glycocalyx and by surface charge of phospholipid in the outer leaflet. The second and third are stimulated by anionic phospholipids which are normally present as components of the inner leaflet.

Sarcoplasmic reticulum

The function of this system has recently been reviewed in detail (Feher & Fabiato, 1990). The SR membrane contains a Ca pump which accumulates Ca and contributes to the process of relaxation. This transport is regulated through phosphorylation processes controlled by phospholamban, calmodulin, protein kinases and phosphatases. The SR also contains a channel responsible for the rapid release of Ca to contribute to contractile activation. The lumina of the lateral cisternae and corbular SR contain a Ca-binding protein, calsequestrin, which contributes to the storage capacity of the system.

Of particular interest from the point of view of Ca movement within the cell is the recent definition of the 'feet structures' of the junctional SR (Inui *et al.*, 1988). These structures seem to be identical to the Ca-release channels and to the ryanodine receptors. The feet span the 100 Å cleft which separates the transverse tubular portion of the sarcolemmal membrane and the SR. The feet are square prisms of about $27 \times 27 \times 14 \, \text{nm}$ dimension and appear to have a central channel from which four radial channels extend to the periphery (Wagenknecht *et al.*, 1989). These channels are proposed to represent the exit routes for Ca into the junctional space. According to this proposal, Ca induces release of Ca from the SR cistern via channels in the feet. It is released into the 100 Å, small volume cleft between the SR and T tubule membranes and, it is proposed, diffuses into the myoplasm. It should be noted, however, that Ca release into the restricted cleft would be expected to increase the Ca concentration in this region to levels higher than in the general myoplasm, perhaps by many-fold. This would place a transiently high Ca concentration at the inner leaflet of the sarcolemmal membrane. This point will be returned to later.

The junctional SR discussed above is only one element of the SR system. Jorgensen *et al.* (1988) indicate that the junctional and corbular SR contain calsequestrin whereas the longitudinal or non-junctional SR does not. The SR with calsequestrin has a relatively high calcium content (12.4 mmol/kg dry wt) while the other has a relatively low content (2.8 mmol/kg dry wt). It was proposed that both corbular and junctional SR are potential sources of Ca release following excitation (Jorgensen *et al.*, 1988). The longitudinal component is assigned the role of Ca-pumping.

In summary, the calsequestrin-containing junctional SR releases its Ca through its attached feet into the narrow SR–T tubule cleft via the mechanism of Ca-induced Ca release. A portion of this Ca is assumed to be that which activates the myofilaments. It is expected that the release into the volume-restricted cleft region might cause a transient increase of Ca concentration in the region much above the level in the general myoplasm. Resequestration of Ca occurs via the Ca pump within the longitudinal elements of the SR.

Mitochondria

The Ca relationships of this organelle have recently been reviewed in detail (Crompton, 1990). It is now clear that Ca serves as a second messenger for the adjustment of mitochondrial ATP synthesis to the energy requirements of the cell. Ca in the mitochondrion is controlled by two transport systems, a uniporter and a Na–Ca carrier. The uniporter transports Ca into the mitochondria passively down the very large electrochemical gradient for Ca (the magnitude of the inner membrane potential is -160 to -200 mV). The charge compensation occurs via extrusion of H^+ by pumps of the respiratory chain. Thus proton donation (e.g. by $H_2PO_4^-$) provides H^+ for extrusion and augments Ca uptake by the uniporter (Langer & Nudd, 1980). Efflux is via Na–Ca exchange with the stoichiometry not yet completely resolved though electroneutral exchange is favoured. The central role of Ca is to regulate oxidative metabolism via its effect on pyruvate dehydrogenase, oxoglutarate dehydrogenase and isocitrate dehydrogenase. These enzymes are control points and their sensitivity to Ca is the means by which the ion regulates oxidation of carbohydrates and fatty acids. Thus, as Crompton (1990) emphasises, the mitochondria transport Ca to regulate their own metabolism. The Ca level in the cell is seen as a guide to its ATP requirements. As Ca increases, energy requirements increase, mitochondrial Ca rises and more ATP is produced.

The mitochondria contain approximately 20% of the cellular Ca (Walsh & Tormey, 1988) under physiological conditions in which diastolic myoplasmic Ca concentration is in the range of 0.1–0.2 μM and systolic levels are transiently no more than 1–2 μM. There is evidence (Allshire *et al.*, 1987), that, if the level of myoplasmic Ca exceeds 1.5–3.0 μM for a prolonged period, mitochondrial Ca overload occurs. It seems that this overload induces an increased permeability of the mitochondrial membrane. This leads to uncoupling, decline in the transmembrane potential and failure of oxidative phosphorylation.

In summary, mitochondrial function is controlled via Ca effects on critical enzymes, thereby relating ATP output to cellular demand. Steady-state Ca levels are maintained by balance of influx through a passive uniporter which responds to the electrochemical gradient and efflux via a Na–Ca exchanger. The mitochondria can increase their Ca uptake and serve as an intracellular buffer system under conditions of increased load until myoplasmic Ca rises to contracture-producing concentrations (1.5–3.0 μM). Persistent levels in this range then lead to mitochondrial damage and shutdown.

Myofilaments

These represent the end-point of Ca regulation. The systems reviewed above, through their operation, determine the level of Ca at the myofilaments. 50% activation of the myofilaments requires that the myoplasmic Ca concentration be increased to 1.2–1.5 μM. In order that this concentration be achieved, Fabiato (1983) has calculated that 50% of maximum force development requires 50–60 μmol Ca/kg wet wt of myocardium. Pierce, Philipson & Langer (1985) indicate that twice this amount is necessary. The large excess of Ca above the activation concentration is due to the extensive buffering systems in the cell – which include Ca-binding sites, the SR and the mitochondria. The pattern of subcellular Ca distribution will determine the amount of Ca which will cycle to the myofilaments with each excitation and, therefore, the magnitude of the contractile response.

Kinetically defined subcellular compartments

With the characteristics of the cellular organelles in mind, the pattern of steady-state Ca exchange in the intact functional cell will be defined, then the exchange pattern will be related to Ca compartments within the cell and finally, to complete the circle, these compartments will be related to function.

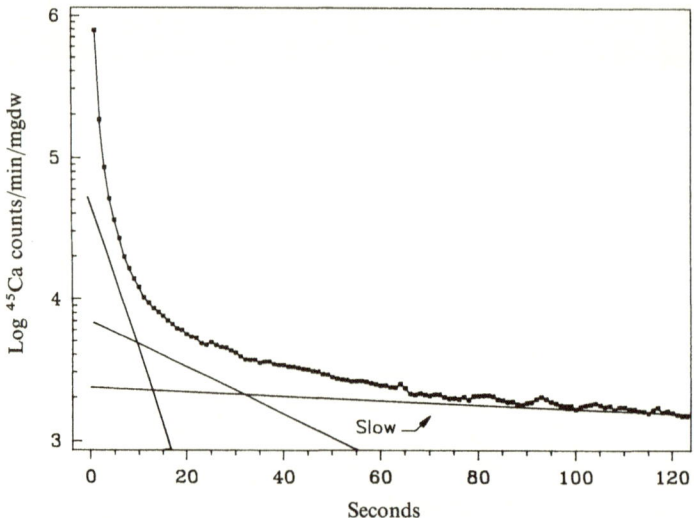

Fig. 1. ^{45}Ca washout from single rat ventricular cells. Washout rate = 2.8 ml/s; effluent counted at 1 s intervals. Upper curve represents cellular washout after blank washout subtraction. Resolution of the curve is shown below. The 'slow' component was defined as a single exponential from 120 s to 30 min with $t_{1/2}$ = 3.6 min. (Full washout not shown.) Sequential curve peeling by computer for the 3–120 s period reveals two further phases, $t_{1/2}$ = 3.5 and 19 s. These constitute the 'intermediate' compartment(s). See text for further discussion. (Reprinted with permission from the *American Journal of Physiology*.)

Pattern of steady–state exchange

A system has recently been developed which permits measurement of ^{45}Ca exchange in single ventricular cells under essentially non-perfusion-limited conditions (Langer, Rich & Orner, 1990). The technique permits continuous on-line measurement of ^{45}Ca exchange in which there is no period of non-recorded wash of ^{45}Ca from the extracellular space before cellular exchange begins to be measured. The high perfusion rate essentially eliminates reflux and, therefore, permits much more accurate quantitation of compartmental size and exchange rates.

The non-perfusion limited ^{45}Ca washout from rat ventricular cells is illustrated in Fig. 1. Prolonged washout (not shown) shows a single monoexponential component from 120 s to 30 min by which time counts have reached background levels. This slow compartment is shown in Fig. 1 and has a $t_{1/2}$ = 3.6 min. It contains 1.6 mmoles Ca/kg dry wt cells. The next segment of the washout curve is defined by a curve-peeling computer program which derives two exponential components with $t_{1/2}$s of 3.5 and 19 s. The intermediate compartment(s) contain 2.1 mmoles Ca/kg dry wt

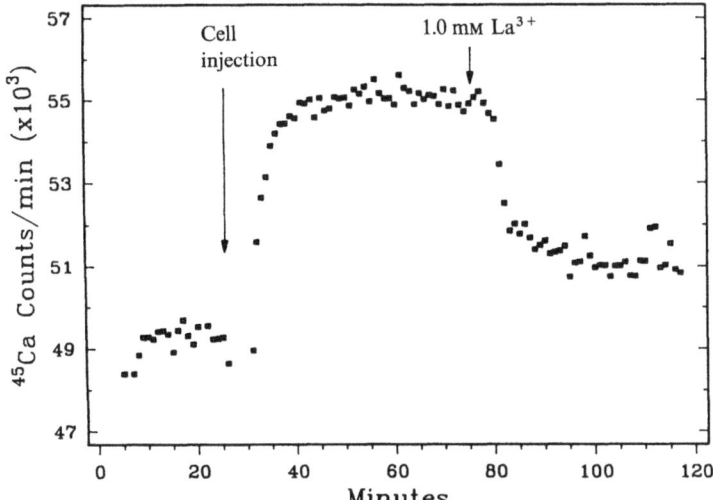

Fig. 2. ^{45}Ca uptake in single rat ventricular cells. Perfusion rate = 10 ml/min; uptake recorded at 1 min intervals. The flow cell is first filled with ^{45}Ca-labelled perfusate. At the 26th min cells were injected and as they label and settle to the surface of the scintillator disc their ^{45}Ca signal becomes obvious. Asymptote is achieved within 15–20 min as cells continue to settle and remains stable until 1.0 mM La^{3+} is added to the ^{45}Ca-labelled perfusate at the 76th min. This produces a ^{45}Ca displacement from the cells of 3800 counts/min. See text for further description. (Reprinted with permission from the *American Journal of Physiology*.)

cells. The initial 2–3 s of washout cannot be defined from the washout curve alone since, despite the rapid flow, the washout in the first two seconds contains isotopic activity derived from the chamber as well as from the cells. The most rapid component is defined by combining results from ^{45}Ca labelling and washout experiments.

Fig. 2 shows ^{45}Ca-labelling of cells as they are injected into the flow cell and settle and adhere to a disc of scintillator material which then is activated by the cells' ^{45}Ca emission. These photons are recorded by a photomultiplier tube in close apposition to the scintillator disc. The details of this on-line method as used for cultured cells have been previously described (Frank *et al.*, 1977). This is a perfusion-limited system since high perfusion rates will wash away the adherent cells. It can be used, however, to define net changes in ^{45}Ca-labelling where response time is not critical. The technique obviates the need for an interposed wash period to clear extracellular ^{45}Ca activity and, therefore, avoids washing away rapidly exchangeable cellular-associated ^{45}Ca. The period up to the 25th min in Fig. 2 (Langer, Rich & Orner, 1990) records the count level of the

Table 1. *Subcellular calcium compartments*

	Rapid	Intermediate	Slow	Inexchangeable
$t_{1/2}$	<1 s	3.5, 19 s	3.6 min	–
Content (mmoles/kg dry wt cells)	2.6	2.1	1.6	1.2

chamber filled with ^{45}Ca before addition of cells. As cells are injected (1.0–1.5 mg dry wt cells) and settle and adhere to the surface of the scintillation disc, they become labelled with ^{45}Ca and their signal is obvious. At the slow 10 ml/min perfusion rate approximately 15 min is required for an asymptotic count level to be achieved. This level remains stable from the 50th through the 76th min which documents that cellular Ca is at steady state and that the cells are not becoming progressively 'leaky'. At 76 min, 1 mM La^{3+} is added to the labelled perfusate and, over the next 15 min, a loss of 3.8×10^3 cpm is recorded. Application of the factor for cellular counting efficiency indicates that this loss represents displacement of 2.6 mmoles Ca/kg dry wt cells.

With this displacement documented, the rapid ^{45}Ca washout technique was used to define the exchange rate of the the La-accessible ^{45}Ca pool. 1 mM La^{3+} was added to the perfusate at the 2 s point of cellular washout. This addition produced *no* discernible displacement of ^{45}Ca into the washout flow. The sensitivity of the washout system is such that, even if 10–20% of the La-displaceable ^{45}Ca pool had remained after 2 s washout, it would have been easily detected. This means that the large 2.6 mmolar La-displaceable Ca pool must exchange, under non-perfusion limited conditions, with a $t_{1/2} < 1$ s.

Finally we (Langer, Rich & Orner, 1990) analysed the cells for the Ca pool which remains unlabelled after 60 min ^{45}Ca labelling. This measures 1.2 mmoles/kg dry wt cells and represents 'inexchangeable' or very slowly exchangeable Ca. The exchange rates and Ca contents of the kinetically defined cellular compartments are summarised in Table 1.

Loci of the compartments

The curve peeling procedure used to define the compartments is arbitrary and, by itself, provides little clue as to the cellular origin of the exchangeable Ca. However, the compartment profile provides a guide for the application of various specific probes in order to study their effects on the defined exchange pattern.

Phosphate

As discussed previously, addition of phosphate donates protons for the mitochondrial transport chain, leads to enhanced H^+ extrusion and increased uptake by the mitochondrial Ca uniporter. Addition of phosphate increases Ca uptake by the ventricular cells. The uptake is significantly suppressed by warfarin, an inhibitor of mitochondrial respiration. Removal of phosphate from the perfusing solution releases the Ca previously taken up (Langer, Rich & Orner, 1990). Therefore manipulation of phosphate in the perfusate provides a probe for mitochondrial Ca. Cells are first labelled with ^{45}Ca in the presence of 10 mM NaH_2PO_4 and ^{45}Ca washout commenced in the presence of the phosphate. During the course of the washout, a phosphate-free solution is abruptly substituted at 3.5, 5.0, 7.5 and 10 min of washout and the peak ^{45}Ca release which follows is measured and plotted versus time. The ^{45}Ca release upon phosphate removal decreased with a $t_{1/2} = 3.3$ min, similar to the 3.6 min $t_{1/2}$ of the slow compartment (Table 1). Therefore it is likely that a significant part of the slow compartment has its origin in the mitochondria.

Caffeine and ryanodine

It is generally agreed that caffeine crosses the sarcolemmal membrane rapidly and induces a release of Ca specifically from the SR (Smith *et al.*, 1988; Rousseau & Meissner, 1989). It is also well documented that ryanodine at concentrations $<10^{-6}$ M induces a Ca leak from the SR, reducing its content (Bers, 1987; Lai & Meissner, 1989). The washout pattern was probed with both these drugs. Caffeine was abruptly added to the washout solution at 4, 6, 8, 10, 15, 20, 40, 60, 120 and 180 s of washout. The addition produced increases in effluent activity which reached a maximum within 1 s and then declined over the next 10 s. Pretreatment of the cells with 10^{-6} M ryanodine for 60 min prior to washout reduced the caffeine-releasable ^{45}Ca by at least 85% at each time point. This substantiates the SR origin of the Ca released by caffeine. The total ^{45}Ca released at each time was plotted semilogarithmically. The resulting curve gave two exponential components with $t_{1/2}$s of 2 and 19 s. This places the SR Ca releasable by caffeine in the intermediate compartment (Table 1).

Lanthanum

La^{3+} addition to Ca^{45} washout at 10 s or at 10 min does not produce any displacement of Ca. This means that neither the intermediate nor the slow compartment is the source of the La-accessible Ca. Neither did La^{3+} addition produce displacement at the 2 s point of washout. Fig. 2 clearly indicates, however, that there is a La-displaceable pool of 2.6 mmoles/kg dry wt. The washout studies indicate, then, that this pool exchanges with a $t_{1/2} < 1$ s and therefore belongs to another compartment designated as 'rapid' (Table 1). The rapidity of its exchange would place it at the sarcolemma or at a cellular site in very rapid equilibrium with sarcolemmal sites.

It is not possible, at this time, to define with any certainty the subcellular locus of this large Ca compartment. Though its cellular origin is unknown, present information indicates that the sodium–calcium exchanger may play a significant role in the exchange of a portion of the 'rapid' compartment. Bridge, Smolley & Spitzer (1990) have clearly identified the current generated by the electrogenic Na–Ca exchanger in guinea pig ventricular cells. In a Ca-loaded cell in which the function of the SR had been removed and the Na–Ca exchange has been inactivated by removal of extracellular Na, reapplication of Na activated a current (i_{Na-Ca}) which developed fully within a few milliseconds and decayed with a $t_{1/2}$ of 235 ms. Crespo, Grantham & Cannell (1990) using single ventricular cells found that, upon activation of the Na–Ca exchanger at -80 mV membrane potential, Ca extrusion via the exchanger operated with a time constant of 0.5 sec ($t_{1/2} = 350$ ms) similar to the rate found by Bridge *et al.* (1990). Therefore these studies indicate that the Na–Ca exchanger is fast enough to account for the exchange of the Ca in the 'rapid' compartment.

The Ca flux via the 'rapid' compartment as measured isotopically and assuming a $t_{1/2} = 1$ s is > 1800 μmoles/kg dry wt cells/s (~ 300 μmols/kg wet cells/s) (Langer, Rich & Orner, 1990). Gruver, Katz & Messineo (1990) using a rapid filtration apparatus, measured ^{45}Ca fluxes from canine sarcolemmal vesicles with millisecond resolution. The system was applied to measure Na-gradient-dependent Ca flux, i.e. Na–Ca mediated flux. A V_{max} of 37 μmol/mg sarcolemmal protein/s was found. Using data from Tibbits *et al.* (1981) a value of 21 mg sarcolemmal protein/gm dry wt cell is derived. If this value is used to extrapolate the measured vesicle flux to the cell a value of almost 800 μmol/kg dry wt cells/s is obtained – within the range for 'rapid' compartment flux.

Studies in progress indicate that, though rapidly exchangeable, the Na–Ca dependent Ca pool is not accessible to displacement by La^{3+}. Thus the kinetically defined 'rapid' compartment seems to originate from diverse loci. The Na–Ca dependent pool is not reduced in size by ryanodine which indicates that its origin is probably not the junctional SR. In the absence of Na–Ca exchange the pool does not exchange via alternative routes, i.e. it does not 'turn over' until the exchange is activated. This indicates a rather discrete compartmentation which, given the rapidity of exchange, would seem to place the pool in close proximity to the sarcolemma but not accessible to extracellularly applied La^{3+}. If its origin could be identified as well as the origin of the La-displaceable Ca, considerable further insight into excitation–contraction coupling processes would be gained.

Calcium exchange and contraction in whole tissue

Having described Ca and contraction relations in the single cell and subcellular loci of exchange, an attempt will be made, in this final section, to place things in the context of function and exchange in the intact whole tissue.

The compartmentation of Ca in a kilogram of wet tissue is as follows (in mmols) (Langer, 1990): vascular: 0.105; interstitium: 0.250; exchangeable cellular: ~ 1.2; 'inexchangeable' cellular: 0.7. These values are for tissue perfused with 1 mM $[Ca]_o$. With these values in mind, the turnover rate in each of the anatomical compartments can be quantified.

Vascular

At physiological rates of perfusion, the turnover of Ca in the vascular space is approximately 25 μmol/s/kg.

Interstitium

250 μmol/kg is the content of 'free' Ca in this space. Kinetic compartmentation studies indicate that at least an equivalent amount is bound to anionic moieties within the interstitium. With 500 μmol/kg content, the turnover of Ca in this space is about 6 μmol/s/kg.

Cell

The values listed in Table 1 for non-perfusion-limited Ca exchange indicate a *trans*-sarcolemmal flux of > 300 μmol/s/kg. This is > 12 times

Tissue model

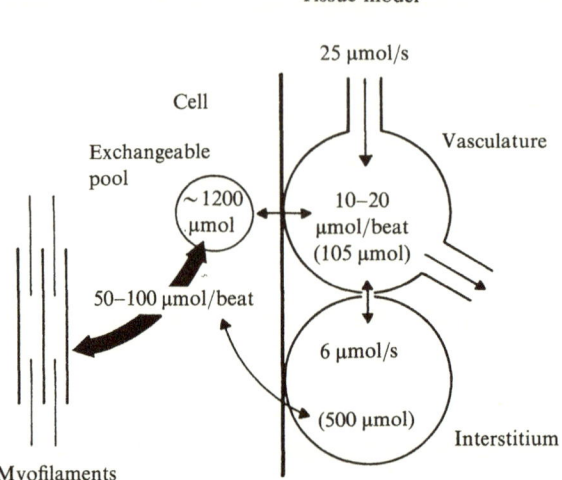

Myofilaments

Fig. 3. Tissue model for Ca exchange. $[Ca]_o$ is 1.0 mM. All values are per kg wet wt tissue. The cell contains an exchangeable Ca pool of 1200 μmol from which 50–100 μmol cycle to the myofilaments with each beat to generate 50% maximum force. With coronary flow at 1500 ml/kg/min vascular flow supplies 25 μmol Ca/s from which 10–20 μmol/beat can be extracted to enter the cell (as measured under brief, non-steady-state conditions). The static content of the vascular space is 105 μmol. Interstitial content is 500 μmol and it exchanges with the vascular space at a rate of 6 μmol/s. It also exchanges with the cellular exchangeable Ca in the tissue. Note that the arrangement of compartments allows for direct vascular-to-cell exchange as well as vascular-to-interstitial exchange. (Reprinted with permission of Raven Press, New York.)

the vascular flux and > 50 times the interstitial flux. This means that the exchange of cellular Ca is markedly perfusion limited when the cells are present within whole tissue perfused at physiological rates of perfusion. The cell stores or buffers a large amount of exchangeable Ca (~ 1200 μmol/kg) in compartments whose inherent exchange rate is masked by perfusion limitation in whole tissue.

Fig. 3 summarises the tissue compartmentation and fluxes discussed above. Since a major theme of this book is interval–force relationships, it is pertinent to discuss the fluxes associated with excitation and contraction in the context of the scheme shown in Fig. 3 (Langer, 1990). The value of 50–100 μmol/beat in the figure represents the amount of Ca estimated to produce 50% of maximum contractile force – which is the level produced at 1 mM $[Ca]_o$ by hearts of a number of mammalian species. Note also that the arrangement of the compartments allows for direct vascular-to-cellular exchange as well as vascular-to-interstitial exchange. There is strong ultrastructural (Frank & Langer, 1974) and kinetic (Philipson & Langer, 1979; Lewartowski, 1983) support for such a shunting of the interstitial space.

Consider, for example, the case where coronary flow is 1500 ml/kg/min, $[Ca]_o$ is 1.0 mM, heart rate is 60/min and developed force is 50% maximum. Each beat requires 50–100 μmol, derived from exchangeable cellular compartments of 1200 μmol content. These compartments are probably represented by the rapid ($t_{1/2} < 1$ s) and intermediate compartments ($t_{1/2} = 3.5$ and 19 s) (Table 1) of the cell. The vasculature exchanges with this labile pool in the amount of 10–20 μmol/beat. Since the vasculature conducts 25 μmol Ca/s through the capillaries, the vascular-to-cell exchange represents 40–80% extraction from the blood. The interstitium contains about 500 μmol which exchanges with the vasculature at a rate of 6 μmol/s. The content of the interstitium also exchanges with the cytosol and could exchange significant amounts of Ca with the exchangeable pool or other portions of the cell. It serves as a significant reservoir of tissue Ca. At 60 beats/min, 3000–6000 (60×50–100) μmol cycle between the exchangeable pool and myofilaments each min. The vascular or interstitial beat-associated fluxes are, at most, 40% of this value. It is, therefore, necessary that the largest fraction of contractile-dependent Ca cycles intracellularly between the exchangeable pool and cytosol under steady-state conditions of contraction.

The functionally defined 'fast' and 'slow pools' defined in the single cell would be expected to be part of the exchangeable pool in Fig. 3. Therefore, this pool is represented by the SR and the loci of the rapid compartment.

Finally, consider the non-steady-state condition of commencing stimulation from a quiescent state. The contractile function is manifested by a positive force staircase in hearts from most species. Using the arterially perfused right ventricular wall of the rabbit at a coronary flow of 1.5 ml/g/min stimulation was initiated at 48/min at $[Ca]_o = 1$ mM (Pierce, Rich & Langer, 1987). The extraction of [45]Ca from the vasculature was measured in the quiescent state and continuously as stimulation was commenced. Maximal uptake rate occurred within 3 beats (3.75 s) and indicated that 42 μmol Ca were removed from the vascular space from a total 94 μmol supplied by the vascular flow during this time. This is a 45% extraction. Lewartowski, Pytkowski & Janczewski (1984) found even higher extraction during initial excitation in guinea pig heart. Thus, there is a very high level of net Ca influx during the first beats after quiescence.

It should be noted that such a high extraction level need not be maintained for more than a few beats as the contractile-dependent exchangeable pool (Fig. 3) is supplemented to a new steady-state level of Ca. An average 14 μmol/kg wet wt net influx for 20 beats will add 280 μmol to the pool. This can then add to the amount cycled to the myofilaments as steady-state contractile force is achieved.

Acknowledgements

This work was supported by grants from the National Heart, Lung and Blood Institute, Castera Endowment and the Laubisch Fund.

References

Allshire, A., Piper, M. H., Cuthbertson, K. S. R. & Cobbold, P. A. (1987). Cytosolic free Ca^{2+} in single rat heart cells during anoxia and reoxygenation. *Biochemistry Journal*, **244**, 381–5.

Bers, D. M. (1985). Ca influx and sarcoplasmic reticulum Ca release in cardiac muscle activation during post rest recovery. *American Journal of Physiology*, **248**, H366–81.

Bers, D. M. (1987). Ryanodine and calcium content of cardiac SR. *American Journal of Physiology*, **253**, C408–15.

Bers, D. M., Bridge, J. H. B. & Spitzer, K. W. (1989). Intracellular Ca^{2+} transients during rapid cooling contractions in guinea-pig ventricular myocytes. *Journal of Physiology*, **417**, 537–53.

Bridge, J. H. B., Smolley, J. R. & Spitzer, K. W. (1990). The relationship between charge movements associated with I_{Ca} and I_{Na-Ca} in cardiac myocytes. *Science*, **248**, 376–8.

Campbell, D. L. & Giles, W. (1990). Calcium currents. In *Calcium and the Heart*, ed. G. A. Langer, pp. 27–84. New York: Raven Press.

Carafoli, E. (1990). Sarcolemmal calcium pump. In *Calcium and the Heart*, ed. G. A. Langer, pp. 109–26. New York: Raven Press.

Crespo, L. M., Grantham, C. J. & Cannell, M. B. (1990). Kinetics, stoichiometry and role of the Na–Ca exchange mechanism in isolated cardiac myocytes. *Nature*, **345**, 618–21.

Crompton, M. (1990). The role of Ca^{2+} in the function and dysfunction of heart mitochondria. In *Calcium and the Heart*, ed. G. A. Langer, pp. 167–98. New York: Raven Press.

Fabiato, A. (1983). Calcium-induced release of calcium from the cardiac sarcoplasmic reticulum. *American Journal of Physiology*, **245**, C1–14.

Feher, J. J. & Fabiato, A. (1990). Cardiac sarcoplasmic reticulum: calcium uptake and release. In *Calcium and the Heart*, ed. G. A. Langer, pp. 199–268. New York: Raven Press.

Frank, J. S. & Langer, G. A. (1974). The myocardial interstitium: its structure and its role in ionic exchange. *Journal of Cell Biology*, **60**, 586–601.

Frank, J. S., Langer, G. A., Nudd, L. M. & Seraydarian, K. (1977). The myocardial cell surface, its histochemistry and the effect of sialic acid and calcium removal on its structure and cellular ionic exchange. *Circulation Research*, **41**, 702–14.

Gruver, C. L., Katz, A. M. & Messineo, F. C. (1990). Canine cardiac sarcolemmal vesicles demonstrate rapid initial Na^+–Ca^{2+} exchange activity. *Circulation Research*, **66**, 1171–7.

Hryshko, L. V., Stiffel, V. & Bers, D. M. (1989). Rapid cooling contracture as an index of sarcoplasmic reticulum calcium content in rabbit ventricular myocytes. *American Journal of Physiology*, **257**, H1369–77.

Hunter, D. R., Haworth, R. A. & Berkoff, H. A. (1981). Measurement of rapidly exchangeable cellular calcium in the perfused beating rat heart. *Proceedings of the National Academy of Science, USA*, **78**, 5665–8.

Inui, M., Wang, S., Saito, A. & Fleischer, A. (1988). Characterization of junctional and longitudinal sarcoplasmic reticulum from heart muscle. *Journal of Biological Chemistry*, **263**, 10843–50.

Jorgensen, A. O., Broderick, R., Somlyo, A. P. & Somlyo, A. V. (1988). Two ultrastructurally distinct calcium storage sites in rat cardiac sarcoplasmic reticulum: an electron microprobe analysis study.*Circulation Research*, **63**, 1060–9.

Lai, F. A. & Meissner, G. (1989). The muscle ryanodine receptor and its intrinsic Ca^{2+} channel activity. *Journal of Bioengineering and Biomembranes*, **21**, 227–46.

Langer, G. A. (1990). Calcium exchange and contractile control. In *Calcium and the Heart*, ed. G. A. Langer, pp. 355–78. New York: Raven Press.

Langer, G. A., Frank, J. S., Nudd, L. M. & Seraydarian, K. (1976). Sialic acid: effect of removal on calcium permeability of cultured heart cells. *Science*, **193**, 1013–15.

Langer, G. A., Frank, J. S. & Philipson, J. D. (1982). Ultrastructure and calcium exchange of the sarcolemma, sarcoplasmic reticulum and mitochondria of the myocardium. *Pharmacological Therapeutics*, **16**, 331–76.

Langer, G. A. & Nudd, L. M. (1980). Addition and characterization of mitochondrial calcium in myocardial tissue culture. *American Journal of Physiology*, **239**, H769–74.

Langer, G. A., Rich, T. L. & Orner, F. B. (1990). Ca exchange under non-perfusion-limited conditions in rat ventricular cells: identification of subcellular compartments. *American Journal of Physiology*, **259**, H592–602.

Lewartowski, B. (1983). Calcium exchange. In *Cardiac Metabolism*, ed. A. J. Drake-Holland & M. I. M. Noble, pp. 101–16. London: John Wiley & Sons.

Lewartowski, B., Pytkowski, B. & Janczewski, A. (1984). Calcium fraction correlating with contractile force of ventricular muscle of guinea-pig heart. *Pflügers Archiv*, **401**, 198–203.

Philipson, K. D. (1990). The cardiac Na^+–Ca^{2+} exchanger. In *Calcium and the Heart*, ed. G. A. Langer, pp. 85–108. New York: Raven Press.

Philipson, K. D. & Langer, G. A. (1979). Sarcolemmal-bound calcium and contractility in the mammalian myocardium. *Journal of Molecular and Cellular Cardiology*, **11**, 857–75.

Pierce, G. N., Philipson, K. D. & Langer, G. A. (1985). Passive calcium-buffering capacity of rabbit ventricular homogenate preparation. *American Journal of Physiology*, **249**, C248–55.

Pierce, G. N., Rich, T. L. & Langer, G. A. (1987). Trans-sarcolemmal Ca^{2+} movements associated with contraction of the rabbit right ventricular wall. *Circulation Research*, **61**, 805–14.

Piper, H. M., Probst, P., Schwarz, P., Hutter, F. J. & Spieckermann, P. G. (1982). Culturing of stable adult cardiac myocytes. *Journal of Molecular and Cellular Cardiology*, **14**, 397–412.

Post, J. A., Langer, G. A., Op den Kamp, J. A. F. & Verkleij, A. J. (1988). Phospholipid asymmetry in cardiac sarcolemma. Analysis of intact cells and 'gas-dissected' membranes. *Biochimica et Biophysica Acta*, **943**, 256–66.

Post, J. A., Ji, S., Leonards, K. S. & Langer, G. A. (1991). Effects of charged amphiphiles on cardiac cell contractility are mediated via effects on calcium current. *American Journal of Physiology*, **260**, H759–69.

Powell, T., Terrar, D. A. & Twist, V. W. (1980). Electrical properties of individual cells isolated from adult rat ventricular myocardium. *Journal of Physiology*, **302**, 131–53.

Rich, T. L., Langer, G. A. & Klassen, M. G. (1988). Two components of coupling calcium in single ventricular cells of rabbits and rats. *American Journal of Physiology*, **254**, H937–46.

Rousseau, E. & Meissner, G. (1989). Single cardiac sarcoplasmic reticulum Ca^{2+}-release channel; activation by caffeine. *American Journal of Physiology*, **256**, H328–33.

Shine, K. I., Serena, S. D. & Langer, G. A. (1971). Kinetic localization of contractile calcium in rabbit myocardium. *American Journal of Physiology*, **221**, 1408–17.

Smith, G. L., Valdeolmillos, M., Eisner, D. A. & Allen, D. G. (1988). Effects of rapid application of caffeine on intracellular calcium concentration in ferret papillary muscles. *Journal of General Physiology*, **92**, 351–68.

Tibbits, G. F., Sasaki, M., Keda, M., Shimade, K., Tsurahara, T. & Nagatomo, T. (1981). Characterization of rat myocardial sarcolemma. *Journal of Molecular and Cellular Cardiology*, **13**, 1051–61.

Wagenknecht, T., Grassucci, R., Frank, J., Saito, A., Inui, M. & Fleischer, S. (1989). Three dimensional architecture of the calcium channel/foot structure of sarcoplasmic reticulum. *Nature*, **338**, 167–70.

Walsh, L. G., & Tormey, J. McD. (1988). Cellular compartmentation in ischemic myocardium: indirect analysis by electron probe. *American Journal of Physiology*, **255**, H929–36.

Yee, H. F., Weiss, J. N. & Langer, G. A. (1989). Neuraminidase selectively enhances transient Ca^{2+} current in cardiac myocytes. *American Journal of Physiology*, **256**, C1267–72.

Part 4

The expression of interval–force phenomena in cardiac muscle

Myocardial excitation and contraction: factors influencing peak force

B. WOHLFART, P. ARLOCK and
S. E. J. N. MÖRNER

A simple model describing the general view of excitation–contraction coupling is shown in Fig. 1. During the plateau phase of the cardiac action potential there is an inflow of calcium through the sarcolemma. The calcium current (I_{si}), as measured during voltage clamp consists of a rapid component followed by a slower inflow (Arlock and Noble, 1985). During the early part of the action potential there is also a small calcium inflow coupled to extrusion of sodium ions. The calcium entry during excitation governs release of more calcium from the sarcoplasmic reticulum. The amount of calcium that reaches the contractile proteins determines force production (see chapter by Yue, pp. 95–109). Calcium is actively pumped back into the sarcoplasmic reticulum during relaxation. The remaining calcium leaves the cell, mainly via sodium–calcium exchange. One calcium ion is thereby coupled to entry of three sodium ions (Eisner & Lederer, 1985; Rasgado-Flores & Blaustein, 1987; Rasgado-Flores, Santiago & Blaustein, 1989). Some calcium also leaves the cell through the sarcolemmal calcium pump. In addition to these events, some calcium may also be reversibly bound to the sarcolemma, being released upon membrane depolarisation and bound again on repolarisation (see Lüllmann & Peters, 1979).

Variations of the interval between contractions strongly affect the calcium metabolism of the myocardial cell (see Lewartowski & Pytkowski, 1987; Schouten et al., 1987; Reiter, 1988). Force production is therefore critically dependent on the excitation interval. The configuration of the action potential is also dependent on the interval and this reflects changes in transmembrane calcium fluxes. This makes interval-force relationships of the heart complex.

Some factors influencing peak force of a given contraction are summarised in Fig. 2. Force production is determined by (1) the shape of the

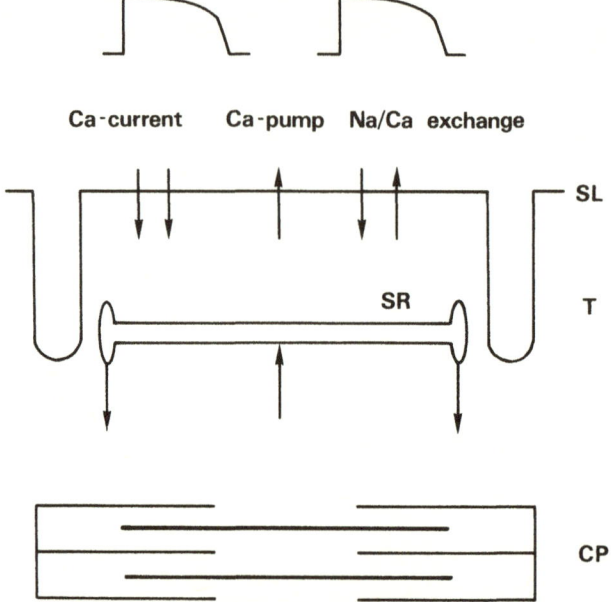

Fig. 1. A simple model of cardiac EC-coupling. Sarcolemma (SL), T-tubules (T), sarcoplasmic reticulum (SR) and contractile proteins (CP) are schematically illustrated.

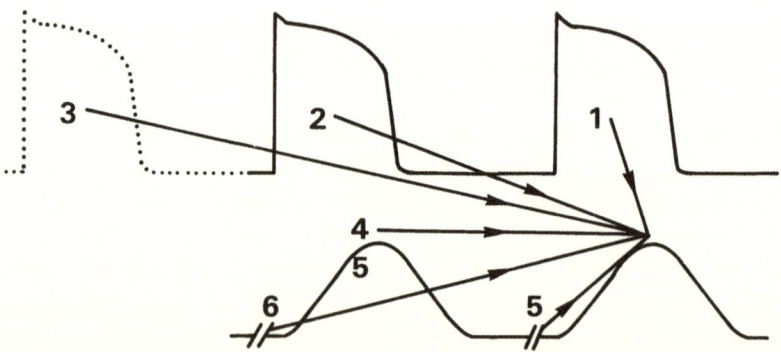

Fig. 2. Factors influencing peak force of a given contraction. Action potentials in upper row and myograms in lower row of the figure. See text for details.

concomitant action potential, (2) the preceding action potential and (3) earlier excitations via a long-term influence. Force is also related to (4) the amplitude of the preceding contraction, (5) the duration of the preceding excitation interval and (6) the pre-preceding excitation interval. These relations are discussed further below.

Force in relation to the concomitant membrane depolarisation

A sudden rise in intracellular calcium concentration induces release of more calcium from the sarcoplasmic reticulum (Fabiato, 1985). The calcium-induced calcium release is a graded process dependent on the kinetics of the rise in calcium. Membrane depolarisation leads to such a rise in intracellular calcium concentration.

With the voltage clamp technique applied to a papillary muscle preparation, it is possible to evaluate relationships between membrane voltage and force production. In the experiment demonstrated in Fig. 3(*a*) (Arlock & Wohlfart, 1990), the preparation was primed with 200 ms clamp pulses at an overall rate of 1.0 Hz.

The holding potential was -70 mV or -40 mV and the cell was clamped to 0 mV until steady state was reached. A single test clamp was then introduced on which the cell was clamped from holding potential to different voltages for 200 ms. It can be seen in the figure that a depolarisation to -30 mV was required in order to get force development. Increases in voltage step amplitude beyond this caused more force production up to an optimum value of about $+15$ mV and force declined again at more positive voltages.

In the experiment demonstrated in Fig. 3(*b*), the duration of the test clamp was varied from about 20 ms up to 500 ms. It can be seen that force production increased for durations between 20 and about 100 ms but was constant for longer durations.

These experiments confirm the idea that calcium-induced calcium release is not only a function of the amount of calcium in the sarcoplasmic reticulum but is indeed a graded process.

Force production related to the previous membrane depolarisation

According to Fabiato (1985), calcium inflow during excitation serves both to trigger calcium release and to load the sarcoplasmic reticulum for subsequent releases. The experiment demonstrated in Fig. 4 is compatible with these ideas. The same experimental protocol as described above was

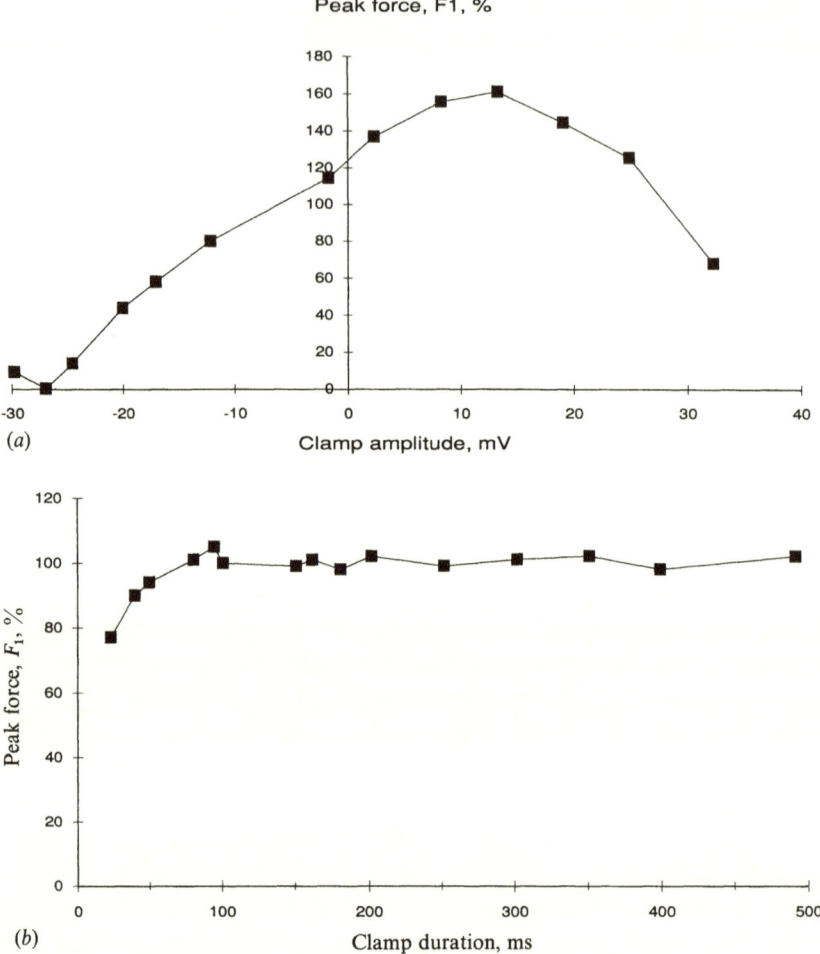

Fig. 3. Peak force related to clamp amplitude (panel (*a*)) and clamp duration (panel (*b*)) of the same cardiac cycle. Peak force is expressed as a percentage of the preceding control beat.

used, but with a second test contraction following the first and activated by a clamp pulse identical in shape and interval to those in the steady-state period. Peak force of the second test contraction is plotted against the duration of voltage clamp on the preceding contraction (clamp 1) in Fig. 4. This relation was studied for different amplitudes of test clamp 1 as indicated in the figure. It can be seen that, for longer durations of clamp 1, more force was produced in contraction 2, the relation becoming steeper for greater clamp amplitudes. A longer duration of membrane depolarisa-

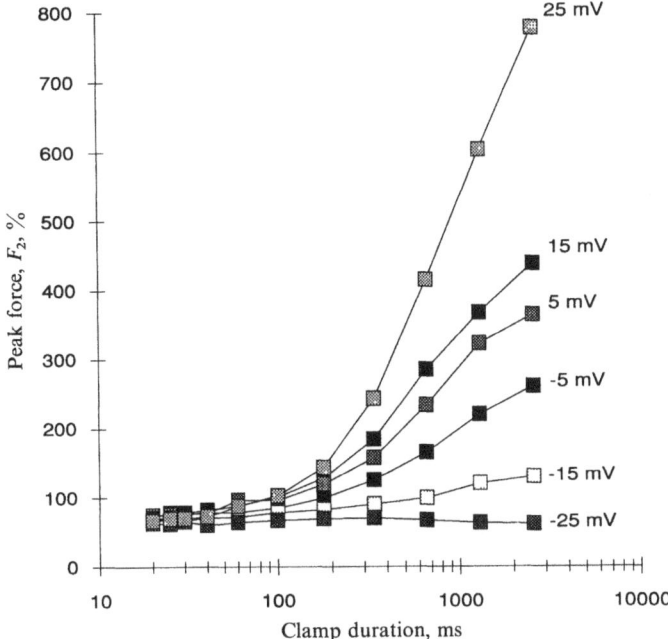

Fig. 4. Peak force of test contraction 2 related to clamp duration and amplitude of the previous cardiac cycle.

tion at greater amplitudes thus creates greater potentiation of the following contraction. This is most likely to be due to a greater calcium entry which loads the sarcoplasmic reticulum more. Calcium enters via second inward current and also via sodium–calcium exchange at the longer clamp durations (Barcenas-Ruiz *et al.*, 1987; Fedida *et al.*, 1987; Egan *et al.*, 1989; Horackova, 1989).

Long-term influences on force production levels

During the action potentials, there is a loading of calcium within the cell. There is also an outflow of calcium both during and between depolarisations. This occurs mainly via the sodium–calcium exchange (Hilgemann, 1986*a,b*; Hilgemann & Noble, 1987). The balance between inflow and outflow determines the net calcium flux over the sarcolemma. A period of high frequency excitation gradually loads the cell with increased levels of activator calcium. This may follow from the cellular accumulation of sodium at high frequencies, affecting the balance of the sodium–calcium exchange and leading to a net accumulation of activator calcium. There is thus a long-term influence of membrane depolarisations on calcium homeostasis.

Amplitude of the preceding contraction (recirculation of activator calcium)

During relaxation, calcium is pumped back to the sarcoplasmic reticulum and some calcium is actively extruded from the cell as outlined earlier. There is thus a competition between these two processes, both of which tend to lower the cytosolic intracellular calcium concentration. It follows that a fraction of the amount of calcium released at excitation is recirculated within the cell. A greater calcium release is thus followed by a greater recirculation than a smaller calcium release. We have previously suggested a simple method to indirectly estimate the recirculating fraction. This can be done by analysing the decay of post-extrasystolic potentiation, using the experimental protocol shown in Fig. 5. If the amplitude of the contraction following the potentiated one (F3 in Fig. 5) is plotted against the amplitude of the potentiated contraction (F2 in Fig. 5), a straight line is obtained (Fig. 6). The slope of this line, always less than one, is a measure of the proportion of activator calcium that recirculates. The slope of this line reflects how much a given increase in contractile potentiation affects the post-potentiated contraction, i.e. the proportion of activator that recirculates. This measure is dimensionless. It is not influenced by the sensitivity of the contractile system to released calcium as long as the sensitivity is not changed between the two analysed contractions. It has been shown to be independent of muscle length (Mörner & Wohlfart,

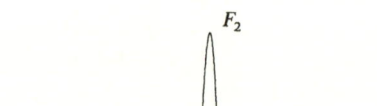

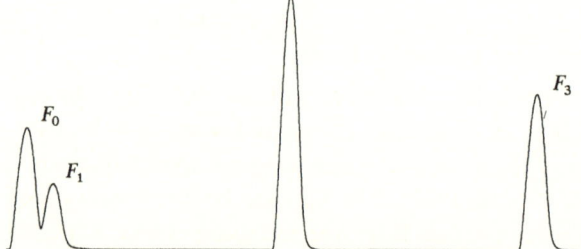

Fig. 5. Isometric recordings of force of an isolated guinea-pig papillary muscle. In the experimental protocol steady-state contractions are denoted 'F0'. Three test contractions are analysed and the interval before contraction 1 is systematically varied.

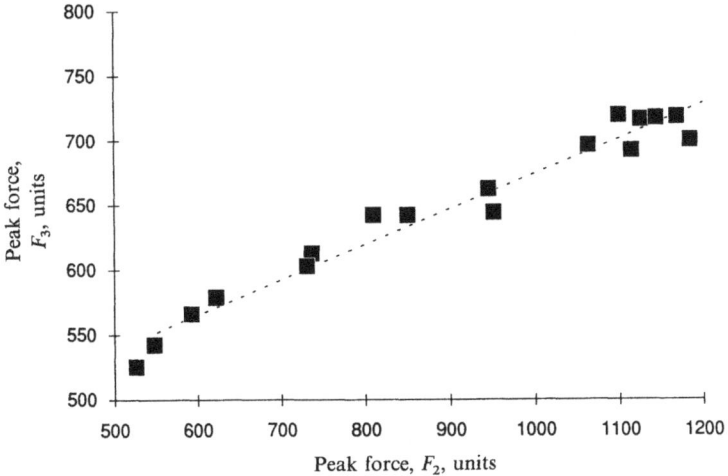

Fig. 6. Peak force of test contraction 3 related to peak force of test contraction 2. The experimental protocol is shown in Fig. 5.

1992). The recirculating fraction of calcium evaluated as the slope of the line can be used as a simple measure of the inotropic state (Seed & Walker, 1988).

Using this method, the recirculation fraction was determined to be 0.2 in the isolated rabbit papillary muscle (Wohlfart, 1979) and 0.7 in rat papillary muscles (Ragnarsdóttir *et al.*, 1982). The technique was also applied to the intact heart using maximum rate of pressure development in the left ventricle as a measure of the contractile state. The recirculation fraction was found to be 0.6 in open chest rabbits (Wohlfart & Elzinga, 1982), 0.7 in closed chest dogs (Elzinga *et al.*, 1981). The fraction is 0.5 in healthy man and 0.4 or below in a group with congestive cardiomyopathy (Seed *et al.*, 1984). The recirculation fraction could also be determined in voltage clamp experiments on isolated ferret and guinea-pig papillary muscles (Arlock & Wohlfart, 1990). In these experiments, potentiation was obtained after voltage steps with increased amplitudes and prolonged durations and the slope was around 0.4. Some pharmacological influences on the slope have also been studied in guinea-pig papillary muscles. The positive inotropic agents, amrinone (Mörner & Wohlfart, 1990) and enoximone (Mörner *et al.*, 1990), both increase the slope (from about 0.35 to 0.52 and 0.46, respectively) whereas the negative inotropic agent BDM (Mörner & Wohlfart, 1991) has no effect on the slope.

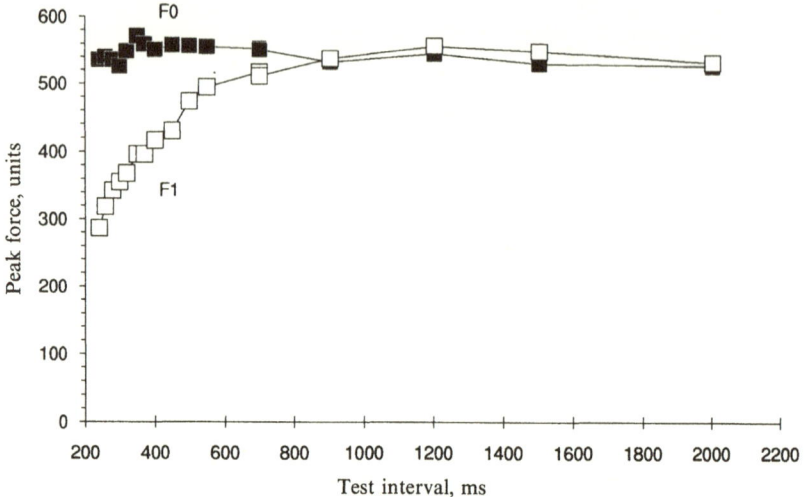

Fig. 7. Peak force of test contraction 1 related to the duration of the stimulus interval preceding contraction 1. Control contractions at 0.5 Hz are denoted F_0.

Preceding excitation interval (mechanical restitution)

After a contraction, there is a gradual recovery in the ability to produce force. This process is referred to as mechanical restitution (see chapter by Jóhannsson in this book, pp. 227–43). In Fig. 7, in which peak force of a guinea-pig papillary muscle has been plotted against the duration of the preceding stimulus interval, F1 represents a mechanical restitution curve. It can be seen that force rises as the interval lengthens.

Mechanical restitution is generally attributed to the recovery of the calcium release mechanism that takes place between releases. The calcium store within the sarcoplasmic reticulum can functionally be divided into an uptake store and a release store (see Wohlfart & Noble, 1982; Schouten *et al.*, 1987; and chapter by Allen in this book). After calcium has been taken up, a certain time is required before this calcium can be released again from the sarcoplasmic reticulum. This time delay can be due to the transport of calcium from the uptake to the release compartment. Another hypothesis is that the calcium release channels within the SR are refractory just after a release, and slowly recover as a function of time. The SR-channels might thus go through the same cycle of events as a population of sarcolemmal ion channels, i.e. activation followed by inactivation and recovery from inactivation.

There are pronounced species differences in mechanical restitution. In

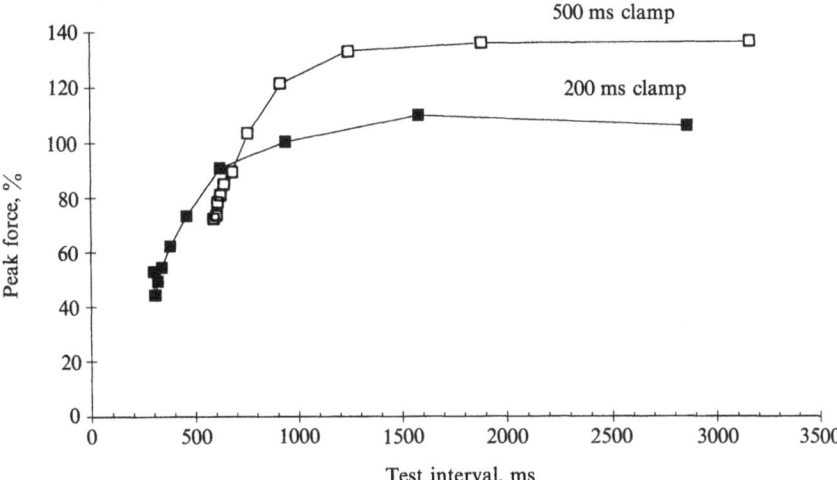

Fig. 8. Mechanical restitution during voltage clamp. Peak force is related to the preceding stimulus interval. Two clamp durations were tested as indicated in the figure.

rabbit and guinea-pig papillary muscles force reaches an optimum value at about 0.8 s (Edman & Jóhannsson, 1976). For longer intervals, there is a decline in force development. The mechanical restitution curve is similar to this in shape in the intact canine (Elzinga *et al.* 1981) and human heart (Pidgeon *et al.*, 1982). In these *in vivo* experiments, force production was evaluated by means of maximum rate of pressure development in the left ventricle, In rat isolated papillary muscles, force continues to rise at intervals longer than one second (Ragnarsdóttir *et al.*, 1982) and the same holds for atrial muscle (Jóhannsson & Ásgrímsson, 1989; see chapter by Jóhannsson). The explanation for this difference is unclear but it seems likely that there is a gradual replenishment of SR with calcium during long intervals.

Mechanical restitution in voltage-clamped ferret papillary muscles has recently been studied (Fig. 8, Arlock, Wohlfart & Noble, 1991). Mechanical restitution was studied after an ordinary clamp pulse of 200 ms duration and also after a 500 ms clamp pulse. The curve obtained after a longer clamp duration was shifted by 300 ms towards longer intervals. This finding is in agreement with the idea that mechanical restitution starts with membrane repolarisation. It therefore seems unlikely that mechanical restitution is due to a process that takes place solely within the SR, such as a time-dependent transport of calcium from an uptake to a release store. It seems plausible that the recovery of the

SR-channel is dependent on a decline of the intracellular calcium concentration, which is retarded until membrane repolarisation. Alternatively, mechanical restitution may be determined by sarcolemmal calcium binding. Trigger calcium for SR release might be bound to the cell membrane at repolarisation and released upon membrane depolarisation (Lüllmann & Peters, 1979).

Pre-preceding excitation (post-extrasystolic potentiation)

Force production is also influenced by the duration of the pre-preceding stimulus interval. When this interval is short, post-extrasystolic potentiation of force occurs (Figs 5 and 9). The contraction that immediately follows the short interval, i.e. the extrasystole, is not fully restituted. Some calcium is left in the SR after the extrasystole and the net cellular outflow of calcium is reduced. The extra calcium accumulated in SR after the extrasystole thus adds to the amount entering the cell during the action potential and causes contractile potentiation. Post-extrasystolic potentiation is critically dependent on the duration of the pre-preceding stimulus interval (F2 in Fig. 9); the smaller the degree of mechanical restitution of the extra contraction, the greater is the ensuing potentiation (Burkhoff *et al.*, 1984; Yue *et al.*, 1985). In rabbit papillary muscle the action potential

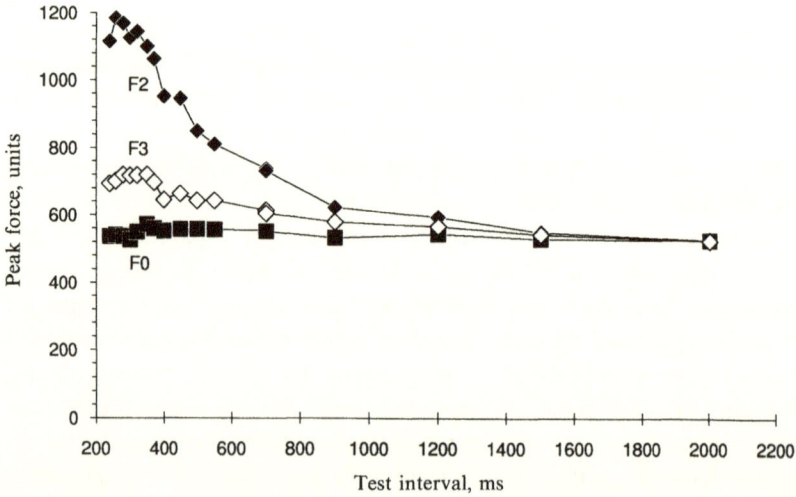

Fig. 9. Post-extrasystolic potentiation of force. Peak force (F2 and F3) related to the interval preceding contraction 1. Contractions labelled as in Fig. 5.

of the extra contraction shows an increased plateau voltage and also a prolonged duration (Wohlfart, 1979). This suggests an increased calcium inflow during the action potential which probably contributes to the potentiation of force. The increased calcium inflow would follow from the greater driving force for calcium over the sarcolemma when intracellular calcium is low as is the case during the premature extra contraction. In other preparations such as the cat papillary muscle (Bass, 1975), the action potential duration associated with the extra contraction is short. However, the short action potential does not exclude an increased calcium inflow. An increased calcium inflow could be masked by the increased potassium outflow during premature action potentials.

The six factors described above together can explain many manifestations of force–interval relationships. Together, they constitute a dynamic system that repeats from contraction to contraction in a recursive manner. Under certain conditions, the system may go into oscillations and mechanical alternans then occurs (Wohlfart, 1982; and see Chapter by Lab & Spencer, pp. 277–82). The precise physiologic background of the six factors described remains, however, to be unravelled.

References

Arlock, P. & Noble, D. (1985). Two components of 'second inward current' in ferret papillary muscle. *Journal of Physiology*, **369**, 88P.

Arlock, P. & Wohlfart, B. (1990). Force production following transient potential changes in voltage-clamped myocardium. *Acta Physiologica Scandinavica*, **140**, 63–72.

Arlock, P., Wohlfart, B. & Noble, M. I. M. (1991). Cardiac cell membrane repolarization is required for onset of mechanical restitution in papillary muscle. *Acta Physiologica Scandinavica*, **142**, 113–18.

Barcenas-Ruiz, L., Beuckelmann, D. J. & Wier, W. G. (1987). Sodium–calcium exchange in heart: membrane currents and changes in $[Ca^{2+}]_i$.*Science*, **238**, 1720–2.

Bass, B. G. (1975). Restitution of the action potential in cat papillary muscle. *American Journal of Physiology*, **228**, 1717–24.

Burkhoff, D., Yue, D. T., Franz, M. R., Hunter, W. C. & Sagawa, K. (1984). Mechanical restitution of isolated perfused canine left ventricle. *American Journal of Physiology*, **246**, H8–16.

Edman, K. A. P. & Jóhannsson, M. (1976). The contractile state of rabbit papillary muscle in relation to stimulation frequency. *Journal of Physiology*, **254**, 565–81.

Egan, T. M., Noble, D., Noble, S., Powell, T., Spindler, A. J. & Twist, V. W. (1989). Sodium–calcium exchange during the action potential in guinea-pig ventricular cells. *Journal of Physiology*, **411**, 639–61.

Eisner, D. A. & Lederer, W. J. (1985). Na–Ca exchange stoichiometry and electrogenicity. *American Journal of Physiology*, **248**, C189–202.

Elzinga, G., Lab, M. J., Noble, M. I. M., Papadoyannis, D. E., Pidgeon, J., Seed, A. & Wohlfart, B. (1981). The action-potential duration and contractile response of the intact heart related to the preceding interval and the preceding beat in the dog and cat. *Journal of Physiology*, **314**, 481–500.

Fabiato, A. (1985). Calcium-induced release of calcium from the sarcoplasmic reticulum. *Journal of General Physiology*, **85**, 189–320.

Fedida, D., Noble, D., Shimoni, Y. & Spindler, A. J. (1987). Inward current related to contractions in guinea-pig ventricular myocytes. *Journal of Physiology*, **385**, 565–89.

Hilgemann, D. W. (1986a). Extracellular calcium transients and action potential configuration changes related to post-stimulatory potentiation in rabbit atrium. *Journal of General Physiology*, **87**, 675–706.

Hilgemann, D. W. (1986b). Extracellular calcium transients at single excitations in rabbit atrium measured with tetramethylmurexide. *Journal of General Physiology*, **87**, 707–35.

Hilgemann, D. W. & Noble, D. (1987). Excitation–contraction coupling and intracellular calcium transients in rabbit atrium: reconstruction of basic cellular mechanisms. *Proceeding of the Royal Society Series B*, **230**, 163–205.

Horackova, M. (1989). Possible role of Na^+–Ca^{2+} exchange in the regulation of contractility in isolated adult ventricular myocytes from rat and guinea pig. *Canadian Journal of Physiology and Pharmacology*, **67**, 1525–33.

Jóhannsson, M. & Ásgrímsson, H. (1989). Short-term effects of stimulus interval changes in guinea-pig and rat atrial muscle. *Acta Physiologica Scandinavica*, **135**, 73–81.

Lewartowski, B. & Pytkowski, B. (1987). Cellular mechanism of the relationship betweenmyocardial force and frequency of contractions. *Progress in Biophysics and Molecular Biology*, **50**, 97–120.

Lüllmann, H. & Peters, T. (1979). Action of cardiac glycosides on the excitation–contraction coupling in heart muscle. *Progress in Pharmacology*, **2**, 1–57.

Mörner, S. E. J. N., Christley, H. M. & Wohlfart, B. (1990). Analysis of the inotropic mechanism of enoximone in guinea pig ventricular muscle. *Cardiovascular Pharmacology*, **16**, 423–9.

Mörner, S. E. J. N. & Wohlfart, B. (1990). Inotropic mechanisms of amrinone in papillary muscles from guinea-pig hearts. *Acta Physiologica Scandinavica*, **139**, 575–81.

Mörner, S. E. J. N. & Wohlfart, B. (1991). The action of 2,3-butanedionemonoxime on the inotropic state in guinea pig myocardium. *Acta Physiologica Scandinavica*, **142**, 211–9.

Mörner, S. E. J. N. & Wohlfart, B. (1992). Myocardial force interval relationships: influence of external sodium and calcium, muscle length, muscle diameter and stimulation frequency. *Acta Physiologica Scandinavica*, in press.

Pidgeon, J., Miller, G. A. H., Noble, M. I. M., Papadoyannis, D. & Seed, W. A. (1982). The relationship between the strength of the human heart beat and the interval between beats. *Circulation*, **65**, 1404–10.

Ragnarsdóttir, K., Wohlfart, B. & Jóhannsson, M. (1982). Mechanical restitution of the rat papillary muscle. *Acta Physiologica Scandinavica*, **115**, 183–91.

Rasgado-Flores, H. & Blaustein, M. P. (1987). Na/Ca exchange in barnacle muscle cells has a stoichiometry of 3 Na^+/1 Ca^{2+}. *American Journal of Physiology*, **252**, C499–504.

Rasgado-Flores, H., Santiago, E. M. & Blaustein, M. P. (1989). Kinetics and stoichiometry of coupled Na efflux and Ca influx. Na/Ca exchange in barnacle muscle cells. *Journal of General Physiology*, **93**, 1219–41.

Reiter, M. (1988). Calcium mobilization and cardiac inotropic mechanisms. *Pharmacological Reviews*, **40**, 189–217.

Schouten, V. J. A., Van Deen, J. K., De Tombe, P. & Verveen, A. A. (1987). Force–interval relationship in heart muscle of mammals. A calcium compartment model. *Biophysical Journal*, **51**, 13–26.

Seed, W. A., Noble, M. I. M., Walker, J. M., Miller, G. A. H., Pidgeon, J., Redwood, D., Wanless, R., Franz M. R., Schoettler, M. & Schaefer, J. (1984). Relationships between beat-to-beat interval and the strength of contraction in the healthy and diseased human heart. *Circulation*, **70**, 799–805.

Seed, W. A. & Walker, J. M. (1988). Relation between beat interval and force of the heartbeat and its clinical implications. *Cardiovascular Research*, **22**, 303–14.

Wohlfart, B. (1979). Relationships between peak force, action potential duration and stimulus interval in rabbit myocardium. *Acta Physiologica Scandinavica*, **106**, 395–409.

Wohlfart, B. (1982). Analysis of mechanical alternans in rabbit papillary muscle. *Acta Physiologica Scandinavica*, **115**, 405–14.

Wohlfart, B. & Elzinga, G. (1982). Electrical and mechanical responses of the intact rabbit heart in relation to the excitation interval. *Acta Physiologica Scandinavica*, **115**, 331–40.

Wohlfart, B. & Noble, M. I. M. (1982). The cardiac excitation–contraction cycle. *Pharmacology and Therapeutics*, **16**, 1–43.

Yue, D. T., Burkhoff, D., Franz, M. R., Hunter, W. C. & Sagawa, K. (1985). Postextrasystolic potentiation of the isolated canine left ventricle: relationship to mechanical restitution. *Circulation Research*, **56**, 340–50.

Mechanical restitution in cardiac muscle

MAGNÚS JÓHANNSSON

Introduction

When a short stimulus interval (a test interval) is inserted into a regular train of stimuli to cardiac muscle, the contraction following the short interval, the extrasystole, is weak (see Fig. 1). When this short interval is successively increased in duration toward the basic interval, the force of the extrasystole is gradually restored: this has been called mechanical restitution.

The first unequivocal observation of mechanical restitution was made by Woodworth (1902) in a dog heart. On page 243 he stated: 'The extra contraction is always weak in comparison with the regular beat, and it is weaker the more closely it follows the preceding regular beat.' The term 'restitution', to describe this phenomenon, was first used by Braveny & Kruta (1958), and has been used by most writers in this field since then.

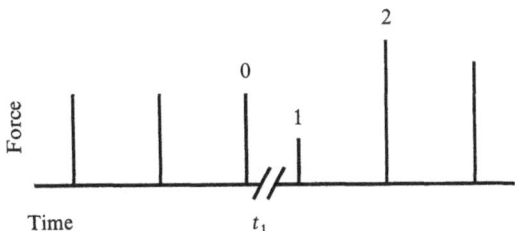

Fig. 1. Pacing protocol to determine mechanical restitution. t_1 is the test interval, which can be varied within the appropriate range. The regular beats are denoted by 0, the first beat after the test interval by 1 and the second beat by 2. In the example shown, the test interval is shorter than the regular interval, therefore beat 1 is weak (mechanical restitution) and beat 2 is strong (post-extrasystolic potentiation).

In the years to follow Braveny and Kruta made several valuable contributions in this area of research (Kruta & Braveny, 1960, 1961, 1963; Braveny, Sumbera & Kruta, 1966).

If the test interval is increased beyond the basic stimulus interval (usually about 1 s), in some muscles the force decreases again; this is the case, for example, in ventricular muscle from rabbit (Edman & Jóhannsson, 1976; Wohlfart, 1979; Wohlfart & Elzinga, 1982), guinea-pig (Rumberger & Reichel, 1972; Hanafy, Kitzing & Rumberger, 1976), cat (Maylie, 1982), man (Fry et al., 1983) and frog (Rumberger & Reichel, 1972). In other myocardial preparations, the force continues to increase; this is the case, for example, in rat ventricular (Ragnarsdóttir, Wohlfart & Jóhannsson, 1982; Vornanen, 1984; Schouten, 1986) and atrial muscle (Ravens & Ziegler, 1980; Jóhannsson & Ásgrímsson, 1989), guinea-pig atrium (Ravens & Ziegler, 1980; Jóhannsson & Ásgrímsson, 1989), rabbit atrium (Rosin & Farah, 1955), cat ventricular (Hisano, Suga & Ninomiya, 1985), canine ventricular (Endoh & Iijima, 1981) and ferret ventricular muscle (Chappell, Henderson & Lewis, 1986). The latter situation is sometimes regarded as a continuation of mechanical restitution but is also sometimes regarded as a separate phenomenon and then usually called post-rest potentiation.

Mechanical restitution is certainly one of the fundamental properties of the myocardium and it can be seen in all kinds of preparations, from single cells (Maylie, 1982; Shimoni, 1987) to the whole heart (Meijler, 1962; Elzinga et al., 1981; Burkhoff et al., 1984; and see chapters by Burkhoff and Hunter, pp. 283–9 and Seed, pp. 317–54, in this book).

Description of mechanical restitution

Mechanical restitution can often be described satisfactorily with exponential functions. Sometimes the best fit is obtained by using an exponential in a single phase:

$$F = A(1 - e^{-(t-t_0)/s_1})$$

In other cases it is necessary to use a biexponential function:

$$F = A(1 - e^{-(t-t_0)/s_1}) + B(1 - e^{-(t-t_0)/s_2})$$

F denotes the force of the test contraction (F_1), t is the test interval, A and B are parameters for contractile force and s_1 and s_2 are time constants. In all cases, there is a certain time lag in the beginning, t_0. Curve fitting has been done on results from a number of atrial and ventricular muscles from rats and guinea-pigs under a variety of experimental conditions. An

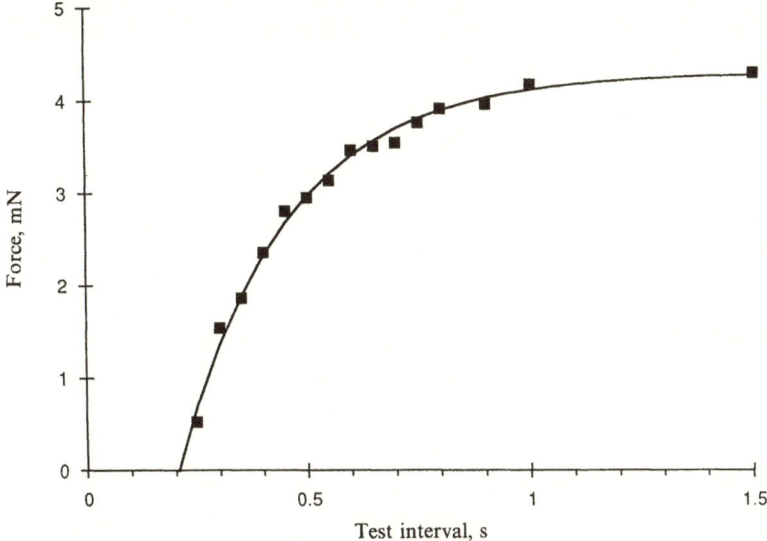

Fig. 2. Mechanical restitution in guinea-pig papillary muscle. The symbols represent peak force (force of contraction 1; see Fig. 1) measured after different test intervals. The line is the calculated curve after fitting with an exponential function ($t_0 = 0.21$ s; $s_1 = 0.25$ s; $A = 4.31$ mN). Basic stimulation intervals of 1 s, Ca concentration 2.0 mM, 32 °C.

acceptable fit was usually obtained using this approach. The curve-fitting programs used were based on non-linear least square methods. The curve fitting was either done on a VAX computer using the NAG Fortran Library, a PC/XT using Enzfitter (a program from Elsevier-BIOSOFT) or a Macintosh using Multifit (Day Computing). All programs gave very similar results, provided the number of experimental points was sufficient (15–20 points for the biexponential function). An example is shown in Fig. 2.

When mechanical restitution ends, force starts to fall again. This fall is sometimes exponential and ends in a contraction which is independent of the former contractile history of the preparation, the rested state contraction. Theoretically, this additional falling phase should be included when mechanical restitution is optimised. The error introduced, by not including the falling phase, is usually very small because the rate of this phase is relatively low compared with the rate of mechanical restitution.

The most common way to determine the contractile ability of an isolated muscle is simply to measure the isometric force (F). Another method is to differentiate the force signal to obtain the first derivative

(dF/dt). The parameters of mechanical restitution were compared in several guinea-pig atrial and ventricular muscles using either F or dF/dt, and the results are very similar. A similar comparison between the restitution of F, dF/dt and the intracellular Ca transient has been made in ferret ventricular myocardium (Wier & Yue, 1986) where all three curves had the same time course. It therefore seems unimportant whether the force or its derivative is used to study restitution.

Ventricular muscle

In isolated mammalian ventricular muscle, papillary muscles and trabeculae, mechanical restitution usually occurs in a single phase and reaches a peak in approximately one second (see above). The most important exceptions are the rat (Ragnarsdóttir *et al.*, 1982) and ferret (Chappell *et al.*, 1986) where mechanical restitution occurs in two phases and has a very late peak (usually 30–100 s). Rat myocardium has better organised sarcoplasmic reticulum (SR) in greater amounts than other mammals (Sommer & Johnson, 1979) and this fact might explain the difference described above.

In rabbit and guinea-pig, mechanical restitution can usually be described with an exponential function in a single phase (Fig. 2). In guinea-pig papillary muscles there is sometimes a dip in the restitution curve (decreased restitution rate) around 0.4 to 0.6 s test interval which can make it difficult to fit with an exponential function. This phenomenon can be seen in Figs. 2 and 4(*a*).

Atrial muscle

In isolated mammalian atrial muscle, atrial strips and trabeculae, mechanical restitution is usually slow and has a late peak. At least in guinea-pig and rat it can be described with an exponential function in two phases (Jóhannsson & Ásgrímsson, 1989; see also Figs. 3 and 4). In several species, e.g. rabbit and guinea-pig, mechanical restitution occurs in a single phase in ventricular, and in two phases in atrial muscle. It has also been found in many cases that atrial cells are richer in SR and have fewer T-tubules than ventricular cells from the same species (Bossen & Sommer, 1984; Van Winkle, 1986). This emphasises the fundamental difference between ventricular and atrial muscle in the same species.

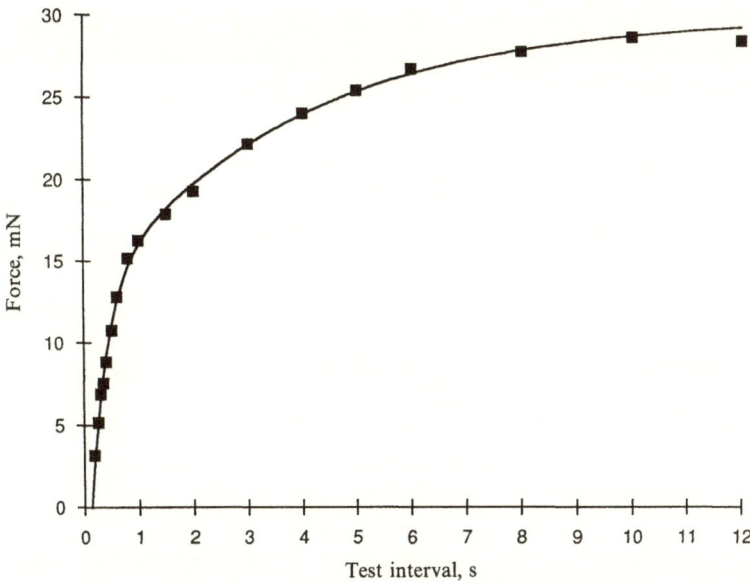

Fig. 3. Mechanical restitution in guinea-pig atrial strip. The symbols represent peak force (force of contraction 1; see Fig. 1) measured after different test intervals. The line is the calculated curve after fitting with an exponential function ($t_0 = 0.13$ s; $s_1 = 0.29$ s; $A = 13.17$ mN; $s_2 = 3.77$ s; $B = 16.74$ mN). Conditions the same as in Fig. 2.

Different species

It is tempting to try to find a relationship between structure and function. Mechanical restitution is found in all types of cardiac muscle, from the frog ventricle to the rat heart. Frog ventricular cells have a small diameter, very little sarcoplasmic reticulum (total SR approx. 0.38 vol.%; Bossen & Sommer, 1984), very long action potentials and activator calcium seems mainly to come directly from the outside with the slow inward current (i_{si}) and possibly also Na–Ca exchange. In this type of muscle, mechanical restitution occurs quickly in a single phase and it seems possible that the rate of restitution is governed by the rate of reactivation of the inward calcium current after the previous beat. At the other end of the spectrum we have rat myocardial cells which are larger, have lots of well organised sarcoplasmic reticulum (total SR approx. 3.5 vol.%; Page & McCallister, 1973), very short action potentials and activator calcium probably originates mostly in the SR. In this type of muscle, mechanical restitution occurs in two clearly separable phases, one fast and another slow. In several species, atrial cells are known to have more and better organised

Table 1. *Values for the parameters of mechanical restitution in guinea-pig and rat myocardium. Mean values and 95% confidence intervals ($\pm t95\%$) of n experiments*

	Guinea-pig ventricular	Guinea-pig atrial	Rat atrial
t_0	0.24 ± 0.02	0.15 ± 0.01	0.13 ± 0.01
s_1	0.20 ± 0.11	0.43 ± 0.04	0.21 ± 0.04
s_2		6.60 ± 0.9	12.10 ± 1.70
A	0.48 ± 0.17	0.51 ± 0.03	0.30 ± 0.07
B		0.49 ± 0.03	0.70 ± 0.07
$A + B$		1.00	1.00
n	$8\text{--}12$	34	15

Temperature $32\,°C$, stimulation rate 1 Hz, 2.0 mM Ca^{2+}. t_0 is the time delay until the beginning of mechanical restitution in s; s_1 and s_2 are the time constants of the exponential phases in s; A and B are the size parameters of the respective phases. In rat atrial and guinea-pig atrial muscle A and B are related to the sum $A + B$. In guinea-pig ventricular muscle, A is scaled to the maximally potentiated twitch after priming with a short period at 4 Hz and a Ca concentration of 4 mM.

SR than ventricular cells (Bossen & Sommer, 1984). It is also known that in several species (rabbit, guinea-pig) restitution occurs in a single phase in ventricular muscle but in two phases in atrial muscle. This might indicate that the second phase of restitution is dependent on a well-developed SR, and further support for this idea comes from the fact that caffeine and ryanodine in relatively low concentrations eliminate the second phase of restitution, leaving the first phase largely unimpaired. Both caffeine and ryanodine strongly affect the function of the SR (see chapter by Allen, pp. 43–65).

The differences between guinea-pig and rat atria are shown in Table 1. As can be seen, the rate of the first phase is about twice as fast but the rate of the second phase is about twice as slow in the rat. The two phases are equal in size in the guinea-pig but the second phase is larger in the rat.

When does restitution start?

When mechanical restitution is plotted, it can be seen that the restitution process does not start at time zero, immediately after a stimulus, but after a certain delay (see Figs. 2, 3 and 4). This lag of time, from a stimulus to the beginning of mechanical restitution, is here denoted t_0. Under normal conditions, t_0 is usually in the range 0.1–0.2 s, which is similar to the duration of the action potential or twitch. It seems reasonable to assume that the beginning of mechanical restitution is determined either by repolarisation of the cell membrane or relaxation of the muscle or by both. This problem is related to the process of excitation–contraction coupling and the origin of activator calcium. A strong correlation between repolarisation and t_0 could mean that activator calcium originated mainly from the sarcolemma (SL) or that calcium originating from the sarcolemma in turn triggered activator calcium from an internal store, probably the SR. A correlation between relaxation and t_0, on the other hand, could mean that activator calcium originated mainly from the internal stores of the sarcoplasmic reticulum and that t_0 and the beginning of mechanical restitution were governed by the handling of calcium by these structures. A possible problem with this interpretation is, however, that mechanical restitution often occurs in two phases. These phases might reflect different processes which might have different times of onset and thus there would be a t_0 for each phase.

As can be seen from Table 1, there is a clear difference in t_0 between guinea-pig ventricular and atrial muscle. On the other hand, no difference can be seen between atrial muscle from guinea-pig and rat even if the difference in action potential duration is appreciable (Jóhannsson & Ásgrímsson, 1989). In these experiments, t_0 decreased slightly with increasing Ca concentration (0.9, 1.8 and 3.6 mM) and with increasing basic stimulation rate (0.2, 0.5, 1 and 2 Hz). These interventions are also well known to decrease the action potential duration and this might indicate a correlation between action potential duration and t_0. The possible correlation between repolarisation and t_0 is further strengthened by the finding in voltage-clamped sheep cardiac Purkinje fibres (Lipsius, Fozzard & Gibbons, 1982) that the time course of restitution was affected by membrane voltage. This question is also discussed in the chapter by Cooper and Noble in this book (pp. 67–91), who provide further evidence that the onset of restitution commences with repolarisation.

Paired-pulse stimulation and restitution

Paired-pulse stimulation of the myocardium causes a marked potentiation of contractions. This is true even when the number of contractions per unit of time is unchanged, e.g. basic stimulus interval of 1000 ms (1 Hz) and paired-pulse stimulation with 300 and 1700 ms intervals. When paired-pulse stimulation is applied, the contraction amplitudes reach a steady state quickly, usually after less than 10 stimulus pairs. When mechanical restitution is determined after a short priming with paired

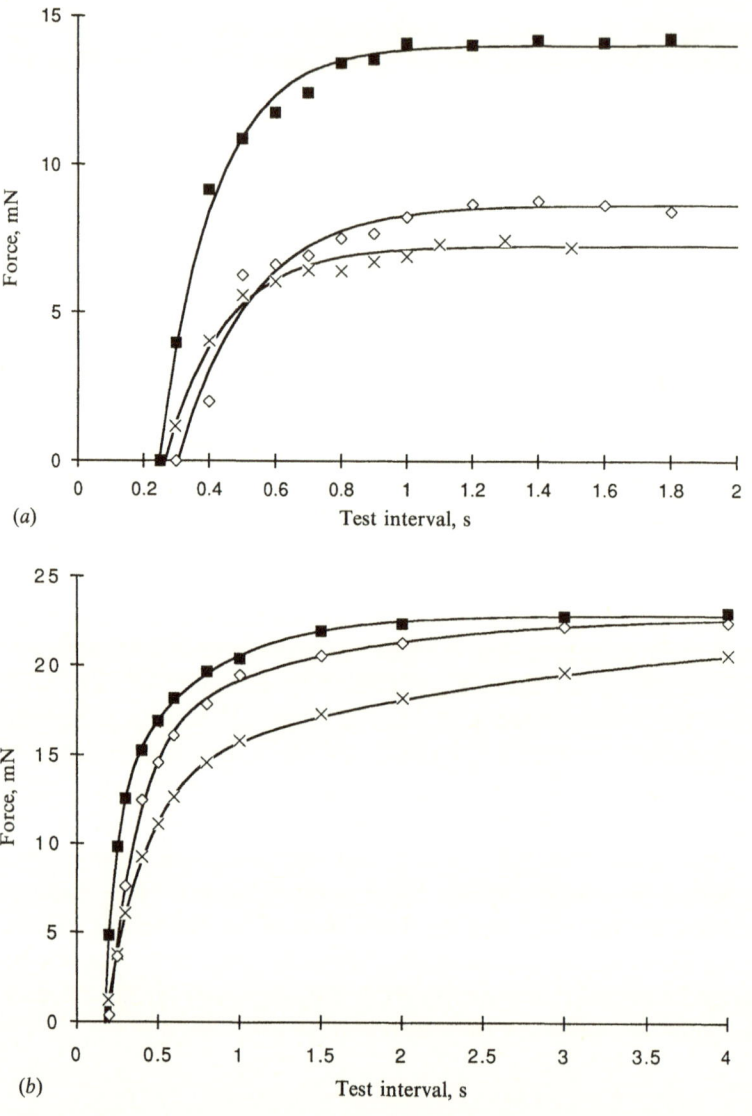

Fig. 4. Mechanical restitution in guinea-pig ventricular and atrial muscle after pacing with paired pulses. In both panels crosses represent the control curves (interval 1 s), open diamonds show restitution after the long interval (1.7 s) and filled rectangles show restitution after the short interval (0.3 s). The lines are the calculated curves after fitting with exponential functions. (a) shows an experiment with papillary muscle. The curves after the long and short interval show a substantial difference in parameter A (Table 1) but the other parameters are similar. (b) shows an experiment with an atrial strip. The curves after the long and short interval are similar, the main difference lies in the time constants.

pulses, this can be done after the short interval (e.g. 300 ms) or the long interval (e.g. 1700 ms). It was found by Wohlfart, 1982, that restitution in rabbit papillary muscles is quite different after the long and short intervals. This has also been compared in guinea-pig papillary muscles and atrial strips. In papillary muscles from guinea-pigs, the findings in rabbit (Wohlfart, 1982) were confirmed (Fig. 4(*a*)). In guinea-pig atrial strips, however, results quite different from those in ventricular muscle are obtained (Fig. 4(*b*)). When the parameters of restitution are analysed after the short and after the long interval, the following is found. In atrial muscle the rate of both phases is about two times higher after the short interval but the size parameters (*A* and *B*) are about the same. In ventricular muscle the main difference is in the size parameter which is about twice as high after the short interval than after the long interval, but restitution rate is about the same (Fig. 4). Here again is a marked difference between guinea-pig ventricular and atrial muscles, i.e. muscles with restitution in one or two phases.

Factors altering restitution

Extracellular calcium

The effects of calcium concentration on the restitution parameters were studied in guinea-pig atria (Jóhannsson & Ásgrímsson, 1989). When calcium concentration was increased from 0.9 to 3.6 mM there was a similar increase in the rate of both phases, whilst the size of parameter *A* increased more than three times and *B* decreased by about 40%. The sum *A* + *B* was relatively insensitive to calcium concentration and was the same at 1.8 and 3.6 mM. In these experiments, a strong, positive linear correlation was found between parameter *A* and the steady-state contractile force.

Similar findings had been reported earlier in rat papillary muscle, where the rate of mechanical restitution was found to increase with increasing Ca concentration (Günther *et al.*, 1984).

Basic stimulation frequency

The parameters of mechanical restitution were studied in guinea-pig and rat atria at various basic stimulation frequencies of 0.2, 0.5, 1 and 2 Hz (Jóhannsson & Ásgrímsson, 1989). Most of the parameters were relatively insensitive to basic stimulation frequency except parameter *A* which steadily increased with frequency. In guinea-pig atria a strong, positive linear correlation was found between parameter A and the steady-state contractile force.

Temperature

Mechanical restitution was studied in several guinea-pig atria at the temperatures 29, 32 and 35 °C. It was found that the sum $A + B$ was insensitive to temperature changes in this range but all the restitution parameters were quite sensitive. With increasing temperature, both parameter A and steady-state force decreased substantially, and parameter B increased by about the same amount. The rate of both phases increased with temperature and had a temperature coefficient (Q_{10}) in the range 2.2 to 3.3. The temperature sensitivity of mechanical restitution is therefore high, and suggests that energy-dependent processes might be involved.

Caffeine

Caffeine in concentrations of 2.5 to 5.0 mM increased the size of parameter A but eliminated the second phase of mechanical restitution in guinea-pig and rat atria. Caffeine in this concentration strongly inhibits the function of the SR but also affects the cell membrane.

Several authors, working with different preparations and species, have previously reported a suppressive effect of caffeine on the late part of mechanical restitution (Endoh & Iijima, 1981; Vornanen, 1984; Bers, 1985; Bouchard et al., 1989; Hryshko et al., 1989).

Ryanodine

At a concentration of 10^{-8} M, ryanodine causes the second phase of mechanical restitution in guinea-pig atrium to disappear. At this concentration, ryanodine has only minor effects on the first phase of restitution and on the steady-state contractile force at 1 Hz stimulation frequency. At a concentration of 10^{-7} M, ryanodine also suppresses the first phase of restitution and the steady-state force. Ryanodine is believed selectively to block the function of the SR.

Ryanodine has previously been reported to increase the rate of restitution in ferret ventricular myocardium (Wier & Yue, 1986). The explanation given by the authors was that calcium entering the cell via i_{si} was no longer buffered by the sarcoplasmic reticulum. Ryanodine has also been reported to suppress or eliminate the late part of mechanical restitution (Bers, 1985; Bouchard *et al.*, 1989).

Calcium antagonists

The effects of Ni^{2+}, D600 and nifedipine on mechanical restitution in guinea-pig and rat atria have been studied and the effects of these different calcium antagonists found to be very similar. In concentrations which lower the steady-state contractile force by 15–50%, the most striking effect of calcium antagonists is to decrease the rate of the first phase of mechanical restitution. The effects on the size parameters, *A* and *B*, are relatively small, and the effects on the rate of the second phase are inconclusive.

The lack of effects on the second phase of restitution is consistent with the findings of Endoh & Iijima, 1981, who were using Mn^{2+} and D600. Verapamil has also been found to diminish the rate of restitution in human myocardium (Fry *et al.*, 1983).

Other interventions

Adrenaline has been shown to increase the rate of mechanical restitution and hypoxia to decrease the rate in human myocardium (Fry *et al.*, 1983). Adrenaline has been found to increase the rate of the first phase of restitution in guinea-pig and rat atria. The calcium agonist BAY K 8644 has been found to depress the late part of restitution (Bouchard *et al.*, 1989; Hryshko *et al.*, 1989). Diazepam (75–150 μM) has been found to increase the rate of restitution in rat atria but to have only small effects on restitution in guinea-pig atria (Jóhannsson & Ásgrimsson, 1989).

The peak of restitution and maximal contractile ability

The peak of restitution in guinea-pig and rat atrium, the sum $A + B$, was found to be insensitive to many inotropic interventions like basic stimulation frequency and calcium concentration above 2 mM (Jóhannsson & Ásgrímsson, 1989). Similar findings have been reported in ferret papillary muscles (Urthaler *et al.*, 1989). It was also seen during long control experiments that parameter *A* steadily decreased by about 10% per hour, parameter *B* steadily increased by about the same amount and thus the sum $A + B$ remained constant. In guinea-pig atria, the force $A + B$ cannot be exceeded by potentiating interventions like increasing the calcium concentration, priming the muscle with stimulation at a high frequency, paired-pulse stimulation or tetanisation in ryanodine and high calcium concentration. Therefore, $A + B$ in guinea-pig and rat atrium seems to represent maximum contractile ability of the muscle. This maximum could be determined by saturation of the contractile proteins or saturation of some Ca transport mechanism in the cell. In guinea-pig ventricular muscle, the situation is quite different; parameter A has a size similar to the steady-state force, which is far less than the force of potentiated twitches after priming with high frequency or paired pulses.

What is mechanical restitution? Models

Mechanical and electrical restitution

Electrical restitution (restitution of action potential duration) has been studied in several species (Gettes & Reuter, 1974; Bass, 1975; Wohlfart, 1979; Jóhannsson & Wohlfart, 1980; Colatsky & Hogan, 1980; Jezek et al., 1982; Schouten, 1986; Seed et al., 1987; Franz et al., 1988; Jóhannsson & Ásgrímsson, 1989). Restitution (recovery from inactivation) of i_{si} has also been studed in several myocardial preparations and it was shown in sheep and pig ventricular trabeculae that restitution of action potential duration and restitution of i_{si} have a very similar time course (Gettes & Reuter, 1974). In some cases, recovery of i_{si} was found to have a similar time course to mechanical restitution (Trautwein, McDonald & Tripathi, 1975; Schulze, 1981) but in general, electrical and mechanical restitution seem to have different time courses. In several cases, electrical restitution has a very fast rise with an overshoot at short intervals but mechanical restitution has a steady, much slower rise (see e.g. Wohlfart, 1979; Jóhannsson & Ásgrímsson, 1989). In a study on anaesthetised dogs (Elzinga et al., 1981), no relationship was found between electrical and mechanical restitution when various pacing protocols were used. Altering thyroid state was found to have profound effects on mechanical restitution in rats without influencing electrical restitution (Poggesi et al., 1987). In the mammalian myocardium, it therefore seems likely that electrical and mechanical restitution occur through separate processes.

Models for excitation–contraction coupling

There is some evidence that activator calcium can, in different species and in different parts of the heart, originate from at least three different sources. These sources are the sarcoplasmic reticulum, binding sites on the sarcolemma and extracellular space. Activator calcium may enter the cell through the calcium channels and with Na–Ca exchange, be released from the sarcolemma by depolarisation and be released from the SR by Ca-induced Ca-release (Chapman, 1979; Wohlfart & Noble, 1982; Wier, 1990; and see chapters by Boyett *et al.*, by Langer and by Lewartowski in this book). All these Ca sources might be of importance and the relative contribution of each one might depend on the species, type of muscle and on various conditions like temperature, Ca concentration, basic contraction frequency and length of the preceding interval.

Mechanical restitution is believed to reflect some of the basic cellular mechanisms that control the contractile force of the myocardium. Restitution, or length of the preceding interval, is one of the five factors of Wohlfart (see chapter by Wohlfart *et al.* in this book) which determine the contractile force from one beat to another. The other factors are size of the preceding beat, length of the pre-preceding interval, length of the preceding action potential and length of the simultaneous action potential.

Models for mechanical restitution

Mechanical restitution theoretically could be governed by several different cellular mechanisms, e.g. (1) Restitution of the contractile elements; this seems highly unlikely because restitution of the intracellular calcium signal (as determined with aequorin) runs in parallel with mechanical restitution (Wier & Yue, 1986; see Figs 4 and 5 of chapter by Yue in this book). (2) Reactivation of i_{Ca}; this might explain the mechanical restitution seen in the primitive myocardium of, for example, frog, which has only very small amounts of SR. In the mammalian myocardium, it seems likely that electrical and mechanical restitution occur through separate processes. An influence of electrical restitution on the time of onset and even the first part of mechanical restitution cannot be ruled out, however. (3) Transfer of Ca from an uptake compartment to a release compartment; this is the model used by most authors, as it offers a simple explanation for mechanical restitution in a single phase. During relaxation, Ca might be taken up by the longitudinal part of the SR (uptake compartment) and then be transferred to the junctional SR where the release takes place (release compartment). It is also possible that the sarcolemma and even the mitochondria have a part in this process. A gradual filling of the release compartment is reflected in mechanical restitution. This model is discussed in more detail in chapters by Allen and by Wohlfart *et al.* in this book. (4) Reactivation of the release mechanism, perhaps Ca channels in the SR; this is usually an alternative to the previous point even if these two mechanisms are not mutually exclusive. Reactivation of Ca channels in the SR might be dependent on changes in intracellular Ca concentration and on repolarisation of the surface membrane. (5) Na–Ca exchange; it seems possible that some of the differences between atrial and ventricular preparations and different species might depend on differences in Na–Ca exchange (see ter Keurs *et al*, 1987) and even the surface membrane Ca pump.

To make things more complicated, these mechanisms might influence each other. Ca-induced Ca release from the SR is not an all or none phenomenon but is governed by the filling of the SR and the size of the Ca signal coming from the cell membrane (Fabiato, 1983). The intracellular Ca transient could influence Ca release from intracellular stores, and could also influence currents through the surface membrane.

Conclusions

1. Mechanical restitution is one of the fundamental processes that determine myocardial contractile force from one beat to the next.
2. Mechanical restitution usually can be described satisfactorily with exponential functions in one or two phases.
3. Restitution occurs in a single phase in muscles which contain small amounts of SR but in two phases in muscles with great amounts of SR.
4. The time course of mechanical restitution can easily be influenced by a variety of interventions.
5. Mechanical restitution is probably determined by more than one mechanism and this differs, both between atrial and ventricular muscle and between species.

References

Bass, B. G. (1975). Restitution of the action potential in cat papillary muscle. *American Journal of Physiology*, **228**, 1717–24.

Bers, D. M. (1985). Ca influx and sarcoplasmic reticulum Ca release in cardiac muscle activation during postrest recovery. *American Journal of Physiology*, **248**, H366–81.

Bossen, E. H. & Sommer, J. R. (1984). Comparative stereology of the lizard and frog myocardium. *Tissue and Cell*, **16**, 173–8.

Bouchard, R. A., Hryshko, L. V., Saha, J. K. & Bose, D. (1989). Effects of caffeine and ryanodine on depression of post-rest tension development produced by Bay K 8644 in canine ventricular muscle. *British Journal of Pharmacology*, **97**, 1279–91.

Braveny, P. & Kruta, V. (1958). Dissociation de deux facteurs: restitution et potentiation dans l'action de l'intervalle sur l'amplitude de la contraction du myocarde. *Archives internationales de Physiologie et de Biochimie*, **66**, 633–52.

Braveny, P., Sumbera, J. & Kruta, V. (1966). After-contractions and restitution of contractility in the isolated guinea-pig auricles. *Archives internationales de Physiologie et de Biochimie*, **74**, 169–78.

Burkhoff, D., Yue, D. T., Franz, M. R., Hunter, W. C. & Sagawa, K. (1984). Mechanical restitution of isolated perfused canine left ventricles. *American Journal of Physiology*, **246**, H8–16.

Chapman, R. A. (1979). Excitation–contraction coupling in cardiac muscle. *Progress in Biophysics and Molecular Biology*, **35**, 1–52.

Chappell, S., Henderson, A. & Lewis, M. (1986). Characterization of the mechanical behaviour of isolated papillary muscle preparations of the ferret. *Journal of Pharmacological Methods*, **15**, 35–49.

Colatsky, T. J. & Hogan, P. M. (1980). Effects of external calcium, calcium channel-blocking agents, and stimulation frequency on cycle length-dependent changes in canine cardiac action potential duration. *Circulation Research*, **46**, 543–52.

Edman, K. A. P. & Jóhannsson, M. (1976). The contractile state of rabbit papillary muscle in relation to stimulation frequency. *Journal of Physiology*, **254**, 565–81.

Elzinga, G., Lab, M. J., Noble, M. I. M., Papadoyannis, D. E., Pidgeon, J., Seed, A. & Wohlfart, B. (1981). The action-potential duration and contractile response of the intact heart related to the preceding interval and the preceding beat in the dog and cat. *Journal of Physiology*, **314**, 481–500.

Endoh, M. & Iijima, T. (1981). Twitch potentiation by rest in canine ventricular muscle: effects of theophylline. *American Journal of Physiology*, **241**, H583–90.

Fabiato, A. (1983). Calcium-induced release of calcium from the cardiac sarcoplasmic reticulum. *American Journal of Physiology*, **245**, C1–14.

Franz, M. R., Swerdlow, C. D., Liem, L. B., Schaefer, J. (1988). Cycle length dependence of human action potential duration in vivo. Effects of single extrastimuli, sudden sustained rate acceleration and deceleration, and different steady-state frequencies. *Journal of Clinical Investigation*, **77**, 1177–84.

Fry, C. H., Walker, J. M., Webb-Peploe, M. M. & Williams, B. T. (1983). Restitution of contractility in vitro of human and guinea-pig ventricular myocardium. *Journal of Physiology*, **339**, 26–7P.

Gettes, L. S. & Reuter, H. (1974). Slow recovery from inactivation of inward currents in mammalian myocardial fibres. *Journal of Physiology*, **240**, 703–24.

Günther, J., Storch, E., Krünes, R. & Scholz, W. (1984). Zur Zeitabhängigkeit der Ca-Bereitstellung im Ratten- und Kaninchenmyokard. *Biomedica Biochimica Acta*, **43**, 995–1004.

Hanafy, M., Kitzing, J. & Rumberger, E. (1976). The influence of calcium and β-sympathomimetics on force–freqency relationship and resting potentiation in guinea pig papillary muscle. *Basic Research in Cardiology*, **71**, 469–81.

Hisano, C., Suga, H. & Ninomiya, I. (1985). Length dependent potentiation and inhibition of post-rest twitch tension development in adult cat and kitten papillary muscles. *Japanese Journal of Physiology*, **35**, 147–58.

Hryshko, L. V., Bouchard, R., Chau, T. & Bose, D. (1989). Inhibition of rest potentiation in canine ventricular muscle by BAY K 8644: comparison with caffeine. *American Journal of Physiology*, **257**, H399–406.

Jezek, K., Pucelik, P., Sauer, J. & Bartak, F. (1982). Basic electrophysiological parameters and frequency sensitivity of the ventricular myocardium of human embryos. *Physiologia Bohemoslovaca*, **31**, 11–19.

Jóhannsson, M. & Ásgrímsson, H. (1989). Short-term effects of stimulus interval changes in guinea-pig and rat atrial muscle. *Acta Physiologica Scandinavica*, **135**, 73–81.

Jóhannsson, M. & Wohlfart, B. (1980). Cellular calcium as a determinant of action potential duration in rabbit myocardium. *Acta Physiologica Scandinavica*, **110**, 241–7.

Kruta, V. & Braveny, P. (1960). Potentiation of contractility in the heart muscle of the rat and some other mammals. *Nature*, **187**, 327–8.

Kruta, V. & Braveny, P. (1961). Restitution de la contractilité du myocarde entre les contractions et les phénomènes de potentiation. *Archives internationales de Physiologie et de Biochimie*, **69**, 645–67.

Kruta, V. & Braveny, P. (1963). Rate of restitution and self-regulation of contractility in mammalian heart muscle. *Nature*, **197**, 905–6.

Lipsius, S. L., Fozzard, H. A. & Gibbons, W. R. (1982). Voltage and time dependence of restitution in heart. *American Journal of Physiology*, **243**, H68–76.

Maylie, J. G. (1982). Excitation–contraction coupling in neonatal and adult myocardium of cat. *American Journal of Physiology*, **242**, H834–43.

Meijler, F. L. (1962). Staircase, rest contractions, and potentiation in the isolated rat heart. *American Journal of Physiology*, **202**, 636–40.

Page, E. & McCallister, L. P. (1973). Quantitative electron microscopic description of heart muscle cells. Application to normal, hypertrophied and thyroxin-stimulated hearts. *American Journal of Cardiology*, **31**, 172–81.

Poggesi, C., Everts, M., Polla, B., Tanzi, F. & Reggiani, C. (1987). Influence of thyroid state on mechanical restitution of rat myocardium. *Circulation Research*, **60**, 142–51.

Ragnarsdóttir, K., Wohlfart, B. & Jóhannsson, M. (1982). Mechanical restitution of the rat papillary muscle. *Acta Physiologica Scandinavica*, **115**, 183–91.

Ravens, U. & Ziegler, A. (1980). Effects of carbachol on contractile force and action potentials of isolated atria at different rates of stimulation. *Journal of Cardiovascular Pharmacology*, **2**, 881–92.

Rosin, H. & Farah, A. (1955). Post-stimulation potentiation of contractility in the isolated auricle of the rabbit. *Americal Journal of Physiology*, **180**, 75–82.

Rumberger, E. & Reichel, H. (1972). The force–frequency relationship: A comparative study between warm- and cold-blooded animals. *Pflügers Archiv*, **332**, 206–17.

Schouten, V. J. A. (1986). The negative correlation between action potential duration and force of contraction during restitution in rat myocardium. *Journal of Molecular and Cellular Cardiology*, **18**, 1033–45.

Schulze, J. J. (1981). Observations on the staircase phenomenon in guinea pig atrium. *Pflügers Archiv*, **391**, 9–16.

Seed, W. A., Noble, M. I. M., Oldershaw, P., Wanless, R. B., Drake-Holland, A. J., Redwood, D., Pugh, S. & Mills, C. (1987). Relation of human cardiac action potential duration to the interval between beats: implications for the validity of rate-controlled QT interval (QTc). *British Heart Journal*, **57**, 32–37.

Shimoni, Y. (1987). The effects of catecholamines on tension reactivation in cardiac muscle. *Proceedings of the Royal Society London, Series B*, **231**, 231–49.

Sommer, J. R. & Johnson, E. A. (1979). Ultrastructure of cardiac muscle. In *Handbook of Physiology, Section 2: The Cardiovascular System, Vol. I: The Heart*, ed. R. M. Berne, N. Sperelakis, & S. R. Geiger, pp. 113–86. Bethesda: American Physiological Society.

ter Keurs, H. E. D. J., Schouten, V. J. A., Bucx, J. J., Mulder, B. M. & De Tombe, P. P. (1987). Excitation–contraction coupling in myocardium: implications of calcium release and Na^+–Ca^{2+} exchange. *Canadian Journal of Physiology and Pharmacology*, **65**, 619–26.

Trautwein, W., McDonald, T. F. & Tripathi, O. (1975). Calcium conductance and tension in mammalian ventricular muscle. *Pflügers Archiv*, **354**, 55–74.

Urthaler, F., Walker, A. A., Reeves, R. C. & Hefner, L. L. (1989). Effects of ryanodine on contractile performance of intact length-clamped papillary muscles. *Circulation Research*, **65**, 1270–82.

Van Winkle, W. B. (1986). The structure of striated muscle sarcoplasmic reticulum. In *Sarcoplasmic Reticulum in Muscle Physiology*, vol. I, ed. M. L. Entman & W. B. Van Winkle, pp. 17–45. Florida: CRC Press, Boca Raton.

Vornanen, M. (1984). Effects of caffeine on the mechanical properties of developing rat heart ventricles. *Comparative Biochemistry and Physiology*, **78C**, 329–34.

Wier, W. G. (1990). Cytoplasmic $[Ca^{2+}]$ in mammalian ventricle: dynamic control by cellular processes. *Annual Review of Physiology*, **52**, 467–85.

Wier, W. G. & Yue, D. T. (1986). Intracellular calcium transients underlying the short-term force–interval relationship in ferret ventricular myocardium. *Journal of Physiology*, **376**, 507–30.

Wohlfart, B. (1979). Relationships between peak force, action potential duration and stimulus interval in rabbit myocardium. *Acta Physiologica Scandinavica*, **106**, 395–409.

Wohlfart, B. (1982). Analysis of mechanical alternans in rabbit papillary muscle. *Acta Physiologica Scandinavica*, **115**, 405–14.

Wohlfart, B. & Elzinga, G. (1982). Electrical and mechanical responses of the intact rabbit heart in relation to the excitation interval. A comparison with the isolated papillary muscle preparation. *Acta Physiologica Scandinavica*, **115**, 331–40.

Wohlfart, B. & Noble, M. I. M. (1982). The cardiac excitation–contraction cycle. *Pharmacology and Therapeutics*, **16**, 1–43.

Woodworth, R. S. (1902). Maximal contraction, 'staircase' contraction, refractory period, and compensatory pause of the heart. *American Journal of Physiology*, **8**, 213–49.

Post-rest potentiation and its decay

URSULA RAVENS

Introduction

Contractile changes due to rate and rhythm changes are endogenous properties of heart muscle (Koch-Weser & Blinks, 1963). When stimulation is initiated in resting ventricular muscle from frog heart, the force of contraction increases within 7 to 8 beats from a low amplitude immediately after rest to the steady-state amplitude during regular pacing. The resemblance of the beat-to-beat increments to a staircase ('Treppe') coined the name for the phenomenon (Bowditch. 1871; see his chapter in this book). The positive staircase found in most mammalian ventricular muscle implies that the ability of the cardiac muscle to develop force *decays* during a period of rest and recovers only upon regular stimulation. In some cardiac tissue, however, the first beat after a prolonged rest is *potentiated* and the potentiated state of contractility decays with subsequent regular beats. The phenomenon of enhanced contractility after prolonged rest is called post-rest potentiation, and its decay during regular stimulation is termed 'negative staircase'.

Thus in heart muscle, stronger or weaker contractions may follow a prolonged period of rest. This chapter will emphasise new results in cardiac myocytes which help to explain these responses. After a brief outline of the basic events in cardiac excitation–contraction coupling, some examples of typical post-rest contraction patterns will be given and then the various cellular mechanisms contributing to post-rest contractions will be discussed.

Cardiac excitation–contraction coupling

Regulation of contractile force depends crucially on the free cellular calcium concentration. Binding of free calcium ions (Ca^{2+}) to troponin

C removes the inhibitory effect of troponin I and thus allows interaction of actin and myosin, the tension-generating step. Upon excitation of the cell membrane, Ca^{2+} ions for activation of contractile proteins are supplied from two sources: (1) they enter the cell during an action potential through voltage-dependent Ca^{2+} channels and possibly also via Na^+/Ca^{2+} exchange and (2) they are released from internal stores, e.g. the sarcoplasmic reticulum (Chapman, 1983). The muscle can relax again upon re-uptake of Ca^{2+} into the cellular stores. There is ample evidence that time is required before these Ca^{2+} ions become re-available for release. Because of their Ca^{2+}-buffering properties, the mitochondria are thought to contribute to the long term regulation of the free cellular Ca^{2+} concentration (Carafoli *et al.*, 1977). The calcium homeostasis of the cell is maintained by outward transport produced by an ATP-driven Ca^{2+} pump and the Na^+/Ca^{2+} exchange mechanism. The contribution of influx and release as sources of Ca^{2+} for the activation of any single contraction is influenced by both rate and rhythm (Wohlfart & Noble, 1982; Lewartowski & Pytkowski, 1987). These calcium fluxes are examined in detail in the chapter by Lewartowski in this book (pp. 173–92).

Typical post-rest contraction patterns

Different patterns of post-rest contractions are observed in various cardiac tissues from several species (Koch-Weser & Blinks, 1963). As shown in Fig. 1, the force developed during the first beat after a prolonged pause *increases* in rat right ventricular strip, human right atrial trabecula, and guinea-pig left atrium. The pattern of decay of post-rest potentiation is typical for heart muscle from a given species: In rat atrium and ventricle, force declines monotonically. In human right atrial trabeculae, the second contraction is similar to the steady-state contraction, i.e. post-rest potentiation has already decayed within the first interval (1 s) of regular stimulation. The post-rest contraction pattern of guinea-pig atrial muscle is composed of an early phase of decay of potentiation to below pre-rest tension, followed by a slow phase of positive staircase.

Post-rest potentiation develops as an exponential function of the duration of the pause (Fig. 2). Exposure to caffeine in a concentration (3 mM) which eventually depletes the sarcoplasmic reticulum of Ca^{2+} because it inhibits re-uptake (Weber & Herz, 1968; Fuchs, 1969) abolishes post-rest potentiation (Figs. 1 and 2) indicating the dominant role of the sarcoplasmic reticulum in this phenomenon (Bers, 1985). Among its multiple actions, caffeine also enhances myocardial Ca^{2+} influx which

Control   Caffeine 3 mM

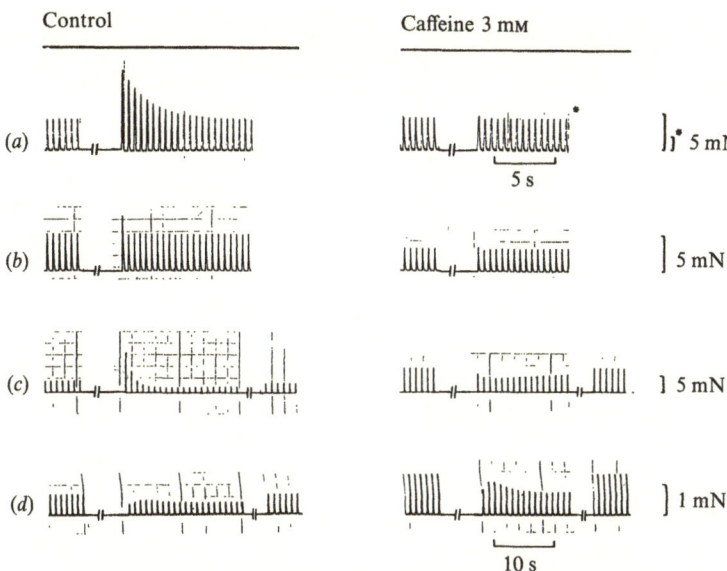

Fig. 1. Force of contraction after a pause of 30 s in different cardiac muscles and the effects of caffeine on potentiation or depotentiation and its decay. Left tracings, control pause: right tracings, after 30 min of exposure to caffeine (3 mM). Recordings from four typical preparations, with calibrations of isometric tension as indicated by the bars. (*a*) Rat right ventricular strips; (*b*) human right atrial trabeculae, (*c*) guinea-pig left atrial strips, and (*d*) guinea-pig right ventricular papillary muscle. The muscles were stimulated with electrical pulses (duration 3 ms, amplitude 10% above threshold, frequency 1 s^{-1} with exception of rat muscle (2 s^{-1})). The asterisk marks the different amplification of the force tracing. The first interruption of the tracings indicates the pause, pre-rest contractions to the left, post-rest contractions to the right of it. The contractions after the second interruption in (*c*) and (*d*) were recorded when stimulation had continued for 3 min after the pause and demonstrate the very slow time course of recovery to pre-rest control.

explains its positive inotropic action during regular stimulation in rat ventricle. By studying post-rest contractions in the presence of caffeine and ryanodine, another tool to impair the calcium release mechanism (Sutko & Kenyon, 1983), Bers (1985) estimated the relative dependence of contractile activation on Ca^{2+} release and on Ca^{2+} influx in various cardiac tissues and found a general sequence which correlates well with the sequence of thresholds for the Ca^{2+}-induced Ca^{2+} release from the sarcoplasmic reticulum reported by Fabiato and Fabiato (1978). This issue is further discussed in the chapters by Allen and by Boyett *et al.* elsewhere in this book.

In the examples in Fig. 1, guinea-pig papillary muscle is an exception

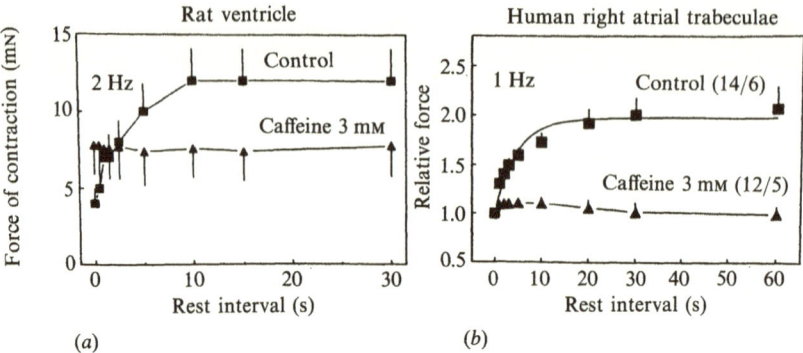

Fig. 2. Effect of caffeine (3 mM) on post-rest potentiation in heart muscle. (a) Force of the first post-rest contraction (mN) of rat ventricular strip plotted against the duration of the pause (s), frequency of regular stimulation 2 s^{-1}. Controls (filled squares) and values after 30 min of exposure to caffeine (3 mM, filled triangles). Mean values $\pm$ standard error of the mean (s.e.m.) from six experiments. (b) Human right atrial trabeculae: force of the first post-rest contraction (expressed as a fraction of the pre-rest control) plotted against the duration of the pause (s), frequency of regular stimulation 1 s^{-1}. Control runs (filled squares) and runs after exposure to caffeine (filled triangles) in the same group of muscles. The figures in parentheses indicate the number of trials/number of trabeculae; mean values $\pm$ s.e.m.

because it does not have a potentiated first beat after a pause (Reiter, Seibel & Karema, 1978). Guinea-pig papillary muscles can be divided into two groups according to their adaptation patterns of force of contraction during the first 20 beats after rest: (1) muscles with an initial phase of rapid force increase lasting about 10 s followed by a second slow phase reaching pre-rest values within 3–5 min (Seibel, 1986), and (2) muscles that show a transient hypercontractility during the early phase of post-rest adaptation. In the latter group, to which the muscle depicted in Fig. 1 belongs, force increases up to the third to eighth beat, decreases again until the tenth to 25th beat and then slowly returns to pre-rest values (Beyer, Hergeröder & Ravens, 1988). The general pattern is not abolished by exposure to caffeine (3 mM) but shifted to higher levels of contraction amplitude.

The first post-rest beat in guinea-pig papillary muscle is characterised by a small amplitude, a delay in the onset of tension development and by a late maximum that coincides with the final phase of repolarisation (Reiter, Vierling & Seibel, 1984). During subsequent beats, an early component develops which is related to Ca^{2+} release from the sarcoplasmic reticulum and is thought to reflect the progressive refilling of this site (Lewartowski, Prokopczuk & Pytkowski, 1978; Beyer *et al.*, 1988). From the linear relationship between the duration of the action potential plateau and the time-to-peak force of the accompanying rested-state contraction, Beresewicz and Reuter (1977) concluded that the electrical activity directly controls the force of contraction of the muscle after rest and proposed that the rested-state contraction was activated by Ca^{2+} influx during the action potential. The decay in contractility during rest reflects the fact that the sarcoplasmic reticulum of guinea-pig papillary muscle does not accumulate Ca^{2+} during the pause, but loses Ca^{2+} instead (Allen, Jewell & Wood, 1976; Bers, 1987). This notion was confirmed in experiments with X-ray microanalysis, in which the calcium content of the sarcoplasmic reticulum was shown to decline with increasing duration of the pause (Wendt-Gallitelli, 1985).

Cellular mechanism determining post-rest contractions

Ca^{2+} transients

In the early studies of force–interval relations of multicellular cardiac preparations, active force production was taken as an indirect estimate of the free cytosolic Ca^{2+} concentration. Since it is unlikely that the Ca^{2+} sensitivity of contractile proteins changes during quiescence, potentiation of the first beat should indicate that more Ca^{2+} is available for this particular contraction. This approach is limited by the fact that the relationship between developed tension and cytosolic Ca^{2+} concentration, which is a non-linear sigmoid function (Solaro *et al.*, 1974), is influenced by sarcomere length (Kentish *et al.*, 1986) and intracellular cAMP levels (Herzig *et al.*, 1981).

For direct measurements of the cellular free Ca^{2+} concentration, the bioluminescent protein aequorin was one of the first calcium detecting agents available (Allen & Blinks, 1978). Technical problems with this method include the necessity to inject several cells (e.g. 40–200, Yue, Marban & Wier, 1986); irreversibility of Ca^{2+} binding to the protein with continuous fading of the response; and the fact that the light and the force signal are not necessarily obtained from the same cells, i.e. superficial cells contribute to the bioluminescent signal and all cells to tension recordings. Furthermore, during repetitive stimulation, the ion concentration in the extracellular space may be difficult to control, particularly in narrow intercellular gaps. Indeed, extracellular K^+ accumulation associated with rapid stimulation of frog ventricular tissue is demonstrated with the use of K^+-selective electrodes (Kline & Morad, 1978).

These problems are elegantly circumvented with the recently developed Ca^{2+}-sensitive dyes (Grynckiewicz, Poenie & Tsien, 1985) and with the technique of obtaining viable single myocytes by enzymatic dissociation procedures (Dow, Harding & Powell, 1981). In myocytes from most mammalian ventricles, peak Ca^{2+} transients and cell shortening correlate well during a train of regular stimuli after rest. This holds true for cardiac cells from species with a positive or negative staircase as well as for those with a first potentiated contraction followed by a positive staircase. Cat ventricular myocytes, for instance, have a positive staircase of cell shortening after rest and this is accompanied by Ca^{2+} transients of increasing amplitude (du Bell & Houser, 1989). When rat myocytes are field-stimulated after rest at a frequency of $0.2\ s^{-1}$ in $1\ mmol/l\ [Ca^{2+}]_o$, both cell shortenings and cytosolic Ca^{2+} transients decline monotonically with similar time courses (Spurgeon et al., 1990).

Force measurement versus unloaded shortening

Since sarcomere length modifies the relation between tension and intracellular calcium ion concentration $[Ca^{2+}]_i$ (Kentish et al., 1986), unloaded shortening may differ from isometric contractions. Post-rest contractions therefore have been compared in strips of right ventricle and isolated myocytes of the rat heart when contractions in response to electrically stimulated action potentials were measured (Fig. 3(a)). Under identical experimental conditions (e.g. temperature, frequency, extracellular $[Ca^{2+}]$), there was no difference in the extent or time course of development of post-rest potentiation between isometric and isotonic contractions.

In single myocytes, comparable data about force and unloaded shortening are rare because of the obvious technical difficulties in attaching a single cell to a force transducer (Brady, Tan & Ricchiuti, 1979; Copelas et al., 1987; Shepherd & Kavaler, 1986; Tarr et al., 1981; Tung, 1986). Furthermore, problems of post-rest potentiation are seldom addressed directly. Nevertheless, a positive force staircase was found in frog ventricular cells (Tung & Morad, 1988) and guinea-pig ventricular myocytes (Shepherd, Vornanen & Isenberg, 1990). In the latter paper, a similar positive staircase was reported for unloaded shortening. Furthermore, after long resting periods, myocyte shortening even exhibits similar late and early components of contraction as described above for papillary muscles during the positive staircase (see Fig. 1 in Isenberg & Wendt-Gallitelli, 1989).

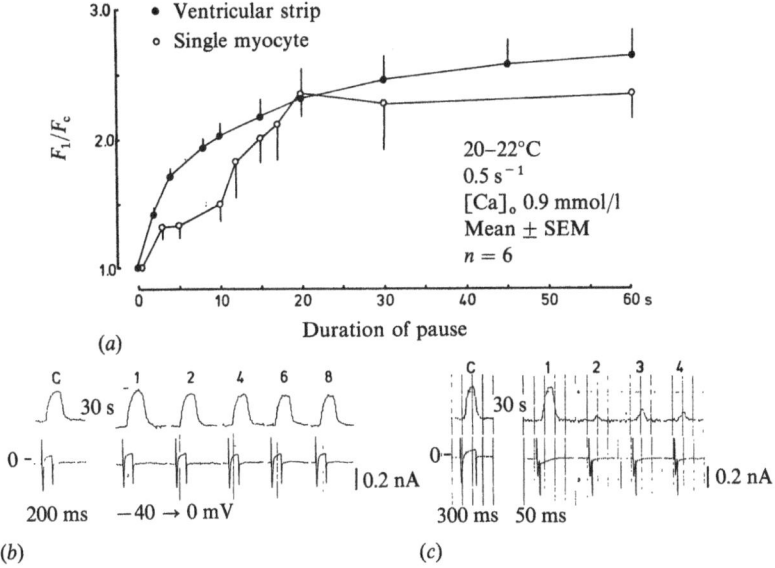

(a)

(b)   (c)

Fig. 3. Post-rest potentiation of contractility in rat heart muscle. (a) Comparison of post-rest potentiation in myocytes isolated enzymatically from adult rat hearts and in strips of ventricular tissue. Ordinate: amplitude of first contraction after rest (F_1) expressed as a factor of the pre-rest control contraction (F_c); abscissa: duration of the period of rest. (For details of cell isolation and experimental procedure, and for recording of contractions, see Ravens, Wang & Wettwer, 1989.) Strips (width 2 mm) of the free wall of the right ventricle were cut and mounted vertically in an organ bath filled with oxygenated Tyrode solution at room temperature (20–22 °C). They were connected to a strain gauge for isometric tension recordings and were stimulated electrically at a frequency of 0.5 s^{-1}. The isolated cells were stimulated in the current clamp mode via a glass electrode conventionally used for single electrode voltage clamp experiments. Extracellular [Ca^{2+}], 0.9 mM. Mean values ± standard error from six experiments. (b) Contractions (upper tracings) and membrane currents (lower tracings) of a rat myocyte before (c) and after interruption of regular clamp steps at a frequency of 0.5 s^{-1} by a pause of 30 s. Voltage clamp pulses from a holding potential, V_h, of −40 mV to 0 mV, duration 200 ms. The numbers indicate clamp pulse after rest. Calibration bar is valid for all tracings, zero current is indicated. (c) Similar to (b) but here the duration of the voltage clamp steps was changed from 300 ms before the pause to 50 ms after the pause. Note the large difference in contraction amplitude between the first and the second contraction.

Ca^{2+} influx via the calcium current (i_{Ca})

Contractile activation and peak calcium current

There is general agreement that i_{Ca} is essential for cardiac excitation–contraction coupling (Mitchell *et al.*, 1985; Fedida *et al.*, 1987), but does the amplitude of i_{Ca} control the size of post-rest contractile activation?

Numerous reports in the literature have attempted to answer this question. In frog atrial muscle, repetitive depolarisations after rest to sufficiently positive potentials induce peak slow inward currents of progressively increasing amplitude which underlie the positive tension staircase (Noble & Shimoni, 1981*a*,*b*). Similar experiments performed in single myocytes of mammalian hearts arrive at the same result and clearly identify calcium ions as the charge carrier for peak inward current (Lee, 1987; Mitra & Morad, 1986; Hryshko & Bers, 1990). Other studies have shown, however, that i_{Ca} declines during the positive staircase of shortening and of intracellular Ca^{2+} transients (DuBell & Houser, 1989). This reciprocal relation between Ca^{2+} transient and i_{Ca} is explained by a negative feedback between the amount of cytosolic calcium and the process which inactivates i_{Ca} (Lee, Marban & Tsien, 1985; DuBell & Houser, 1989; Arlock & Wohlfart, 1990). As pointed out by Schouten and Morad (1989), the discrepancies between the results from various groups are resolved when the holding potential at which the studies are carried out is considered: i_{Ca} seems to increase with frequency only when the membrane potential is held negative to -60 mV.

Contractile activation and clamp pulse duration

Cell shortening of rat heart cells in response to regular clamp steps is apparently near its maximum when the experimental conditions used in Fig. 3(*b*) are chosen (clamp step from -40 mV to 0 mV, 200 ms duration, frequency 0.5 s^{-1}, $[Ca^{2+}]_o$ 0.9 mmol/l), because a pause of 30 s at the holding potential causes only an insignificant post-rest potentiation. Furthermore, no significant change in i_{Ca} can be detected between the first and the eighth clamp pulse after the pause. In Fig. 3(*c*), the duration of the clamp step was varied from 300 ms before to 50 ms after the pause (30 s). The first short clamp step still causes full contractile activation but lower amplitudes were obtained with the subsequent clamp steps. Again, there was no significant change in i_{Ca} after rest, although peak i_{Ca} in response to the short clamp step was reduced (which we consider an artefact due to the low frequency response of the pen writer). In any case, since calcium currents of similar peak amplitude (first and fourth clamp step in Fig. 3(*c*)) produce both low and high amplitude contractions, it is concluded that i_{Ca} can have only a triggering function, especially for the first beat. The decline in steady-state contraction with shorter clamp pulses indicates that the duration of the calcium influx is very important for the loading of the sarcoplasmic reticulum with calcium.

When even shorter clamp pulses are applied, i.e. <5 ms, contractile activation fails altogether (data not shown).

The role of Na^+/Ca^{2+} exchange in post-rest potentiation

Under physiological conditions, Na^+/Ca^{2+} exchange translocates Ca^{2+} ions out of the cells against their electrochemical gradient, utilising the inwardly directed concentration gradient for Na^+ ions as an energy source (Reuter, 1984; see also Ravens & Wettwer, 1989). Because of a stoichiometry of 3 Na^+ to 1 Ca^{2+} (Reeves & Hale, 1984), the countertransport is electrogenic with a reversal potential in the negative potential range, but positive to the resting potential (Mullins, 1979; Sonn & Lee, 1988). Therefore, net Ca^{2+} extrusion is favoured significantly by more negative potentials. It is still a matter of debate whether Na^+/Ca^{2+} exchange actually contributes to Ca^{2+} influx at the positive potentials during the action potential plateau (for a comprehensive discussion of this topic see Hilgemann, 1988). The properties of the Na^+/Ca^{2+} exchanger are also discussed by Boyett *et al.* in their chapter in this book).

Since Na^+/Ca^{2+} exchange operates in the Ca^{2+} efflux mode at the resting potential of normal polarised cells, it may determine the amount of Ca^{2+} available for filling the sarcoplasmic reticulum during a period of rest. In hearts with rest decay of contraction, the Ca^{2+} content of the sarcoplasmic reticulum declines during a pause (Allen *et al.*, 1976; Beresewicz & Reuter, 1977; Lewartowski *et al.*, 1978; Reiter *et al.*, 1984; Wendt-Gallitelli, 1985; DuBell & Houser, 1990). In these muscles, experimental interventions that cause a shift in transmembrane Na^+ and/or Ca^{2+} gradients, so as to retard Ca^{2+} efflux via Na^+/Ca^{2+} exchange, increase the amplitude of post-rest contractions above those elicited by rhythmic stimulation (Sutko, Bers & Reeves, 1986).

Ca^{2+} release

Release of Ca^{2+} from the cardiac sarcoplasmic reticulum is induced by a sudden increase in the intracellular Ca^{2+} concentration (Fabiato & Fabiato, 1978; Fabiato, 1981) which is supplied by i_{Ca} (Beuckelmann & Wier, 1988; Näbauer *et al.*, 1989). Post-rest contractions depend in varying degree on Ca^{2+} released from the sarcoplasmic reticulum (Bers, 1985). As in skeletal muscle, the sarcoplasmic reticulum of cardiac muscle contains a high conductance Ca^{2+} channel that is activated by Ca^{2+} and also by caffeine and ryanodine (Rousseau *et al.*, 1986; Rousseau, Smith &

Meissner, 1987; Rousseau & Meissner, 1989). These latter two drugs diminish the contribution of the sarcoplasmic reticulum to post-rest potentiation (Bers, 1985; MacLeod & Bers, 1987).

Concluding remarks

Post-rest potentiation is not restricted to multicellular preparations but is also observed in single heart cells. Myocytes are valuable models for the study of regulation of contractile activation because they allow the simultaneous measurement of cellular Ca^{2+} transients, i_{Ca} and contraction in stringently controlled ionic and metabolic conditions. Though not directly relevant in a clinical setting, post-rest potentiation has fascinated many generations of investigators of heart function and has yielded valuable information for our understanding of excitation–contraction coupling.

References

Allen, D. G. & Blinks, J. R. (1978). Calcium transients in aequorin-injected frog cardiac muscle. *Nature,* **273,** 509–13.

Allen, D. G., Jewell, B. R. & Wood, E. H. (1976). Studies of the contractility of mammalian myocardium at low rates of stimulation. *Journal of Physiology,* **384,** 1–17.

Arlock, P. & Wohlfart, B. (1990). Force production following transient potential changes in voltage clamped myocardium. *Acta Physiologica Scandinavica,* **140,** 63–72.

Beresewicz, A. & Reuter, H. (1977). The effects of adrenaline and theophylline on action potential and contraction of mammalian ventricular muscle under 'rested-state' and 'steady-state' stimulation. *Naunyn-Schmiedeberg's Archives of Pharmacology,* **301,** 99–107.

Bers, D. M. (1985). Ca influx and sarcoplasmic reticulum Ca release in cardiac muscle activation during postrest recovery. *American Journal of Physiology,* **248,** H366–81.

Bers, D. M. (1987). Ryanodine and the calcium content of cardiac SR assessed by caffeine and rapid cooling contractures. *American Journal of Physiology,* **253,** C408–15.

Beuckelmann, D. J. & Wier, G. (1988). Mechanism of release of calcium from sarcoplasmic reticulum of guinea-pig cardiac cells. *Journal of Physiology,* **405,** 233–55.

Beyer, T., Hergeröder, W. & Ravens, U. (1988). Effects of bivalent cations on post-rest adaptation in guinea-pig heart muscle. *General Physiology and Biophysics,* **7,** 329–44.

Bowditch, H. P. (1871). Über die Eigenthümlichkeiten der Reizbarkeit, welche die Muskelfasern des Herzens zeigen. *Berichte der Königlich-Sächsischen Gesellschaft der Wissenschaften,* **23,** 652–89.

Brady, A. J., Tan, S. T. & Ricchiuti, N. V. (1979). Contractile force measured in unskinned isolated adult rat heart fibres. *Nature,* **282,** 728–9.

Carafoli, E., Crompton, M., Malmström, K., Sigel, E., Salzmann, M., Chiesi, M. & Affolter, H. (1977). Mitochondrial calcium transport and the intracellular calcium homeostasis. In *Biochemistry of Membrane Transport*, ed. G. Semenza & E. Carafoli, pp. 535–51. Berlin: Springer-Verlag.

Chapman, R. A. (1983). Control of cardiac contractility at the cellular level. *American Journal of Physiology*, **245**, H535–52.

Copelas, L., Briggs, M., Grossman, W., Morgan, J. P. (1987). A method for recording isometric tension development by isolated cardiac myocytes: transducer attachment with fibrin glue. *Pflügers Archiv*, **408**, 315–17.

Dow, J. W., Harding, N. G. L. & Powell, T. (1981). Isolated cardiac myocytes. I. Preparation of adult myocytes and their homology with the intact tissue. *Cardiovascular Research*, **15**, 483–514.

du Bell, W. H. & Houser, S. R. (1989). Voltage and beat dependence of Ca^{2+} transient in feline ventricular myocytes. *American Journal of Physiology*, **257**, H746–59.

du Bell, W. H. & Houser, S. R. (1990). Rest decay of calcium transients and contractility in feline ventricular myocytes. *American Journal of Physiology*, **259**, H395–402.

Fabiato, A. (1981). Myoplasmic free calcium concentration reached during the twitch of an intact isolated cardiac cell and during calcium-induced release of calcium from the sarcoplasmic reticulum of a skinned cardiac cell from the adult rat or rabbit ventricle. *Journal of General Physiology*, **78**, 457–97.

Fabiato, A. & Fabiato, F. (1978). Calcium-induced release of calcium from the sarcoplasmic reticulum of skinned cells from adult human, dog, cat, rabbit, rat, and frog hearts and from fetal and new-born rat ventricles. *Annals of the New York Academy of Sciences*, **307**, 473–84.

Fedida, D., Noble, D., Shimoni, Y. & Spindler, A. J. (1987). Inward current related to contraction in guinea-pig ventricular myocytes. *Journal of Physiology*, **385**, 565–89.

Fuchs, F. (1969). Inhibition of sarcotubular calcium transport by caffeine. Species and temperature dependence. *Biochimica et Biophysica Acta*, **172**, 566–70.

Grynckiewicz, G., Poenie, M. & Tsien, R. W. (1985). A new generation of Ca^{2+} indicators with greatly improved fluorescence properties. *Journal of Biological Chemistry*, **260**, 886–9.

Herzig, J. W., Köhler, G., Pfizer, G., Rüegg, J. C. & Woffle, G. (1981). Cyclic AMP inhibits contractility of detergent-treated glycerol extracted cardiac muscle. *Pflügers Archiv*, **391**, 208–12.

Hilgemann, D. W. (1988). Numerical approximations of sodium–calcium exchange. *Progress in Biophysics and Molecular Biology*, **51**, 1–45.

Hryshko, L. V. & Bers, D. M. (1990). Ca current facilitation during postrest recovery depends on Ca entry. *American Journal of Physiology*, **259**, H951–61.

Isenberg, G. & Wendt-Gallitelli, M. F. (1989). Cellular mechanisms of excitation contraction coupling. In *Isolated Adult Cardiomyocytes, Volume II, Electrophysiology and Contractile Function*, ed. H. M. Piper & G. Isenberg, pp. 213–48. Florida: CRC Press, Boca Raton.

Kentish, J. C., Ter Keurs, H. E. D. J., Riccardi, L., Bucx, J. J. & Noble, M. I. M. (1986). Comparison between the sarcomere length–force relations of intact and skinned trabeculae from rat right ventricle. *Circulation Research*, **58**, 755–68.

Kline, R. P. & Morad, M. (1978). Potassium efflux in heart muscle during activity: extracellular accumulation and its implications. *Journal of Physiology*, **280**, 537–58.

Koch-Weser, J. & Blinks, J. R. (1963). The influence of the interval between beats on myocardial contractility. *Pharmacological Reviews*, **15**, 601–52.

Lee, K. S. (1987). Potentiation of the calcium-channel currents of internally perfused mammalian heart cells by repetitive depolarization. *Proceedings of the National Academy of Sciences, USA*, **84**, 3941–5.

Lee, K. S., Marban, E. & Tsien, R. W. (1985). Inactivation of calcium channels in mammalian hearts: joint dependence on membrane potential and intracellular calcium. *Journal of Physiology*, **364**, 395–411.

Lewartowski, B., Prokopczuk, A. & Pytkowski, B. (1978). Effects of inhibitors of slow calcium current on rested state contraction of papillary muscles and post rest contractions of atrial muscle of the cat and rabbit hearts. *Pflügers Archiv*, **377**, 167–75.

Lewartowski, B. & Pytkowski, B. (1987). Cellular mechanism of the relationship between myocardial force and frequency of contractions. *Progress in Biophysics and Molecular Biology*, **50**, 97–120.

MacLeod, K. T. & Bers, D. M. (1987). Effects of rest and ryanodine on changes of extracellular [Ca] in cardiac muscle from rabbits. *American Journal of Physiology*, **253**, C398–470.

Mitchell, M. R., Powell, T., Terrar, D. A. & Twist, V. W. (1985). Influence on a change in stimulation rate on action potentials, currents and contractions in rat ventricular cells. *Journal of Physiology*, **364**, 113–39.

Mitra, R. & Morad, M. (1986). Two types of calcium channels in guinea pig ventricular myocytes. *Proceedings of the National Academy of Sciences, USA*, **83**, 5340–4.

Mullins, L. J. (1979). The generation of electric currents in cardiac fibers by Na/Ca exchange. *American Journal of Physiology*, **236**, C103–10.

Näbauer, M., Callewaert, G., Cleeman, L. & Morad, M. (1989). Regulation of calcium release is gated by calcium current, not gating charge, in cardiac myocytes. *Science*, **244**, 800–3.

Noble, S. & Shimoni, Y. (1981a). The calcium and frequency dependence of the slow inward current 'staircase' in frog atrium. *Journal of Physiology*, **310**, 57–75.

Noble, S. & Shimoni, Y. (1981b). Voltage-dependent potentiation of the slow inward current in frog atrium. *Journal of Physiology*, **310**, 77–95.

Ravens, U., Wang, X.-L. & Wettwer, E. (1989). Alpha adrenoceptor stimulation reduces outward currents in rat ventricular myocytes. *Journal of Pharmacology and Experimental Therapeutics*, **250**, 364–70.

Ravens, U. & Wettwer, E. (1989). Modulation of sodium/calcium exchange: a hypothetical positive inotropic mechanism. *Journal of Cardiovascular Pharmacology*, **14 (Suppl. 3)**, S30–5.

Reeves, J. P. & Hale, C. C. (1984). The stoichiometry of the cardiac sodium-calcium exchange system. *Journal of Biological Chemistry*, **259**, 7733–9.

Reiter, M., Seibel, K., Karema, E. (1978). The inotropic action of noradrenaline on rested-state contractions of guinea-pig ventricular muscle. *Life Science*, **22**, 1149–58.

Reiter, M., Vierling, W. & Seibel, K. (1984). Excitation–contraction coupling in rested-state contractions of guinea-pig ventricular myocardium. *Naunyn-Schmiedeberg's Archives of Pharmacology*, **325**, 159–69.

Reuter, H. (1984). Exchange of calcium ions in the mammalian myocardium. Mechanisms and physiological significance. *Circulation Research*, **34**, 599–604.

Rousseau, E. & Meissner, G. (1989). Single cardiac sarcoplasmic reticulum Ca^{2+} release channel: activation by caffeine. *American Journal of Physiology*, **256**, H328–33.

Rousseau, E., Smith, J. S., Henderson, J. S. & Meissner, G. (1986). Single channel and ^{45}Ca^{2+} flux measurements of the cardiac sarcoplasmic reticulum calcium channel. *Biophysical Journal*, **50**, 1009–14.

Rousseau, E., Smith, J. S. & Meissner, G. (1987). Ryanodine modifies conductance and gating behavior of single Ca^{2+} release channel. *American Journal of Physiology*, **253**, C364–8.

Schouten, V. J. A. & Morad, M. (1989). Regulation of Ca^{2+} current in frog ventricular myocytes by the holding potential, c-AMP and frequency. *Pflügers Archiv*, **415**, 1–11.

Seibel, K. (1986). The slow phase of the staircase in guinea-pig papillary muscle, influence of agents acting on transmembrane sodium flux. *Naunyn-Schmiedeberg's Archives of Pharmacology*, **334**, 92–9.

Shepherd, N. & Kavaler, F. (1986). Direct control of contraction force of single frog atrial cells by extracellular ions. *American Journal of Physiology*, **251**, C653–61.

Shepherd, N., Vornanen, M. & Isenberg, G. (1990). Force measurements from voltage-clamped guinea-pig ventricular myocytes. *American Journal of Physiology*, **258**, H452–9.

Solaro, R. J., Wise, R. M., Shiner, J. S. & Briggs, F. N. (1974). Calcium requirements for cardiac myofibrillar activation. *Circulation Research*, **34**, 525–30.

Sonn, J. K. & Lee, C. O. (1988). Na$^+$–Ca^{2+} exchange in regulation of contractility in canine Purkinje fibers. *American Journal of Physiology*, **255**, C278–90.

Spurgeon, H. A., Stern, M. D., Baartz, G., Raffaeli, S., Hansford, R. G., Talo, A., Lakatta, E. G. & Capogrossi, M. C. (1990). Simultaneous measurement of Ca^{2+}, contraction and potential in cardiac myocytes. *American Journal of Physiology*, **258**, H574–86.

Sutko, J. L., Bers, D. M. & Reeves, J. P. (1986). Postrest inotropy in rabbit ventricle: Na$^+$–Ca^{2+} exchange determines sarcoplasmic reticulum Ca^{2+} content. *American Journal of Physiology*, **250**, H654–61.

Sutko, J. L. & Kenyon, J. L. (1983). Ryanodine modification of cardiac muscle responses to potassium-free solutions: evidence for inhibition of sarcoplasmic reticulum calcium release. *Journal of General Physiology*, **82**, 385–404.

Tarr, M., Trank, J. W., Goertz, K. K. & Leifer, P. (1981). Effect of initial sarcomere length on sarcomere kinetics and force development in single frog atrial cardiac cells. *Circulation Research*, **49**, 767–72.

Tung, L. (1986). An ultrasensitive transducer for measurement of isometric contractile force from single heart cells. *Pflügers Archiv*, **407**, 109–15.

Tung, L. & Morad, M. (1988). Contractile force of single heart cells compared with muscle strips of frog ventricle. *American Journal of Physiology*, **255**, H111–20.

Weber, A. & Herz, R. (1968). The relationship between caffeine contracture of intact muscle and the effect of caffeine on reticulum. *Journal of General Physiology*, **52**, 750–9.

Wendt-Gallitelli, M. F. (1985). Presystolic calcium loading of the sarcoplasmic reticulum influences time to peak force of contraction. X-ray microanalysis of rapidly frozen guinea-pig ventricular muscle preparations. *Basic Research in Cardiology*, **80**, 617–25.

Wohlfart, B. & Noble, M. I. M. (1982). The cardiac excitation–contraction cycle. *Pharmacology and Therapeutics*, **16**, 1–43.

Yue, D. T., Marban, E. & Wier, G. W. (1986). Relationship between force and intracellular $[Ca^{2+}]$ in tetanized mammalian heart muscle. *Journal of General Physiology*, **87**, 223–42.

Post-extrasystolic potentiation and its decay

HENK E. D. J. TER KEURS

Introduction

Post-extrasystolic potentiation is a prominent property of mammalian myocardium, particularly when the latter contains an elaborate sarcoplasmic reticulum. The sarcoplasmic reticulum is an intracellular calcium store with a large capacity, allowing for accumulation of calcium that enters the cell across the sarcolemma and thereby potentiation of force development. Conversely, interruption of the process that leads to addition of calcium to the store should lead to decay of potentiation. This chapter will therefore discuss post-extrasystolic potentiation and the decay of post-extrasystolic potentiation in the light of calcium transport by the sarcoplasmic reticulum and the sarcolemma. Fig. 1 shows a typical example of a longitudinal electron microscopic section through a rapidly fixed trabecula of the right ventricle of a rat heart. The cell border is delineated by a glycoprotein layer overlying the sarcolemma, which invaginates at regular intervals along the cell near the Z-lines of the myofibrils. The resultant transverse tubuli make contact with a longitudinal compartment contained in a lipid membrane, called the sarcoplasmic reticulum. This compartment has been shown to wrap around the myofibrils; its longitudinal component contains a Ca^{2+} ATP-ase which drives calcium into the sarcoplasmic reticulum, while its terminal region contains calcium channels (which can be recognised by their high affinity for ryanodine) involved in calcium release from the contact site (terminal cisterna) with the T-tubuli. Of the intracellular space, 60% is occupied by the contractile proteins arranged in myofibrils which contain the contractile unit: the sarcomere. The remainder of the cell volume is virtually completely occupied by rows of mitochondria adjacent of the sarcomeres (See Fig. 1).

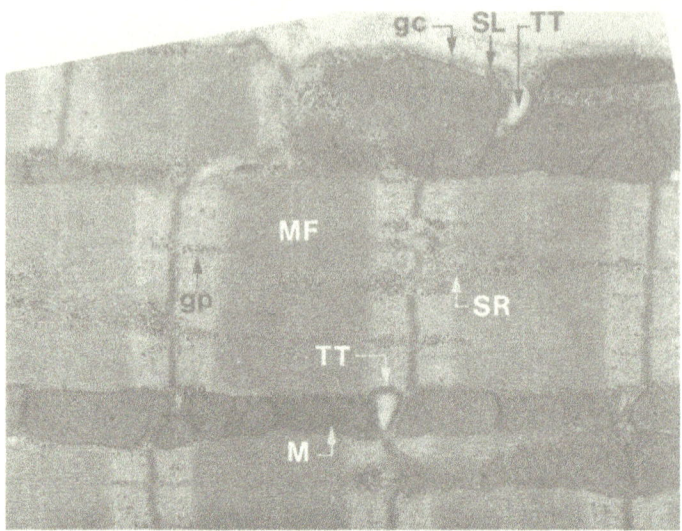

Fig. 1. Longitudinal electron microscopic section of a cardiac cell of the rat. The close spatial interrelationships between the surface membrane (SL) with its surface layer of glyocalyx (gc), the T-tubuli (TT) and the sarcoplasmic reticulum (SR) are prominent. The sarcoplasmic reticulum is seen to envelop the myofibrils (MF), which constitute the major (60%) organelle in the cell; the mitochondria (M) occupy another 40% of the intracellular space. The granules (gp) are glycogenolytic particles.

A functional model of excitation–contraction coupling

It is well accepted that, during excitation–contraction coupling, calcium entry into the cell through the surface membrane and the T-tubuli triggers release of calcium from the sarcoplasmic reticulum. The released calcium activates the contractile machinery and is subsequently partially seques-tered by the sarcoplasmic reticulum together with the calcium that entered the cell during the action potential (Fabiato & Fabiato, 1975; Morad & Cleeman, 1987; Valdeolmillos *et al.*, 1989). The remainder of the calcium leaves the cell through the surface membrane, partly in exchange for Na^+, and partly transported by the Ca^{2+} pump. Calcium efflux through the membrane must balance the influx during the action potential in the steady state. It takes some time before the sequestered calcium can again be released from the sarcoplasmic reticulum. Calcium is probably mostly extruded through the cell membrane by the low affinity, high capacity, Na^+/Ca^{2+} exchanger during systole, while the low capacity high affinity Ca^{2+} pump extrudes calcium during the diastolic interval. These proper-ties can be summarised in a model of the cardiac cell such as that in Fig. 2.

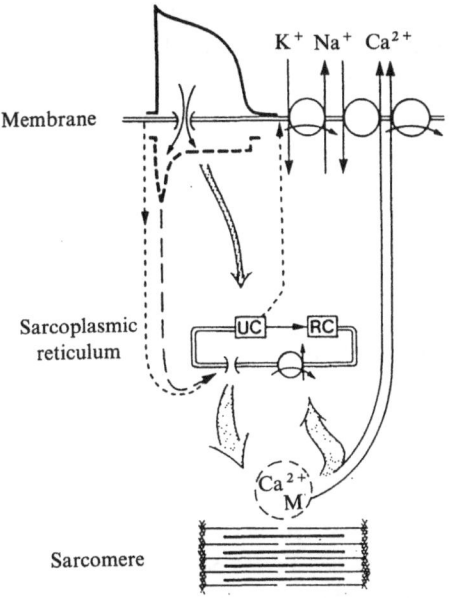

Fig. 2. Diagram of the excitation–contraction coupling system in the cardiac cell. During the action potential, calcium enters the cells as a rapid influx followed by a maintained component of the slow inward current (heavy dashed line). Calcium entry does not lead directly to force development as the calcium ions that enter are rapidly bound to binding sites on the sarcoplasmic reticulum that envelops the myofibrils. The rapid influx of calcium is thought to induce release of calcium from a release compartment (RC) in the sarcoplasmic reticulum, by triggering opening of calcium channels in the terminal cisternae, thus activating the contractile filaments to contract. Relaxation follows because the cytosolic calcium is sequestered again in an uptake compartment (UC) of the sarcoplasmic reticulum and partly extruded through the cell membrane by the Na^+/Ca^{2+} exchanger and by the low capacity high affinity Ca^{2+} pump. The force of contraction is thus determined by the circulation of calcium from the sarcoplasmic reticulum to the myofilaments and back to the sarcoplasmic reticulum, and by the amount of calcium that has entered during the preceding action potential. The relaxation rate of the twitch depends on the rate of calcium dissociation from the myofilaments and on the rates of calcium sequestration and extrusion. It is important to note that the process of Na^+/Ca^{2+} exchange is electrogenic so that calcium extrusion through the exchanger leads to a depolarising current.

This model is comparable to the mathematical model by Schouten *et al.* (1987), in which their exchange compartment has been replaced by the collection of ion-exchangers in the sarcolemma. It is of interest here to consider the amounts of Ca^{2+} that are transported by the transport mechanisms of the sarcoplasmic reticulum and the sarcolemma. The force of contraction of the quietly beating heart is probably only a fraction of the maximal force that can be generated by the contractile filaments. This fraction is probably near 40% (Fabiato, 1981; Kentish *et al.*, 1986). This implies that approximately 40% of the low affinity sites of troponin-C are saturated with Ca^{2+} ions; these sites bind one Ca^{2+} ion each. Simultaneously, another 10 μM of Ca^{2+} is bound to calmodulin, so that the required release of Ca^{2+} is ~ 40 μM (Solaro *et al.*, 1974; Robertson, Johnson & Potter, 1981).

Extrasystole and post-extrasystolic potentiation

An essential component of post-extrasystolic potentiation is that calcium release after a cardiac cycle requires a period of recovery; this underlies mechanical restitution (chapter by Jóhannsson in this book). The full mechanical restitution curve of a human cardiac trabecula is shown in Fig. 3; the figure illustrates that after initial recovery a further increase in force may occur at high extracellular $[Ca^{2+}]$ (rest potentiation), while force eventually declines to a low residual level with increasing intervals (rest depression). Rest potentiation depends on the Na^+ and Ca^{2+} gradients across the cell membrane (Bers, 1985; Schouten, 1985; ter Keurs *et al.*, 1987). The initial recovery of the twitch is usually exponential and has a time constant of several hundreds of milliseconds, as is reflected by the mechanical restitution curve; recovery of force of the twitch mirrors recovery of Ca^{2+} transient (Wier & Yue, 1986; and chapter by Yue in this book). It has been assumed that the recovery is caused by a time-consuming process that transports calcium from the uptake region in the sarcoplasmic reticulum – presumably the longitudinal compartment – back to the terminal cisternae where release is mediated by the ryanodine-sensitive (Sutko *et al.*, 1979) calcium channels of the sarcoplasmic reticulum. As mentioned in the chapter by Yue, pp. 95–109, this explanation suffers from the weakness that the diffusion distance is less than 1 μM; even if diffusion of calcium ions alternated with binding to calsequestrin, the terminal cisternae should be replenished within 100 milliseconds. Alternatively, recovery of the twitch may reflect recovery of the calcium channels themselves following previous release. The latter explanation is supported by recent observations on rapid cooling contractions. Cooling of isolated mammalian myocardial muscle to near 0 °C in less than one second causes a contracture (Bers, Bridge & Spitzer, 1989). It has been suggested that sudden cooling locks the calcium release channels in the sarcoplasmic reticulum in an open state (Sitsapesan *et al.*, 1990).

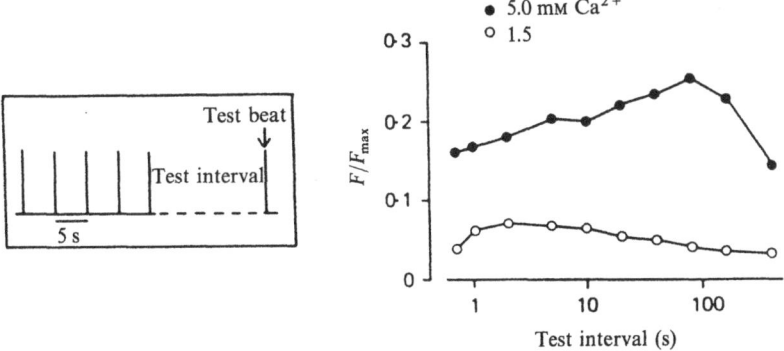

Fig. 3. Mechanical restitution of an isolated trabecula from the human heart at extracellular $[Ca^{2+}]$ of 1.5 mM (open circles) and 5.0 mM (filled circles). Temperature 30 °C. The protocol of stimulation is depicted in the inset. After initial recovery of the twitch a phase of rest potentiation is prominent at high extracellular $[Ca^{2+}]$; rest depression follows the initial recovery for force both at high and at low calcium levels in the superfusate. F_{max} is force following maximal extrasystolic potentiation. (From Quaegebeur, Schouten & ter Keurs, (1986), with permission.)

So, cooling appears to affect the same channels that are normally involved in the twitch, though no action potential is generated. The magnitude of the rapid cooling contracture has been shown to provide a measure of the total calcium content of the sarcoplasmic reticulum (Bers *et al.*, 1989). In contrast to the increase in amplitude of the twitch which is elicited at short – but increasing – intervals after a steady-state twitch, the magnitude of the contracture induced by rapidly cooling of cardiac muscle at short intervals after a steady-state twitch appears to be constant (Banijamali *et al.*, 1991); this observation supports the hypothesis that the early recovery of force following the last twitch is due to time-dependent recovery of the SR calcium release channels.

The inward current of calcium which occurs during the action potential (i_{si}) has been shown to recover considerably faster than the twitch (Josephson, Sanchez-Chapula & Brown, 1984; Tseng, 1988); it is, therefore, unlikely that recovery of the extrasystolic twitch is due to recovery of the slow inward current. On the other hand, the combination of a rapid recovery of i_{si} and a slow recovery of the calcium channels in the sarcoplasmic reticulum would explain part of the potentiating effect of an early extrasystole, as this will lead to an enhanced calcium influx during the action potential of the extrasystole, because calcium entry through calcium channels of the sarcolemma will not be opposed by a rise of

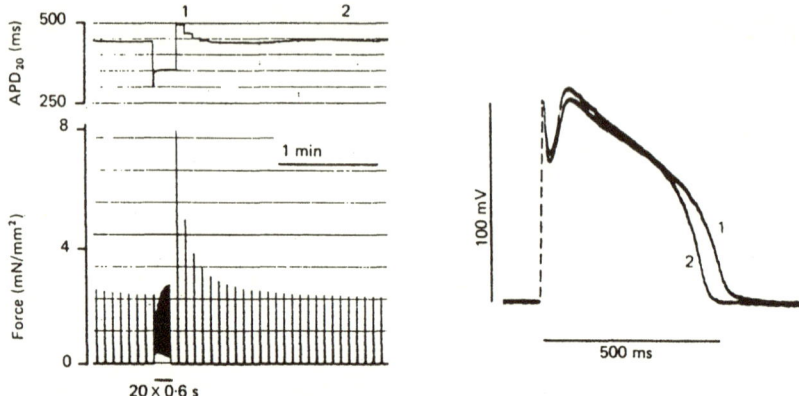

Fig. 4. The effect of a short train of stimuli at 1.7 Hz on isometric force and action potential duration of a trabecula from human heart at 30 °C and an external calcium concentration of 5 mM. Action potential duration was measured between upstroke and the moment that membrane potential had returned to 20% of the action potential amplitude (APD20). The numbers of the action potentials at the right correspond to those on the trace of APD20. (From Quaegebeur, Schouten & ter Keurs (1986), with permission.)

intracellular calcium due to calcium induced calcium release from the sarcoplasmic reticulum. Similarly, the driving force for calcium extrusion through Na^+/Ca^{2+} exchange will be reduced at low intracellular calcium concentration; hence calcium extrusion during the extrasystole is diminished and more of the calcium that has entered the cell through the slow inward current will be sequestered in the sarcoplasmic reticulum than during the normal beat. As a consequence of the increased calcium entry, reduced calcium extrusion, and reduced calcium release from the sarcoplasmic reticulum during the extrasystole, the amount of calcium what will be present in the sarcoplasmic reticulum after the extrasystole must be increased. This evidently leads to potentiation of the post-extrasystolic contraction, which will manifest itself in an increase of twitch force if this beat is elicited at a time when the calcium transport systems have recovered (i.e. if it is fully restituted). Post-extrasystolic potentiation of a trabecula from human heart by a series of extrasystoles is illustrated in Fig. 4.

The contribution of the aforementioned three factors, reduced calcium release from the sarcoplasmic reticulum, increased calcium entry as well as reduced calcium extrusion through the sarcolemma explains why the force of the post-extrasystolic beat can be substantially larger than the *deficit* in force of the extrasystole. The maximum force developed during the potentiated post-extrasystolic beat is limited by the maximal calcium content of the sarcoplasmic reticulum (Schouten *et al.*, 1990*a*). Maximal force that can be attained by post-extrasystolic potentiation amounts to approximately 70% of the maximal force that can be developed when the sarcoplasmic reticulum is bypassed, for example, by exposure to Sr^{2+} ions or when the muscles or cells are skinned and directly exposed to Ca^{2+} ions (Fabiato, 1981; Kentish *et al.*, 1986). It is not known exactly why the apparent content of the sarcoplasmic reticulum is limited; one possibility is that at higher calcium levels in the sarcoplasmic reticulum spontaneous release of calcium may occur – so-called calcium overload induced calcium release (Allen *et al.*, 1985; Kort & Lakatta, 1988). Alternatively, there may be a genuine limitation of the calcium content by saturation of the calcium binding sites, such as calsequestrin, in the sarcoplasmic reticulum.

The maximal amount of calcium that can be accumulated during post-extrasystolic potentiation depends on the calcium binding and uptake system of the longitudinal component of the sarcoplasmic reticulum, as well as on the rate of calcium loss from the sarcoplasmic reticulum. Substances that depress calcium uptake or enhance calcium loss from the sarcoplasmic reticulum, such as caffeine and ryanodine (Banijamali *et al.*, 1991), also decrease the degree of post-extrasystolic potentiation.

Decay of post-extrasystolic potentiation

When contractility of the heart is potentiated by extrasystoles, return to the steady state is characterised by a nearly exponential decay of contractility (see Fig. 4). This behaviour has been observed in the myocardium of most mammalia, including man. The characteristics are qualitatively similar in intact hearts and in isolated muscle (Elzinga *et al.*, 1981; Wohlfart, 1979). The decay process was analysed in detail by Wohlfart (1979), who has shown that a strong linear correlation exists between the force of successive contractions of isolated muscle preparations. The behaviour of the intact heart appeared, in studies in which contractility was measured as the maximal rate of pressure development (LV dP/dt_{max}) in the ventricle at controlled end diastolic volume, to be similar to that of isolated papillary muscles. Figs. 5 and 6 illustrate the decay of LV dP/dt_{max} in the left ventricle of a dog following potentiation by paired pacing, i.e. by recurrent extrasystoles.

It has also been shown that the force of contraction depends on the duration of the plateau phase of the action potential of the preceding beat.

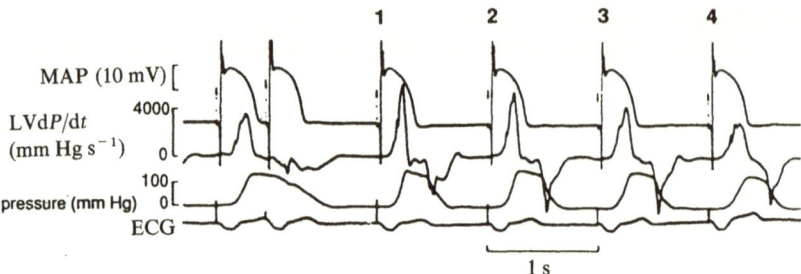

Fig. 5. Post-extrasystolic potentiation and its decay in the dog heart. Top trace: monophasic action potential in the right ventricle measured with a contact electrode catheter. The second trace is the first derivative of left ventricular pressure, and the third trace left ventricular pressure itself. The fourth trace is a low gain ECG showing pacing artefacts and ventricular QRST complexes. The post-extrasystolic beats are numbered 1 through 4. (From ter Keurs et al., 1990, with permission.)

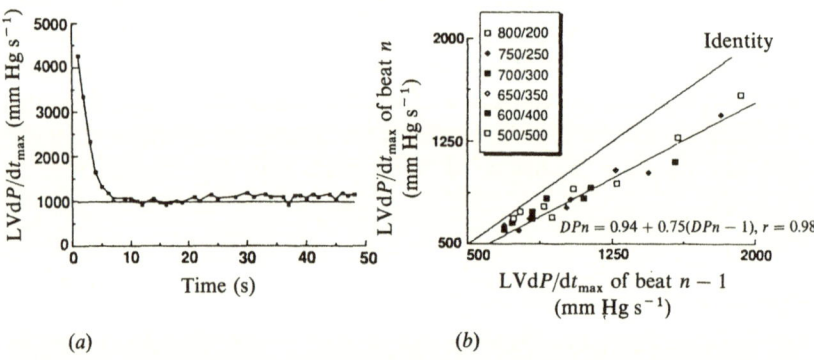

Fig. 6. Panel (a) shows a linear plot of LV dP/dt_{max} for successive beats over a period of 50 s following potentiation. Note that LV dP/dt_{max} decays to a minimum and then rises to a steady-state value. Panel (b) shows a plot of LV dP/dt_{max} of beat n against that of beat $n - 1$ following potentiation induced by stimulation at varied priming intervals and varied extrasystolic coupling intervals (see inset key). The regression line lies below the line of identity and has a slope of 0.75. (From ter Keurs et al., 1990, with permission.)

Therefore, the force of beat n can be described by the following equation:

$$DP_n = B_{DP}(DP_{n-1}) + B_{AP}(AP_{n-1} - D) \qquad [1]$$

in which DP is the contractile force or LV dP/dt_{max} of a beat; n is the rank number of a beat; B_{DP} is the proportionality with which DP of a beat depends on DP of the preceding beat; B_{AP} reflects the proportionality with which DP of a beat depends on the duration of the preceding action potential (AP_{n-1}) (Wohlfart, 1979; Drake-Holland et al., 1983); D is thought to reflect a time during the action potential which does not contribute to contractility.

The effect of action potential duration disappears when decay of potentiation is measured at intervals between the test beats of one second or more. In that case, the action potential has a nearly constant duration during the decay of potentiation and eqn. [1] can be rewritten (ter Keurs *et al.*, 1990) as:

$$DP_n = DP_1 \times e^{\ln B_{DP} \times n} + DP_{as} \qquad [2]$$

in which: DP_1 is LV dP/dt_{max} of the first potentiated beat, $\ln B_{DP}$ is the exponential decay constant, DP_{as} is the asymptotic value to which DP decays, and the other terms have the same meaning as in eqn. [1].

Analysis of the decay of potentiation (Fig. 5) by regression to either eqn. [1] or [2] yielded similar results. The value of B_{DP} for studies in dog heart (ter Keurs *et al.*, 1990), in rat right ventricular trabeculae (Schouten *et al.*, 1987) and also in human myocardium (Seed *et al.*, 1984) is approximately 0.6 to 0.7; this value is independent of the preceding heart rate between 80 and 150 per minute (ter Keurs *et al.*, 1990). Figs. 4 and 5 show that, following the decay toward DP_{as}, DP increases again to a value commensurate with the new steady-state frequency of stimulation; this phenomenon gives rise to a transient undershoot of DP. DP_1 increases with stimulus frequency and with a decrease of the interval preceding the extrasystole. The undershoot of LV dP/dt_{max} before return to steady state is larger with a larger DP_1. The decline of LV dP/dt_{max} of the first six beats with time is exponential and can be fitted reliably by eqn. [2]. The rate constant appears independent of the preceding stimulus frequency or the interval preceding the extrasystole; DP_{as} appears inversely proportional to DP_1.

'Recirculating' activator calcium

The linearity of the relationship between the forces of successive post-extrasystolic contractions is striking, and suggests that a constant fraction (B_{DP}) of the calcium that elicits contraction reappears during the following contraction (Wohlfart, 1979; Drake-Holland *et al.*, 1983; ter Keurs *et al.*, 1990; see also chapter by Wohlfart *et al.*, pp. 213–25). The 'recirculating fraction' of activator calcium $(RF) = 1 - EF$, where EF is the extruded fraction. This relationship only holds at a limited range of intervals between the post-extrasystolic beats. Evidently, if the interval is too short the release system will not have recovered. At intervals longer than a few seconds, rest potentiation or rest depression occur; this suggests that the recirculation and extrusion that are assessed by RF and EF probably occur mostly during systole. If this is true, it is understandable that Ca^{2+} extruded through the Na^+/Ca^{2+} exchanger (EF) would be proportional to the amount of calcium that is released during activation. Likewise, one would expect the rate of calcium transport by the sarcoplasmic reticulum (RF) to follow the enzyme kinetics of the Ca^+ ATP-ase and to be proportional to the cytosolic Ca^{2+} concentration. The hypothesis that a substantial amount of Ca^{2+} is extruded through Na^+/Ca^{2+} exchange during the action potential of the concurrent beat is indeed rather strong, as has been shown by measurement of the duration of the late phase of the action potential (Schouten, ter Keurs & Quaegebeur, 1990*b*) by Ca^{2+} transients in the interstitium (Hilgemann, 1986), as well as by manipulation of the Na^+ and Ca^{2+} gradients across the cell membrane (Bers & Bridge, 1989).

The degree of potentiation and RF

A constant relationship between both EF and RF and the systolic Ca^{2+} concentration would predict an exponential decay of post-extrasystolic contractility toward the steady-state level, but does not explain the undershoot of DP that is observed in Fig. 4. The undershoot is observed with a heart rate of 1 Hz both before potentiation and during the decay of potentiation. Changes of action potential duration can therefore not have played a role (Drake *et al.*, 1982). Possible explanations for the undershoot are the presence of a feedback system which enhances Ca^{2+} removal or reduces Ca^{2+} entry. In either case, the feedback system must exhibit a lag time to explain the undershoot of DP below the control level. Ca^{2+}/calmodulin dependent activation of the sarcolemmal Ca^{2+} pump by oligomerisation of the pump complex could have such an effect (Dixon & Haynes, 1989). Although this effect may be sufficiently large (up to 20 fold), it is not known whether the off-rate of the effect on the pump by this mechanism is sufficiently slow to cause oscillations in Ca^{2+} handling. A simultaneous (but smaller) acceleration of Ca^{2+} pumping by the sarcoplasmic reticulum through calmodulin (James *et al.*, 1989) would keep the recirculation fraction constant. Reduction of Ca^{2+} entry would have the same effect (Lee, Marban & Tsien, 1985), again provided that this feedback lags behind increase of cytosolic $[Ca^{2+}]$. It is unlikely that the latter effect would result from a reduction of the duration of the action potential at higher contractility, because it has been shown that action potential duration is independent of DP (Drake *et al.*, 1982). The eventual return of DP to its steady-state level would in the above situation reflect the dissipation of the effect of feedback of an increased cytosolic $[Ca^{2+}]$ on the balance of Ca^{2+} fluxes into, and out of, the cardiac cell.

The heart rate and RF

In the intact dog heart, *RF* appeared to be unaffected by the degree of potentiation or the preceding steady frequency of activations (ter Keurs *et al.*, 1990). Apparently, the relative rates of calcium re-uptake by the sarcoplasmic reticulum and calcium extrusion through the sarcolemma are constant under these conditions.

The observation that the apparent recirculation fraction is constant at increased stimulus frequency in the intact dog heart is also remarkable. One could again predict that the rate of calcium transport by the sarcoplasmic reticulum would follow the cytosolic Ca^{2+} concentration. The positive inotropic effect of an increase of the stimulus frequency should lead to enhanced re-uptake through this mechanism and possibly by stimulation of the SR-pump. The extrusion rate through the sarcolemma, on the other hand, depends on intracellular Ca^{2+}, but more strongly on the intracellular Na^+ concentration because of the $3Na^+$: $1Ca^{2+}$ stoichiometry. The Na^+ concentration is determined by the balance of Na^+ influx through the Na^+ channel and the Na^+/Ca^{2+} exchanger and Na^+ extrusion through the Na^+/K^+ pump, and increases during increased rates of stimulation (Cohen, Fozzard & Sheu, 1982). The increase in intracellular Na^+ may be substantial as one would expect an influx of ~ 40 μM per beat (i.e. ignoring the Na^+ current and assuming a stoichiometry of the exchanger of $3Na^+:1Ca^{2+}$ (Eisner & Lederer, 1989), and an extrusion fraction of $1/3$ (Schouten *et al.*, 1987), and release of 40 μM Ca^{2+} per beat (Solaro *et al.*, 1974; Robertson, Johnson & Potter, 1981; Fabiato, 1981; Kentish *et al.*, 1986)). The resultant increase of the Na^+ concentration in the cytosol will be mitigated by acceleration of the Na^+/K^+ pump, but should still lead to a reduction of the rate of calcium efflux through the Na^+/Ca^{2+} exchanger; hence, the recirculating fraction of calcium should increase. An increase of the recirculating fraction from 0.65 to 0.80 has indeed been found in isolated rat myocardium, which exhibits a high level of contractility, when the frequency of stimulation is increased from 0.01 Hz to 1.2 Hz (Schouten *et al.*, 1987). The observation in the dog heart that the recirculation fraction of calcium is independent of the heart rate requires activation of a sarcolemmal extrusion mechanism in parallel to the Na^+/Ca^{2+} exchanger. As outlined in the previous section it may be that feedback activation of the sarcolemmal Ca^{2+} pump serves this role. This would explain the transient undershoot of contractility and would be consistent with the observation that DP during the undershoot is inversely proportional to the degree of potentiation. The subsequent recovery of contractility, at a heart rate lower than the rate preceding the extrasystole, would be enhanced as a result of the simultaneous gradual increase of the action potential duration upon return to a lower stimulus frequency (Drake *et al.*, 1982).

The decay of post-extrasystolic potentiation in the diseased heart

It has been shown that the Ca^{2+} ATP-ase activity of the sarcoplasmic reticulum in the failing heart is depressed (Ito, Sutko & Chidsey, 1974). This may be due to a decrease of the number of Ca^{2+} binding and Ca^{2+} transport sites or to a decrease of the activity of the ATPase, and probably both. The effect of a decline of the Ca^{2+} uptake capacity of the sarcoplasmic reticulum would be a decrease of the rate of uptake of Ca^{2+}. The above described model of excitation–contraction coupling predicts that this would cause a higher Ca^{2+} level due to less effective buffering, particularly during the slow inward current. Relaxation should be delayed, and because a larger fraction of the Ca^{2+} is now extruded through Na^+/Ca^{2+} exchange, prolongation of the action potential would ensue (see Fig. 4) (Schouten *et al.*, 1990b). Reduced Ca^{2+} uptake by the sarcoplasmic reticulum would further lead to a decrease of the amount of Ca^{2+} stored and thereby to a reduction of the contribution of Ca^{2+} release from the sarcoplasmic reticulum to the force of contraction. This effect might be overcome by enhanced Ca^{2+} entry, but would eventually become noticeable as a negative inotropic effect. Before the negative inotropic effect became noticeable, the reduction of Ca^{2+} uptake by the sarcoplasmic reticulum would be recognised as a reduction of the fraction of recirculating $Ca^{2+}:RF$.

These predictions are indeed borne out in studies of the failing heart and in experiments on cardiac muscle isolated from failing hearts during cardiac transplant surgery. Morgan's group in Boston has studied muscles isolated from the hearts of patients with end-stage heart failure (Gwathmey *et al.*, 1987). Muscles were loaded with the Ca^{2+} sensitive photo-luminescent protein aequorin and the light emitted following electrical stimulation was measured simultaneously with the *trans*-membrane action potential and force development. Fig. 7 illustrates dramatic differences

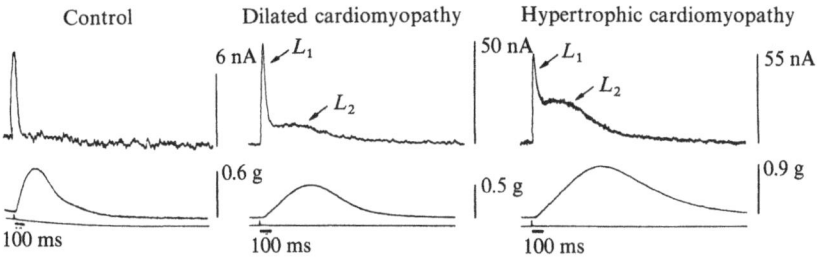

Fig. 7. Upper tracings: light (in nA current from a photomultiplier) emitted by aequorin during activation of human cardiac muscle of normal hearts and of cardiomyopathic hearts. Middle tracing: isometric tension in grams. The lower trace shows the stimulus artefact. It is clear that the light transient from the cardiomyopathic muscles consists of two components (L1 and L2), where the light from the normal muscle is composed of only component L1. Furthermore, twitch tension in the cardiomyopathic muscles was prolonged with a marked delay of relaxation. (From Gwathmey *et al.*, 1987, with permission.)

between muscle obtained from healthy hearts that could not be transplanted and muscles from failing hearts. The Ca^{2+} transient, as reflected by the transient emission of light by aequorin, indeed is biphasic in cardiomyopathic hearts and shows a secondary elevation (L2) which occurs during the plateau of the prolonged action potential (Gwathmey *et al.*, 1987). The observation that the first light transient could be abolished by ryanodine and the second transient by verapamil suggests that the first transient reflects Ca^{2+} release from the sarcoplasmic reticulum and the second transient depends on Ca^{2+} entry through i_{si}. This hypothesis was further supported by the observation that L2 is enhanced at elevated external $[Ca^{2+}]$. The dependence of L2 on $[Ca^{2+}]_o$ was much stronger in cardiomyopathic muscle than in control muscle, which is consistent with the hypothesis that the cardiomyopathic muscles rely more strongly on i_{si} and have a lower intracellular Ca^{2+} buffering capacity.

The study by Morgan and collaborators on Ca^{2+} transients in muscle isolated from normal and from cardiomyopathic hearts is consistent with the hypothesis that abnormal intracellular Ca^{2+} handling underlies cardiac contractile failure. The prediction that reduction of the capacity of the sarcoplasmic reticulum for Ca^{2+} uptake should lead to a decrease of the fraction (RF) of Ca^{2+} that recirculates from beat to beat in the cell was tested by Seed *et al.*, (1984). In the latter study it was observed that B_{DP} was approximately 30% higher in patients with normal left ventricular function than in a group of patients with abnormal left ventricular function. Furthermore it appeared that there was an inverse correlation between B_{DP} and the degree of potentiation of the first post-extrasystolic beat (DP_1). The latter observation is consistent with the analysis of factors (see above) that contribute to Ca^{2+} entry during the extrasystole and to the magnitude of the ensuing post-extrasystolic potentiation. We have seen that depressed Ca^{2+} re-uptake by the sarcoplasmic reticulum in the failing heart is expected to lead to a decrease of B_{DP}, logically with a concomitant reduction of Ca^{2+} release from the sarcoplasmic reticulum during the extrasystole. Therefore, a large reduction of Ca^{2+} re-uptake (i.e. a small B_{DP}) allows very little Ca^{2+} release during the extrasystole and virtually unopposed Ca^{2+} entry through i_{si}. As a result, there is a large degree of post-extrasystolic potentiation. Although these observations require further corroboration because the groups of patients in both studies are rather heterogeneous, it appears that the results are qualitatively consistent with current models of excitation–contraction coupling (see Fig. 2) and with the assumption that Ca^{2+} re-uptake by the sarcoplasmic reticulum in the failing heart is depressed (Ito et al., 1974).

An interesting potential explanation for the observation that the fraction of recirculated Ca^{2+} is reduced, irrespective of the exact nature of the original disease, is that failure of excitation–contraction coupling in the myocytes ultimately results from the effect of a common pathway of influences on the myocardium. One mechanism that would be consistent with a concept of a common pathway is an increased adrenergic drive during the phase of subclinical heart failure. The adrenergic drive would succeed in maintaining cardiac output and blood pressure at a level required by the control systems of the circulation. Eventually a long-standing adrenergic drive might lead to adaptation of the cardiac myocyte in the form of a depression of sarcoplasmic reticulum function. It has been seen that this reduces the contribution of activation of the contractile apparatus by Ca^{2+} release from the sarcoplasmic reticulum, and makes activation of the cardiac cell more dependent on Ca^{2+} entry through the slow inward current. Increase of i_{si} to a maximum implies that further increase of contractility by adrenergic mechanisms must become impossible; a state in which the regulatory mechanisms have become self-defeating. Drugs which reduce the adrenergic drive on the heart should delay the development of such uncontrollable failure. The rapid and reproducible induction of heart failure by rapid pacing of an otherwise perfectly normal dog heart (Armstrong et al., 1986) may provide an experimental model in which this concept can be tested.

Study of the recirculating fraction of Ca^{2+} in the clinical situation is of potential importance because it allows insight into the derailment of mechanisms that subserve contraction of the cardiac cell, while the recirculating fraction of Ca^{2+} is independent of the multitude of mechanisms in the heart and in the vascular system that influence the mechanical performance of the heart as a pump.

Summary

A model of excitation–contraction coupling is presented which can be used to explain several aspects of post-extrasystolic potentiation and its decay. A key aspect is the presence of the sarcoplasmic reticulum in the myocyte. This compartment accumulates calcium ions by an active process, and releases calcium upon calcium influx into the cell during the action potential as a result of calcium-induced calcium release. The sequence of calcium release followed by re-uptake into the sarcoplasmic reticulum causes a fraction of the activator calcium to recirculate from beat to beat. Time-dependent recovery of the calcium release channels is responsible for the shortfall of calcium release during the occurrence of an early extrasystole, simultaneously allowing larger *trans*-membrane calcium entry and reduced calcium extrusion across the cell membrane during the extrasystole. The increased net calcium entry into the cell during the extrasystole allows extra uptake of calcium into the sarcoplasmic reticulum and is manifested as potentiation of calcium release and subsequent force development during the post-extrasystolic beat. Because a fraction of the calcium that is released during this beat recirculates, the potentiation decays exponentially. The constant of decay of post-extrasystolic potentiation is determined by the fraction of calcium recirculating from beat to beat. The latter is determined by the relative rates of calcium re-uptake in the sarcoplasmic reticulum and calcium extrusion through the cell membrane, and amounts to approximately 60% of all released calcium in normal mammalian cardiac muscle. Reduction of the uptake capacity of the sarcoplasmic reticulum leads to changes in kinetics of intracellular calcium transport, slowed relaxation kinetics of the twitch and reduced twitch force as well as to a decrease of the recirculating fraction. As the recirculating fraction of activator calcium can be estimated in the intact heart, it may serve as a measure of intracellular calcium turnover in the clinical situation.

Acknowledgements

This work was supported by the Alberta Heritage Foundation for Medical Research of which the author is a Medical Scientist. The author thanks Dr H. Benediktsson for his assistance with the electronmicroscopic study of the cardiac trabeculae.

References

Allen, D. G., Eisner, D. A., Pirolo, J. S. & Smith, G. L. (1985). The relationship between intracellular calcium and contraction in calcium-overloaded ferret papillary muscles. *Journal of Physiology*, **364**, 169–82.

Armstrong, P. W., Stopps, T. P., Ford, S. E. & De Bold, A. J. (1986). Rapid ventricular pacing in the dog: pathophysiologic studies of heart failure. *Circulation*, **74**, 1075–84.

Banijamali, H. S., Gao, W.-D., MacIntosh, B. R. & ter Keurs, H. E. D. J. (1991). The force–interval relationships of twitches and cold contractures in rat cardiac trabeculae: the effect of ryanodine. *Circulation Research*, **69**, 937–48.

Bers, D. M. (1985). Ca influx and sarcoplasmic reticulum release in cardiac muscle activation during postrest recovery. *American Journal of Physiology*, **248**, H366–81.

Bers, D. M. & Bridge, J. H. B. (1989). Relaxation of rabbit ventricular muscle by Na–Ca exchange and sarcoplasmic reticulum calcium pump. *Circulation Research*, **65**, 334–42.

Bers, D. M., Bridge, J. H. B. & Spitzer, K. W. (1989). Intracellular calcium transients during rapid cooling contractures in guinea-pig ventricular myocytes. *Journal of Physiology*, **417**, 537–53.

Cohen, C. J., Fozzard, H. A. & Sheu, S-S. (1982). Increase in intracellular sodium activity during stimulation in mammalian cardiac muscle. *Circulation Research*, **50**, 651–62.

Dixon, D. A. & Haynes, D. H. (1989). Kinetic characterization of the Ca^{2+}-dumping ATPase of cardiac sarcolemma in four states of activation. *Journal of Biological Chemistry*, **264**, 13612–22.

Drake, A. J., Noble, M. I. M., Schouten, V., Seed, A., ter Keurs, H. E. D. J. & Wohlfart, B. (1982). Is action potential duration of the intact dog heart related to contractility or stimulus rate? *Journal of Physiology*, **331**, 499–510.

Drake-Holland, A. J., Noble, M. I. M., Pieterse, M., *et al.* (1983). Cardiac action potential and contractility in the intact dog heart. *Journal of Physiology*, **345**, 75–85.

Eisner, D. A. & Lederer, W. J. ((1989). The electrogenic sodium-calcium exchange. In *Sodium–calcium Exchange*, ed. T. J. A. Allen, D. Noble & H. Reuter, pp. 178–207, University Press: Oxford.

Elzinga, G., Lab, M. J., Noble, M. I. M., Papadoyannis, D., Pidgeon, J., Seed, A. & Wohlfart, B. (1981). The action potential duration and contractile response of the intact heart related to the preceding interval and the preceding beat in the dog and cat. *Journal of Physiology*, **314**, 481–500.

Fabiato, A. (1981). Myoplasmic free calcium concentration reached during the twitch of an intact isolated cardiac cell and during calcium-induced release of calcium from the sarcoplasmic reticulum of a skinned cardiac cell from the adult rat or rabbit ventricle. *Journal of General Physiology*, **78**, 457–97.

Fabiato, A. & Fabiato, F. (1975). Contractions induced by a calcium-induced release of calcium from the sarcoplasmic reticulum of single skinned cardiac cells. *Journal of Physiology*, **249**, 469–95.

Gwathmey, J. K., Copelas, L., MacKinnon, R., Schoen, F. J., Feldman, M. D., Grossman, W. & Morgan, J. P. (1987). Abnormal intracellular calcium handling by myocardium from patients with end-stage heart failure. *Circulation Research*, **61**, 70–6.

Hilgemann, D. W. (1986). Extracellular calcium transients and action potential configuration changes related to post-stimulatory potentiation in rabbit atrium. *Journal of General Physiology*, **87**, 675–706.

Ito, Y., Sutko, J. & Chidsey, C. A. (1974). Intracellular calcium and myocardial contractility. V. Calcium uptake of sarcoplasmic reticulum fragments in hypertrophied and failing rabbit hearts. *Journal of Molecular and Cellular Cardiology*, **6**, 237–47.

James, P., Inui, M., Tada, M., Chiesi, M. & Carafoli, E. (1989). Nature and site of phospholamban regulation of the Ca^{2+} pump of sarcoplasmic reticulum. *Nature*, **342**, 90–2.

Josephson, J., Sanchez-Chapula, J. & Brown, A. M. (1984). A comparison of calcium currents in rat and guinea-pig single ventricular cells. *Circulation Research*, **54**, 144–56.

Kentish, J. C., ter Keurs, H. E. D. J., Ricciardi, L., Bucx, J. J. J. & Noble, M. I. M. (1986). Comparison between the sarcomere length–force relations of intact and skinned trabeculae from rat right ventricle: influence of calcium concentrations on these relations. *Circulation Research*, **58**, 744–68.

Kort, A. A. & Lakatta, E. G. (1988). Spontaneous sarcoplasmic reticulum calcium release in rat and rabbit cardiac muscle: relation to transient and rested-state twitch tension. *Circulation Research*, **63**, 969–79.

Lee, K. S., Marban, E. & Tsien, R. W. (1985). Inactivation of calcium channels in mammalian heart cells: joint dependence on membrane potentials and intracellular calcium. *Journal of Physiology*, **364**, 395–411.

Morad, M. & Cleeman, L. (1987). Role of Ca^{2+} channel in development of tension in heart muscle. *Journal of Molecular and Cellular Cardiology*, **19**, 527–53.

Quaegebeur, J. M., Schouten, V. J. A. & ter Keurs, H. E. D. J. (1986). Mechanical restitution in isolated human myocardium. *Journal of Physiology*, **377**, 120P.

Robertson, S. P., Johnson, J. D. & Potter, J. D. (1981). The time-course of Ca^{2+} exchange with calmodulin, troponin, parvalbumin and myosin in response to transient increases in Ca^{2+}. *Biophysical Journal*, **34**, 559–69.

Schouten, V. J. A. (1985). Excitation–contraction coupling in heart muscle. PhD thesis, Leiden State University, The Netherlands.

Schouten, V. J. A., Bucx, J. J. J., de Tombe, P. P. & ter Keurs, H. E. D. J. (1990*a*). Sarcolemma, sarcoplasmic reticulum, and sarcomere as limiting factors in force production in rat heart. *Circulation Research*, **67**, 913–22.

Schouten, V. J. A., ter Keurs, H. E. D. J. & Quaegebeur, J. M. (1990*b*). Influence of electrogenic Na/Ca exchange on the action potential in human heart muscle. *Cardiovascular Research*, **24**, 758–67.

Schouten, V. J. A., van Deen, J. K., de Tombe, P. & Verveen, A. A. (1987). Force-interval relationship in heart muscle of mammals. *Biophysical Journal*, **51**, 13–26.

Seed, W. A., Noble, M. I. M., Walker, J. M., Miller, G. A. H., Pidgeon, J., Redwood, D., Wanless, R., Franz, M. R., Schoettler, M. & Schaefer, J. (1984). Relationships between beat-to-beat interval and the strength of contraction in the healthy and diseased human heart. *Circulation*, **70**, 903–10.

Sitsapesan, R., Montgomery, R. A. P., MacLeod, K. T. & Williams, A. J. (1990). Increased open probability of sheep cardiac sarcoplasmic reticulum calcium release channels induced by low temperatures. *Journal of Physiology*, **426**, 21P.

Solaro, R. J., Wise, R. M., Shiner, J. S. & Briggs, F. N. (1974). Calcium requirements for cardiac myofibrillar activation. *Circulation Research*, **34**, 525–30.

Sutko, J. L., Willerson, J. T., Templeton, G. H., Jones, L. R. & Beach, H. R. (1979). Ryanodine: its alteration of cat papillary muscle contractile state and responsiveness to inotropic interventions and a suggested mechanism of action. *Journal of Pharmacology and Experimental Therapeutics*, **209**, 37–47.

ter Keurs, H. E. D. J., Schouten, V. J. A., Bucz, J. J., Mulder, B. M. & de Tombe, P. P. (1987). Excitation–contraction coupling in myocardium: implications of calcium release and Na^+–Ca^{2+} exchange. *Canadian Journal of Physiology and Pharmacology*, **65**, 619–26.

ter Keurs, H. E. D. J., Gao, W. D., Bosker, H., Drake-Holland, A. J. & Noble, M. I. M. (1990). Characterisation of decay of frequency induced potentiation and postextrasystolic potentiation. *Cardiovascular Research*, **11**, 903–10.

Tseng, G-N. (1988). Calcium current restitution in mammalian ventricular myocytes is modulated by intracellular calcium. *Circulation Research*, **63**, 468–82.

Valdeolmillos, M., O'Neill, S. C., Smith, G. L. & Eisner, D. A. (1989). Calcium-induced calcium release activates contraction of intact cardiac cells. *Pflüger's Archiv*, **413**, 676–8.

Wier, W. G. & Yue, D. T. (1986). Intracellular calcium transients underlying the short-term force–interval relationship in ferret ventricular myocardium. *Journal of Physiology*, **376**, 507–30.

Wohlfart, B. (1979). Relationships between peak force, action potential duration and stimulus interval in rabbit myocardium. *Acta Physiologica Scandinavica*, **106**, 395–409.

The cellular basis of pulsus alternans

MAX J. LAB and C. IAN SPENCER

Prevalence

The earliest observations of mechanical alternans, defined as alternating large and small amplitude pressure or force while the heart rate is steady, were made in the clinical setting in man (see chapter by Seed, pp. 317–54). It has been experimentally studied in isolated intact hearts or ventricles (Guntheroth *et al.*, 1969; Noble & Nutter, 1970; McGaughey *et al.*, 1985), and in superfused myocardium (Mitchell, Sarnoff & Sonnenblick, 1963; Braveny, 1964; Nayler & Robertson, 1965; Lu, Lange & Brooks, 1968; Spear & Moore, 1971; Wohlfart, 1982) and continues to be so (Lab & Lee, 1990; Orchard *et al.*, 1991). The latter authors have been able to demonstrate electromechanical alternans in single isolated ventricular myocytes (Fig. 1).

Brief characteristics

Isolated myocardium can be predisposed to mechanical alternans by stimulation at a rate faster than a certain threshold (Badeer *et al.*, 1967; Lu *et al.*, 1968; Spear & Moore, 1971). The actual initiation of alternans often requires an interruption such as a pause or premature stimulus. At steady-state frequencies just below the alternans threshold, the pause or extra stimulus gives rise to transient alternans (Wohlfart, 1982), which decays over the subsequent beats. A number of interventions are known to act individually, or in combination, to lower the alternans threshold; examples are hypothermia and hypocalcaemia (Badeer *et al.*, 1967; Lu, *et al.*, 1968; Spear & Moore, 1971), and also hypercapnic acidosis (Lab & Lee, 1990; Orchard *et al.*, 1991) and the K^+ channel blocking drug 4-aminopyridine (Wohlfart, 1982).

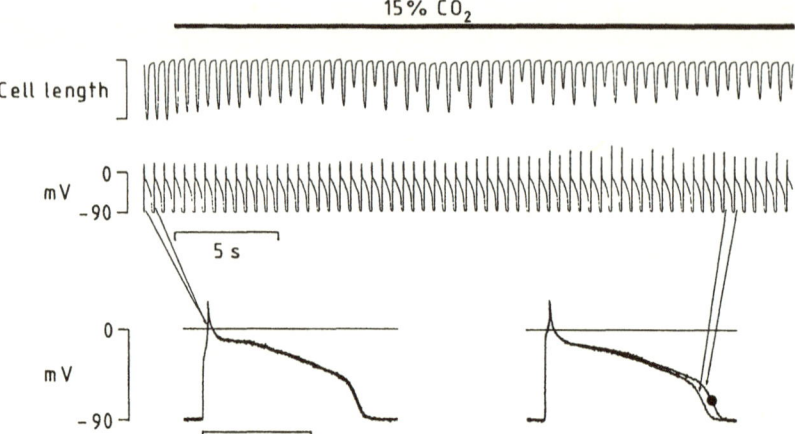

Fig. 1. Alternation of contraction strength and action potential duration in an isolated ferret ventricular myocyte. *Top panel*: Cell length and membrane potential from a myocyte generating action potentials, before and during exposure to acidosis. *Bottom panel*: Superimposed action potentials from consecutive beats under control conditions (*left*) and during acidosis-induced alternans (*right*; the action potential that accompanied the large contraction is marked with a black dot). Stimulation rate, 2 Hz. (Reproduced by permission of Orchard *et al.*, 1991 and the American Heart Association, Inc.)

Mechanisms

Many mechanisms have been proposed to account for mechanical alternans. In particular, there has been a long debate as to whether mechanical alternans is the consequence of alternations in end-diastolic muscle fibre properties (e.g. length or degree of relaxation), or whether it is an intrinsic length-independent property of the myocardium.

Alternating mechanical parameters

Most earlier studies addressing this problem led to phenomenological explanations including what has been called alternating 'deletion and potentiation' of contractility (Wiggers, 1927; Guntheroth *et al.*, 1969), and alternation in the extension of series elasticity in the muscle (Mitchell *et al.*, 1963). It has been suggested that failure of complete mechanical relaxation of the large contractions partially inhibits contractility on the alternate beats which consequently relax more fully, and then the following beat is again large and so on (Spear & Moore, 1971). It is, however, difficult to reconcile any of these theories with the current evidence for in-phase alternation of the calcium transient in mechanical alternans (Kihara & Morgan, 1987; Lab & Lee, 1990) which points to an intracellular basis for the phenomenon. Examples of more specifically intracellular mechanisms for alternans include alternation of action potential duration, and alternation in intracellular Ca^{2+}-cycling involving the sarcoplasmic reticulum (SR). These will be dealt with below.

Alternation of the action potential duration

Alternation of action potential duration (see Fig. 1) due to incomplete restitution of alternate beats could vary the calcium currents to alter SR loading and thus produce mechanical alternans. The evidence against the action potential being the primary cause of mechanical alternans is mounting. The relation between action potential duration and alternans has been studied directly and, in cases where both mechanical and electrical alternans were present, the large beat of mechanical alternans has been associated with both prolonged (Spear & Moore, 1971; Boyett & Jewell, 1978) and shortened (Spear & Moore, 1971; Wohlfart, 1982; Lu *et al.*, 1968) action potentials. Mechanical alternans may also be be found in the absence of alternation in electrical activity (Nayler & Robertson, 1965; Spear & Moore, 1971; Brooks, Gilbert & Janse, 1964; Badeer *et al.*, 1967) as was also the case in the voltage clamped myocytes of Orchard *et al.* (1991). Any electrical alternation that was observed accompanying mechanical alternans would be the result of alternation in $[Ca]_i$ (Kihara & Morgan, 1987; Lab & Lee, 1990) and thus alternation of a calcium activated current (Orchard *et al.*, 1991).

Calcium oscillations

It has been suggested that alternans is a result of synchronised spontaneous calcium releases from the SR as a manifestation of excessive calcium loading of the myocytes (Capogrossi & Lakatta, 1985). It is quite probable that, with the exception of lowering extracellular calcium, interventions which lower the alternans threshold such as increasing the stimulation frequency (for review see Lewartowski & Pytkowski, 1987), lowering the temperature (Blinks & Koch-Weser, 1963; Langer & Brady, 1969; Shattock & Bers, 1987) and hypercapnic acidosis (Allen & Orchard, 1983; Orchard, 1987), do load the myocytes with calcium. This being the case, oscillations which are synchronised with steady-state stimulation should affect the general shapes of restitution curves obtained from alternating muscles. The occurrence of oscillations at stimulus intervals close to the steady state may be expected to give a 'hump' in the restitution curve for the contraction following the small alternans beat. The evidence so far is that this is not so and restitution following both sizes of contraction has an essentially monotonic timecourse (Braveny, 1964; Mahler & Rogel, 1970; Spencer, Lab & Seed, 1991).

Restitution

In hypotheses relating to the cellular metabolism of calcium, it has been suggested that, for instance, the small contraction resulting from an extra stimulus or abrupt increase in stimulation frequency leads to mechanical alternans because the following contraction restitutes more rapidly giving rise to a large contraction and this process continues (Mahler & Rogel, 1970). It has also been suggested that conditions which promote alternans do so by slowing down mechanical restitution, which produces a weak beat (Orchard *et al.*, 1991). This is accompanied by increased transmembrane calcium entry, causing the next contraction to be large, which inhibits calcium entry, and so on. Work from our own laboratory (Spencer *et al.*, 1991) suggests that the rate of mechanical restitution is the same following the large and small contractions in alternating myocardium, and also that, under certain conditions, alternans is associated with more rapid restitution than when the muscle is stimulated at lower steady-state frequencies under the same conditions (unpublished observations from our laboratory). The work of Wohlfart (1982) suggests that the larger is a contraction, the larger is the amount of calcium which is retained by the myocardium to be released intracellularly on the subsequent beat. In this way, mechanical alternans is subject to damping.

Although mechanical alternans is clearly the result of alternation in the size of the intracellular calcium transient, the underlying cause of this calcium alternans is still unclear. It appears that the genesis of alternans results from the failure of those intracellular mechanisms which at low rates of stimulation tend to equalise the force of successive contractions.

References

Allen, D. G. & Orchard, C. H. (1983). The effects of changes of pH on intracellular Ca^{2+} transients in mammalian cardiac muscle. *Journal of Physiology*, **335**, 555–67.

Badeer, H. S., Ryo, U. Y., Gassner, W. F., Kass, E. J., Cavaluzzi, J., Gilbert,

J. L. & Brooks, C. McC. (1967). Factors affecting pulsus alternans in the rapidly driven heart and papillary muscle. *American Journal of Physiology*, **213**, 1095–101.

Blinks, J. R. & Koch-Weser, J. (1963). Physical factors in the analysis of the actions of drugs on myocardial contractions. *Pharmacological Reviews*, **15**, 531–99.

Boyett, M. R. & Jewell, B. R. (1978). A study of the factors responsible for rate-dependent shortening of the action potential in mammalian ventricular muscle. *Journal of Physiology*, **285**, 359–80.

Braveny P. (1964). The relation of alternating contractility of the heart to the inotropic effects of rhythm. *Archives Internationales de Physiologie et de Biochimie*, **72**, 553–65.

Brooks, C. McC., Gilbert, J. L. & Janse, M. J. (1964). Failure of integrated cardiac action at supernormal heart rates. *Proceedings of the Society for Experimental Biology and Medicine*, **117**, 630–4.

Capogrossi, M. C. & Lakatta, E. G. (1985). Frequency modulation and synchronisation of spontaneous oscillations in cardiac cells. *American Journal of Physiology*, **248**, H412–8.

Guntheroth, W. G., Morgan, C., McGough, G. A. & Scher, A. M. (1969). Alternate deletion and potentiation as the cause of pulsus alternans. *American Heart Journal*, **78**, 669–81.

Kihara, Y. & Morgan, J. P (1987). Abnormal intracellular calcium handling is the primary cause of pulsus alternans. *Circulation*, **76**, IV–331.

Lab, M. J. & Lee, J. (1990). Alternation in force and intracellular calcium concentration during rapid stimulation of ferret papillary muscle. *Circulation Research*, **66**, 585–95.

Langer, G. A. & Brady, A. J. (1968). The effects of temperature upon contraction and ionic exchange in rabbit ventricular myocardium. *Journal of General Physiology*, **52**, 683–713.

Lewartowski, B. & Pytkowski, B. (1987). Cellular mechanism of the relationship between myocardial force and frequency of contractions. *Progress in Biophysics and Molecular Biology*, **50**, 47–120.

Lu, H.-H., Lange, G. & Brooks, C. McC. (1968). Comparative studies of electrical and mechanical alternation in heart cells. *Journal of Electrocardiology*, **1**, 7–17.

Mahler, Y. & Rogel, S. (1970). Interrelation between restitution time constant and alternating contractility in dogs. *Clinical Science*, **39**, 625–39.

McGaughey, M. D., Maughan, W. L., Sunagawa, K. & Sagawa, K. (1985). Alternating contractility in pulsus alternans studied in the isolated çanine heart. *Circulation*, **71**, 357–62.

Mitchell, J. H., Sarnoff, S. J. & Sonnenblick, E. H. (1963). The dynamics of pulsus alternans: alternating end-diastolic fibre length as a causative factor. *Journal of Clinical Investigation*, **42**, 55–60.

Nayler, W. G. & Robertson, P. G. (1965). Mechanical alternans and the staircase phenomenon in dog papillary muscle. *American Heart Journal*, **70**, 494–8.

Noble, R. J. & Nutter, D. O. (1970). The demonstration of alternating contractile state in pulsus alternans. *Journal of Clinical Investigation*, **49**, 1166–77.

Orchard, C. H., McCall, E., Kirby, M. S. & Boyett, M. R. (1991). Mechanical alternans during acidosis in ferret heart muscle. *Circulation Research*, **68**, 69–76.

Orchard, C. H. (1987). The role of the SR in the response of ferret and rat heart muscle to acidosis. *Journal of Physiology*, **384**, 431–49.

Shattock, M. J. & Bers, D. M. (1987). Inotropic response to hypothermia and the temperature dependence of ryanodine action in isolated rabbit and rat ventricular muscle: implications for E–C coupling. *Circlation Research*, **61**, 761–71.

Spear, J. F. & Moore, E. N. (1971). A comparison of alternation in myocardial action potentials and contractility. *American Journal of Physiology*, **220**, 1708–16.

Spencer, C. I., Lab, M.J. & Seed, W. A. (1991). Restitution of mechanical force during alternans in isolated guinea-pig papillary muscles. *Journal of Physiology*, **438**, 18P.

Wiggers, C. J. (1927). The dynamics of ventricular alternation. *Annals of Clinical Medicine*, **5**, 1022–7.

Wohlfart, B. (1982). Analysis of mechanical alternans in rabbit papillary muscle. *Acta Physiologica Scandinavica*, **115**, 405–14.

Applicability of myocardial interval–force relationships to the whole ventricle: studies in isolated perfused hearts

DANIEL BURKHOFF and WILLIAM C. HUNTER

Myocardial force–interval relationships characterise alterations in contractile strength accompanying either transient or sustained changes in the interval between beats. Force–interval relationships are a direct consequence of interval-dependent calcium release to the myofilaments (Wier & Yue, 1986). Therefore, fundamental mechanisms of cardiac excitation–contraction coupling underlie force–interval relationships. While the precise relationship between indices of force–interval behaviour and the properties of subcellular processes are not totally understood at present, it has been proposed that abnormalities in force–interval relationships may reveal aberrations of subcellular processes accompanying or even causing some forms of heart disease. Consistent with this idea, results of several studies have suggested that altered force–interval relationships may be identified in hearts with various disease processes in which other abnormalities in calcium handling have also been identified (Anderson *et al.*, 1976; Anderson *et al.*, 1977; Cohn, 1980; Seed et al., 1984; Gwathmey *et al.*, 1987; Yue & Sagawa, 1987; Burkhoff *et al.*, 1988; Phillips *et al.*, 1990).

Potential problems in studying ventricular force–interval relationships

In addition to the uncertainty regarding how indices of force–interval behaviour relate to fundamental mechanisms of excitation–contraction coupling, other potental limitations arise when considering the interpretation of force–interval studies of intact ventricles (Fig. 1). Ventricular force–interval relations have as their basis the force–interval properties of the muscles which comprise the chamber. It is not surprising, therefore, that qualitative similarities between ventricular and muscle force–interval relationships are readily apparent. However, the quantitative relationship

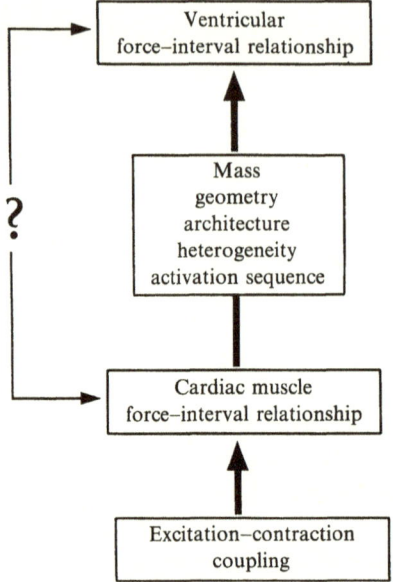

Fig. 1. Factors which determine the quantitative relationship between muscle and ventricular force–interval behaviour.

between muscle and ventricular properties is dependent upon several complex structural features of the chamber. These include:

1. the number of muscle cells comprising the chamber (mass)
2. the varying muscle fibre orientations within the ventricular wall (architecture)
3. the overall shape of the chamber (geometry)
4. the finite time required for all the cells to become activated during a contraction (activation sequence), and
5. the possibility that muscle force–interval behaviour varies from one part of the ventricle to another (heterogeneity of muscle properties).

Besides the issue of having to relate global to regional properties, other problems arise when relating ventricular and muscle force–interval relations. One example is the long-standing problem of assessing contractile strength in the intact ejecting ventricle. Changes in preload volume and afterload pressure which accompany alterations in the interval between beats may ultimately limit the use of simple indexes of contractile strength such as dP/dt_{max} (Burkhoff et al., 1984b; Burkhoff, 1985). This problem was overcome in the studies described here by constraining the hearts to contract isovolumically. The availability of techniques to measure ventricular volume continuously in the clinical setting, currently under development (Baan *et al.*, 1984), may facilitate the use of newer, less load-sensitive indexes of contractile strength such as the end-systolic pressure–volume relationship for quantifying force–interval relations (Burkhoff, 1985).

To what extent can the measurement of force–interval relationships from intact ventricles *quantitatively* reflect the force–interval relationships of the muscles that make up the ventricle? Insight into this question can be gained from comparison of:

1. right and left ventricular force–interval relationships (Burkhoff *et al.*, 1984*a*)
2. force–interval relationships measured with different activation sequences (Burkhoff & Sagawa, 1986), and
3. force–interval relationships measured from the left ventricle and an *in situ* right ventricular papillary muscle (Hunter *et al.*, unpublished observations).

Experimental approaches

The isolated, blood perfused canine heart (at 37 °C) enables the physiologically perfused myocardium to be studied under controlled haemodynamic conditions. The results of a number of studies (Burkhoff *et al.*, 1984*a*; Burkhoff, 1985; Burkhoff & Sagawa, 1986; Hunter *et al.*, unpublished observations) suggest that, despite the many complex factors involved in relating muscle and ventricular properties, it appears reasonable at least for normal canine ventricles to equate the ventricular force–interval relation to that of the muscle cells that make up the chamber.

In all of the studies, force–interval behaviour of the hearts was appraised by measuring mechanical restitution curves and post-extrasystolic potentiation curves. Hearts were paced at a constant priming rate (for 10 to 15 beats) and an extrasystolic stimulation introduced at a test pulse interval. This was followed by a second test stimulation introduced at a fixed interval which was between 700 and 1200 ms. Mechanical restitution curves were obtained by plotting the contractile response on the extrasystolic stimuli as a function of test pulse interval. The value of the test pulse interval was varied between 300 and 2000 ms from one run to the next. Post-extrasystolic potentiation curves were obtained by plotting the post-extrasystolic response as a function of test pulse interval.

Contractile strength on test beats was quantified by maximal developed pressure (P_{max}) and maximal rate of rise of pressure (dP/dt_{max}) and, for the case of the papillary muscles, maximal developed force (F_{max}). In all cases, each index of contractile strength was normalised by the strength of the steady-state contractions that preceded the test beat.

Right versus left ventricular force–interval relationships

Comparisons between right and left ventricular force–interval relationships from isolated hearts can be used to assess, indirectly, the influence of muscle mass and ventricular chamber geometry on the global expression of the force–interval relationships. Both chambers were constrained to contract isovolumically. Both chambers exhibited alterations in contractile strength with changes in pacing interval that are typical of cardiac muscle. In order to adjust for differences in absolute pressure generating capabilities, related predominantly to differences in muscle mass, P_{max} and dP/dt_{max} of extra- and post-extrasystolic contractions were normalised to their respective values on the preceding steady-state contractions in the respective ventricle. Typical examples of right and left ventricular mechanical restitution curves and post-extrasystolic potentiation curves are shown in Fig. 2(a) and 2(b). As shown, right and left ventricular normalised dP/dt_{max} values were nearly superimposable on both extra- and post-extrasystolic contractions. In order to quantify the degree of similarity, the normalised right ventricular responses were plotted as a function of the normalised left ventricular responses on all the test beats. These data points fell very close to the line of identity (dotted line, Fig. 2(c)).

The degree of similarity between right ventricular and left ventricular force–interval relationships was quantified by applying linear regression analysis to these data. Mean ($\pm$ S.D.) results from these studies revealed that $dP/dt_{max,RV} = 0.96 \pm 0.05 \, dP/dt_{max,LV} + 4.79 \pm 3.79\%$ (with r^2 ranging between 0.986 and 0.999), where $dP/dt_{max,RV}$ and $dP/dt_{max,LV}$ are the normalised maximal rate of rise of right and left ventricular pressures on test beats, respectively. Similar results were obtained if normalised P_{max} was used as the index of contractile strength instead of dP/dt_{max}. $P_{max,RV} = 0.96 \pm 0.05 \, P_{max,LV} + 4.24 \pm 4.31\%$ (with r^2 ranging between 0.987 and 0.999).

Thus despite the marked differences in right and left ventricular mass, geometry, and potential difference in muscle properties, the force–interval relations of the two chambers are practically indistinguishable.

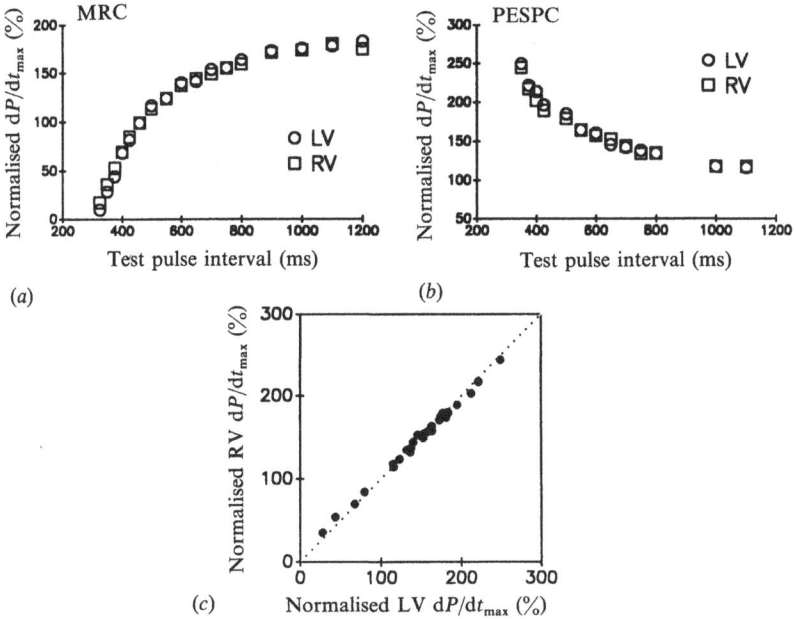

Fig. 2. Mechanical restitution curves (MRC, panel (*a*)) and post-extrasystolic potentiation curves (PESPC, panel (*b*)) measured from the right (RV) and left (LV) ventricles of a single isolated heart. The degree of similarity between the force–interval relations of the RV and LV was quantified by plotting the normalised responses of the RV as a function of the responses of the LV (panel (*c*)). These data points fell very close to the line of identity (dotted line). (Adapted from Burkhoff *et al.*, 1984*a*.)

Influence of pacing site on the force–interval relationships

The influence of activation sequence on the global expression of the force–interval relation can be assessed by measurement of mechanical restitution curves and post-extrasystolic potentiation curves from iso-volumically contracting isolated left ventricles, with the hearts paced from five different sites, namely the atrium, right ventricular endocardium, right ventricular free wall, left ventricular free wall and left ventricular apex. The order in which each of the pacing sites was tested was randomised from one experiment to the next. Representative pressure and surface electrocardiographic recordings (Fig. 3) reveal that the absolute strength of the steady-state, extrasystolic and post-extrasystolic contractions varied with pacing site. Similarly, absolute values of dP/dt_{max} were also influenced by pacing site. A separate analysis (Burkhoff, Oikawa & Sagawa 1986) indicated that there was an inverse relationship between steady-state

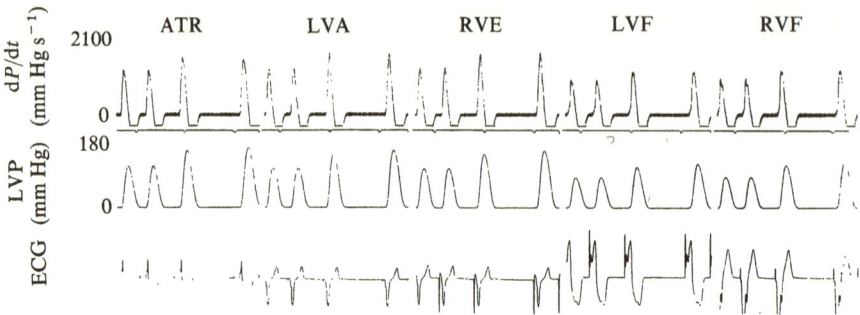

Fig. 3. Left ventricular pressure (LVP), the first derivative with respect to time of LVP (dP/dt) and surface electrogram (ECG) obtained from a representative heart in which the interval between beats was altered with the heart paced from various sites. Absolute strength on steady-state and test beats varied inversely with the duration of the QRS complex. ATR: atrium, LVA: left ventricular apex, RVE: right ventricular endocardium, LVF: left ventricular free wall epicardium, RVF: right ventricular free wall epicardium. (From Burkhoff et al., 1986 with permission.)

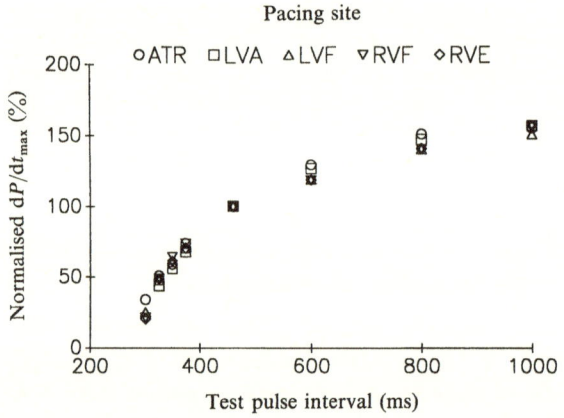

Fig. 4. Mechanical restitution curve obtained from a single heart while pacing from the five different sites on the heart. With contractile strength quantified by maximal rate of pressure rise, normalised to that of the steady-state contractions, the MRC was fairly insensitive to activation sequence. Key: as for Fig. 3. (Adapted from Burkhoff et al., 1986.)

contractile strength and the duration of the QRS deflection of the surface electrocardiogram.

Typical mechanical restitution curves from a single ventricle obtained while pacing from each of the five sites on the heart are shown in Fig. 4

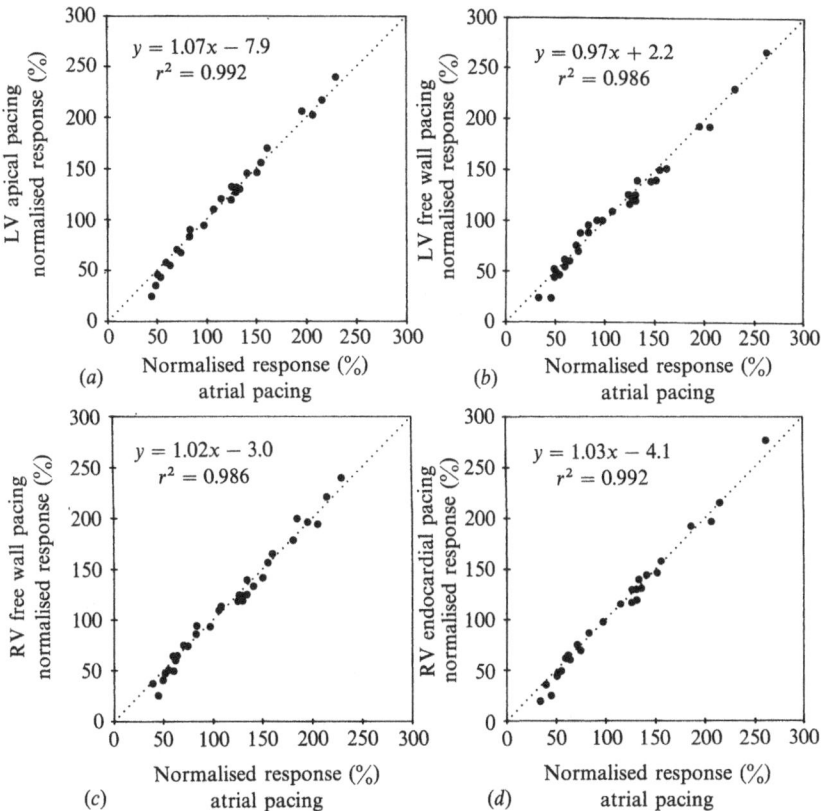

Fig. 5. Normalised extrasystolic and post-extrasystolic dP/dt_{max} responses obtained with ventricular pacing were compared to those obtained with atrial pacing at corresponding test pulse intervals. Summary of results obtained from six ventricles. Similarity between responses was quantified by linear regression analysis, the results of which are presented in each panel. Dotted lines are lines of identity. (From Burkhoff *et al.*, 1986 with permission.)

(steady-state heart rate of 130 beats/min). When dP/dt_{max} values on the test beats were normalised by dP/dt_{max} on the preceding steady-state contractions obtained with the same pacing site, the mechanical restitution curves became very similar.

Results from six hearts studied in this series were summarised by plotting normalised dP/dt_{max} on test beats obtained with ventricular pacing as a function of normalised dP/dt_{max} on test beats with the same values of test pulse interval measured during atrial pacing (Fig. 5). In each case, the normalised responses on test beats were very similar between atrial and ventricular pacing (regression analyses summarised in each panel of the figure). A comparable degree of similarity was noted if normalised P_{max} was used in the analysis instead of dP/dt_{max}.

Thus, when contractile strengths of test beats are normalised by the strength of steady-state contractions (with both having the same activation sequence), the ventricular force–interval relationship was relatively insensitive to changes in activation sequence.

Ventricular versus *in situ* right ventricular papillary muscle force–interval relationships

In order to make a more direct comparison between muscle and ventricular properties, force–interval relationships were compared simultaneously in the left ventricle and from an *in situ* right ventricular papillary muscle. It was reasoned that, if these force–interval relationships were different, it could be a consequence of any number of the factors summarised in Fig. 1. However, if the force–interval relationships were the same, it would support the idea that these structural factors do not distort the global expression of the muscle force–interval relationship.

Typical experimental recordings are shown in Fig. 6. There is a striking similarity between the contours of the ventricular isovolumic pressure tracing and the isometric force tracing from the right ventricular papillary muscle. The mechanical restitution curves and post-extrasystolic potentiation curves from one experiment, when quantified by normalising peak pressure and force (see Fig. 7), reveal the near identity of the left ventricular and right ventricular papillary muscle force–interval relations.

The similarity between left and right ventricular papillary muscle force–interval relations were quantified by plotting the normalised right ventricular papillary muscle force on test beats versus normalised left ventricular pressure and applying linear regression analysis. The pooled results from eight ventricles showed that: $P_{max,LV} = 1.00\, F_{max,RVPM} + 0.5\%$ ($r^2 = 0.983$), where $P_{max,LV}$ is the normalised developed pressure of the left ventricle and $F_{max,RVPM}$ is the normalised peak force of the right ventricular papillary muscle.

Thus, despite the marked complexity in ventricular structure, activation sequence and possible heterogeneity of muscle properties throughout the ventricle, the left ventricular force–interval relationship is indistinguishable from that of right ventricular papillary muscle of the same heart.

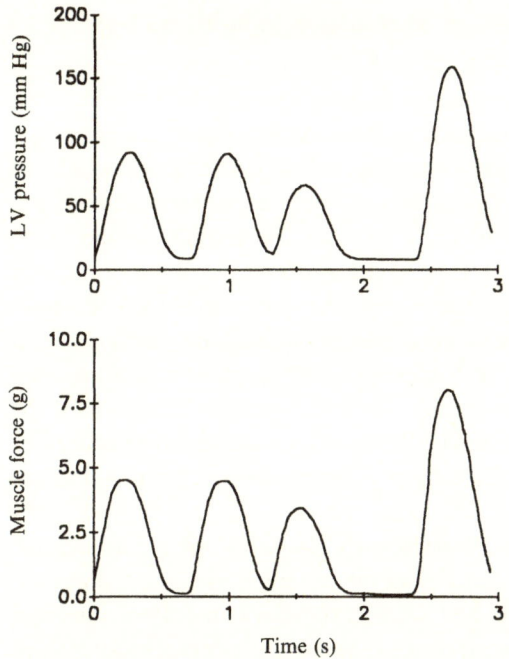

Fig. 6. Typical experimental recordings of isovolumic left ventricular pressure and right ventricular papillary muscle force obtained while varying the interval between beats.

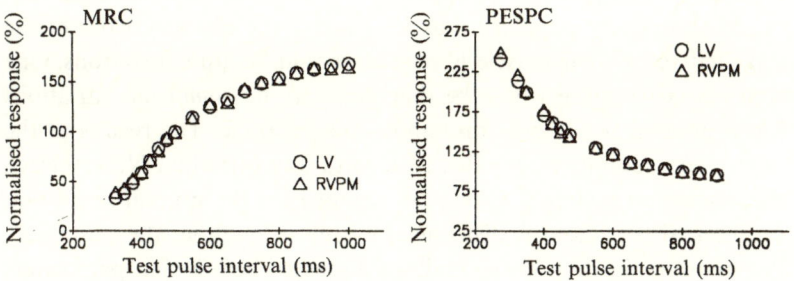

Fig. 7. Mechanical restitution curves (MRC) and post-extrasystolic potentiation curves (PESPC) measured simultaneously from an isovolumically contracting left ventricle and an isometrically contracting *in situ* right ventricular papillary muscle.

What is the meaning of force–interval relationships measured from papillary muscle or the ventricle?

In order to interpret force–interval relationships measured from the intact ventricle within the same framework as muscle force–interval relations, it must be determined how muscle force–interval properties are transformed into ventricular properties. The results of three experiments have been discussed which support the idea, at least for the normal canine heart, that the complex structural factors of the ventricle do not significantly distort the global expression of the muscle fibre force–interval behaviour. Right and left ventricles have different muscle masses and vastly different geometries yet, when *normalised* indexes of contractile strength are used to quantify responses to test stimuli, the force–interval relations of the two chambers are indistinguishable. When activation sequence is drastically altered by pacing the heart from different sites, absolute strength varies, but the *normalised* contractile response on extra- and post-extrasystolic contractions is not significantly altered. There are no significant differences between the force–interval relations measured simultaneously from the left ventricle and from a papillary muscle of the right ventricle. In each case, any dependence of the force–interval relationships on structural features of the ventricle *cancelled out* when contractile strength of test stimuli were *normalised* by the contractile strength on the preceding steady-state contractions measured under the same conditions.

The problem introduced by the potential of heterogeneous muscle force–interval properties deserves further mention. Any measure of global ventricular function reflects an average behaviour of all its muscle cells. If there were large regional differences in force–interval behaviour, then how could the equivalence of the left ventricular and papillary muscle force–interval relationships be explained? One possibility would be that the right ventricular papillary muscles possess the characteristics of the average left ventricular muscle fibre. This would be quite fortuitous. One alternative explanation would be that there are no *significant* variations in force–interval behaviour throughout the ventricle. The results of the present study cannot resolve this issue with any certainty. Nevertheless, in the discussion to follow it will be assumed for the normal heart that force–interval behaviour is distributed evenly throughout the ventricle.

The main implication of the findings discussed here is that parameters which characterise force–interval relations measured from the intact ventricle may accurately and quantitatively characterise muscle properties. Two specific examples follow:

Implications for mechanical restitution

First, mechanical restitution curves measured from isovolumically contracting isolated dog hearts can be characterised by three parameters:

1. time constant of restitution (τ)
2. plateau value, referred to as maximum contractile response (CR_{max}) and,
3. a minimum test pulse interval at which a contraction can be elicited (t_0).

An example of how the mechanical restitution curve is altered by increasing the pacing rate during the priming period from 70 to 130 beats/min is shown in Fig. 8(a) (Burkhoff et al., 1984b). With the higher steady-state heart rate, CR_{max} increases (the curve increases in amplitude), t_0 decreases (the curve shifts towards the left) and the time constant of mechanical restitution is unaffected. 't_0' has been hypothesised to reflect a period of the cardiac cycle during which calcium is sequestered in an unreleasable storage site within the sarcoplasmic reticulum (Gibbons & Fozzard, 1971; Kaufmann et al., 1974; and see chapters by Wohlfart et al. and by Jóhannsson in this book), whilst τ reflects the time constant with which calcium can move (either functionally or physically) from its unreleasable state to a releasable state (Kaufmann et al., 1974; Wohlfart, 1979, 1982). The plateau of the mechanical restitution curve reflects the total amount of calcium available for release from the sarcoplasmic reticulum if enough time is allowed between beats (Edman & Jóhannsson, 1976; Wohlfart, 1979, 1982; Burkhoff et al., 1984b; Yue et al., 1985). According to the hypothesis set forth above, it follows that the values obtained for each of these parameters, and the nature of their variations with priming frequency, are *quantitatively* indicative of the corresponding measurement at the muscle level and ultimately reflect fundamental aspects of excitation– contraction coupling.

Implications for recirculation fraction

A second example is the beat-dependent decay of contractile strength following an abrupt decrease in pacing rate. In the example of Fig. 8(b), pacing rate was decreased abruptly from 130 to 60 beats per minute. At the point when heart rate is decreased, there is an initial increase (pause potentiation), followed by a beat-by-beat decrease in contractile strength. The linear relationship between developed pressure on a given beat DP_k and the developed pressure on the following beat DP_{k+1} for each beat

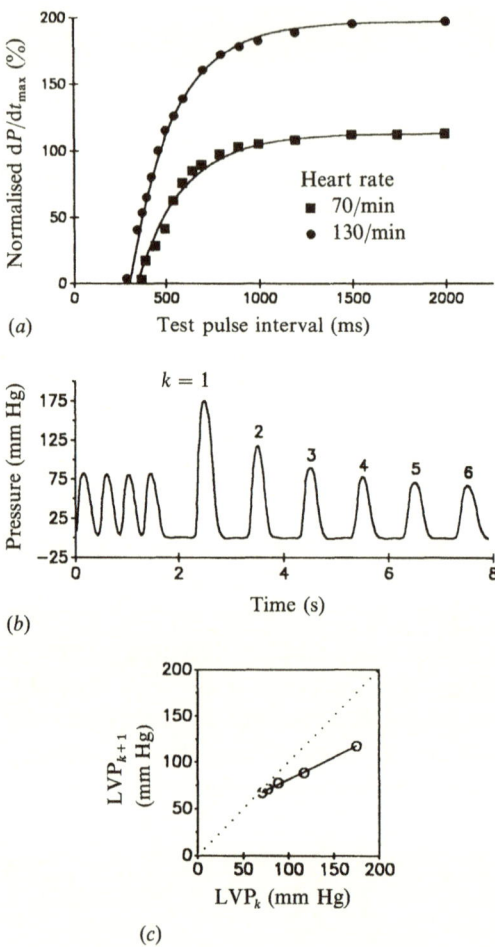

Fig. 8. Examples highlighting how parameters which characterise force–interval relations measured from intact ventricles can be interpreted within the framework of excitation–contraction mechanisms. (*a*) The influence of steady-state pacing (two rates) on the mechanical restitution curve. (*b*) Alterations in developed pressure measured following a switch in pacing rate from 130/min to 60/min (*k* signifies the beat number after the switch in rate). (*c*) Plot of peak pressure (LVP) on beat *k* + 1 as a function of LVP on beat *k* for the contractions following the switch in pacing rate in panel (*b*). The regression slope is called the *recirculation fraction*. The line of identity is indicated by dots.

in the series (Fig. 8(c)) indicates, as is true for isolated muscle (Wood, Heppner & Weidmann, 1969; Morad & Goldman, 1973; Wohlfart, 1979), that contractile strength decays in a beat-dependent monoexponential manner. This permits calculation of an exponential decay constant which has been referred to as the *recirculation fraction* (see pp. 266–7). The recirculation fraction is believed to quantify the fraction of calcium released to the myofilament that is sequestered by the sarcoplasmic reticulum (Morad & Goldman, 1973). Here, too, it is asserted that the value obtained for the recirculation fraction quantitatively reflects the value of this parameter for the ventricular muscle cells.

Implications for the human heart

One limitation of the experiments described is that all studies were performed in normal canine hearts. Human hearts are obviously larger, may have a different geometry and the activation time is longer. In most forms of human heart disease, these factors become even more disparate from the canine heart. Furthermore, human heart disease may introduce obvious inhomogeneities of muscle properties. Thus, questions may still arise regarding quantitative equivalence of muscle and ventricular force–interval relations in the clinical setting.

In one previous study, force–interval relations were measured from explanted diseased human hearts, obtained at the time of orthotopic heart transplant, with various forms of end-stage cardiomyopathy (Yue & Sagawa, 1987; Burkhoff *et al.*, 1988). The left ventricles of these hearts were fitted with balloons and studied in a manner similar to the way the canine hearts were studied. In addition, thin trabeculae were excised and studied in a muscle bath. Striking similarities were identified in the force–interval relationships measured from the ventricle (Fig. 9) and from the muscle (Fig. 10). This included the heart of one patient with idiopathic restrictive cardiomyopathy which demonstrated no change in contractile strength on extrasystoles and no post-extrasystolic potentiation. In contrast, the force–interval behaviour of ventricles and isolated muscles from hearts with idiopathic dilated cardiomyopathy exhibited expected variations in force with changes in pacing interval. These observations were obtained in both intact ventricle and in the isolated muscle. The findings from the restrictive cardiomyopathic heart were interpreted as suggesting a marked abnormality in sarcoplasmic reticular function. Further support for this hypothesis was obtained from the findings that addition of ryanodine (a specific sarcoplasmic reticulum blocker) eliminated the

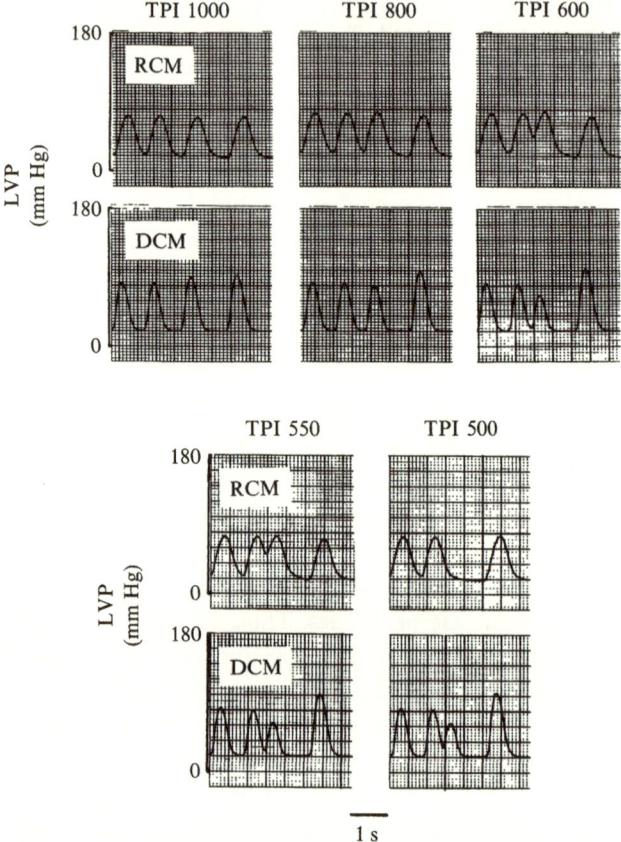

Fig. 9. Left ventricular pressure (LVP) measured from two isolated, isovolumic-ally contracting human hearts while the interval between beats was varied. RCM: end-state idiopathic restrictive cardiomyopathy. DCM: end-state idiopathic dilated cardiomyopathy. TPI: test pulse interval, which precedes the third beat on each record. (From Burkhoff *et al.*, 1988, with permission.)

force–interval relationship in muscle from the dilated cardiomyopathic heart (Fig 10, middle panel), but had almost no effect on the muscle from the restrictive cardiomyopathic heart (not shown here; see Yue & Sagawa, 1987). Other observations which could be ascribed to sarcoplasmic reticular dysfunction were identified in these hearts (see Yue & Sagawa, 1987; Burkhoff *et al.*, 1988). While these findings cannot serve to address the quantitative similarity between muscle and ventricular properties in human hearts, they do indicate, for a case of markedly abnormal behaviour, that the same conclusion regarding force–interval properties

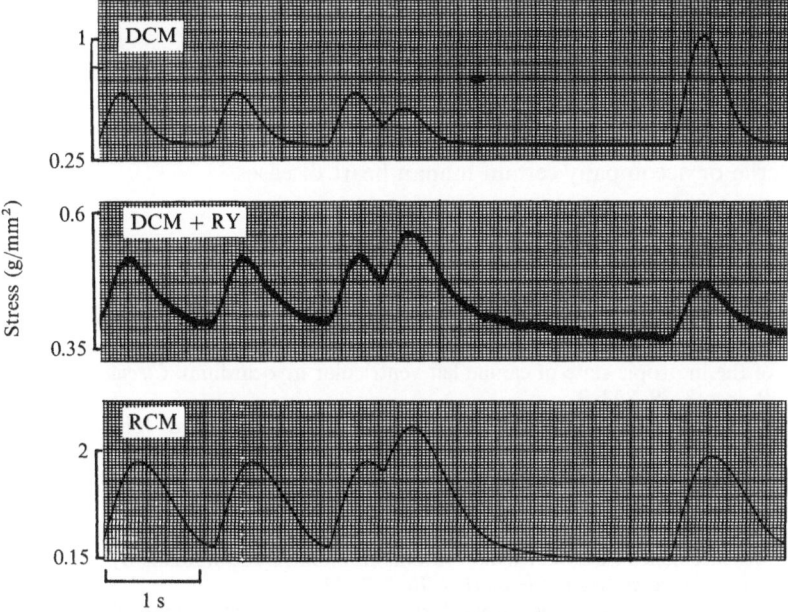

Fig. 10. Muscle stress measured from isometrically contracting thin trabeculae of human myocardium taken from one patient with idiopathic restrictive cardiomyopathy (RCM) and from one patient with idiopathic dilated cardiomyopathy (DCM). The middle panel shows the effect of ryanodine in DCM. (Adapted from Yue & Sagawa, 1988.)

can be obtained from the intact ventricle with its complex structural characteristics and from isolated muscle.

Conclusion

The problem of relating global ventricular properties to the properties of the muscles within the wall of the chamber is not unique to the interpretation of the force–interval relationship. Yet, in this regard, it may be simpler to extract such information from measurements of force–interval relations than other aspects of cardiac physiology since many of the complex factors appear to cancel out when normalised indexes of contractile strength are used to assess the ventricular responses. This contrasts with the immense task of attempting to relate ventricular pressure–volume characteristics to muscle force–length properties in absolute terms. Therefore, the ventricular force–interval relationship may offer a means of assessing certain aspects of cardiac muscle excitation–

contraction coupling in the clinical setting, that are independent of the structural features of the heart.

As understanding of the mechanisms which underlie force–interval relations improves, the clinical evaluation of such relations may result in new research tools for uncovering abnormalities in cellular processes that underlie or accompany certain human heart diseases.

References

Anderson, P. A. W., Rankin, J. S., Arentzen, C. E., Anderson, R. W. & Johnson, E. A. (1976). Evaluation of the force–frequency relationship as a descriptor of the inotropic state of canine left ventricular myocardium. *Circulation Research*, **39**, 832–9.

Anderson, P. A. W., Manring, A., Arentzen, C. E., Rankin, J. S. & Johnson, E. A. (1977). Pressure-induced hypertrophy of cat right ventricle: an evaluation with the force–interval relationship. *Circulation Research*, **41**, 582–8.

Baan, J., van der Velde, E. T., DeBruin, H. G., Smeenk, G. J., Koops, J., Van Dijk, A. D., Temmerman, D., Senden, J. & Buis, B. (1984). Continuous measurement of left ventricular volume in animals and humans by conductance catheter. *Circulation*, **70**, 812–23.

Burkhoff, D. (1985). The myocardial force–interval relationship studied in isolated canine hearts (PhD Thesis). Baltimore: The Johns Hopkins University.

Burkhoff, D., Flaherty, J. T., Yue, D. T., Herskowitz, A., Oikawa, R. Y., Sugiura, S., Franz, M. R., Baumgartner, W. A., Schaefer, J., Reitz, B. A. & Sagawa, K. (1988). *In vitro* studies of isolated supported human hearts. *Heart and Vessels*, **45**, 185–96.

Burkhoff, D., Oikawa, R. Y. & Sagawa, K. (1986). Influence of pacing site on canine left ventricular contraction. *American Journal of Physiology*, **251**, H428–35.

Burkhoff, D. & Sagawa, K. (1986). Influence of pacing site on canine left ventricular force–interval relationship. *American Journal of Physiology*, **250**, H414–18.

Burkhoff, D., Yue, D. T., Franz, M. R., Hunter, W. C. & Sagawa, K. (1984a). Quantitative comparison of the force–interval relationships of the canine right and left ventricles. *Circulation Research*, **54**, 468–73.

Burkhoff, D., Yue, D. T., Franz, M. R., Hunter, W. C. & Sagawa, K. (1984b). Mechanical restitution of isolated perfused canine left ventricles. *American Journal of Physiology*, **246**, H8–16.

Cohn, P. F. (1980). Editorial: Evaluation of inotropic contractile reserve in ischemic heart disease using postextrasystolic potentiation. *Circulation*, **61**, 1071–5.

Edman, K. A. P. & Jóhannsson, M. (1976). The contractile state of rabbit papillary muscle in relation to stimulation frequency. *Journal of Physiology*, **254**, 565–81.

Gibbons, W. R. & Fozzard, H. A. (1971). Voltage dependence and time dependence of contraction in sheep cardiac Purkinje fibers. *Circulation Research*, **28**, 446–60.

Gwathmey, J. K., Copelas, L. MacKinnon, R., Schoen, F. J., Feldman, M. D., Grossman, W. & Morgan, J. P. (1987). Abnormal intracellular calcium handling in myocardium from patients with end-stage heart failure. *Circulation Research*, **61**, 70–6.

Kaufmann, R., Bayer, R., Furniss, T., Krause, H. & Tritthart, H. (1974). Calcium-movement controlling cardiac contractility II. Analog computation of cardiac excitation–contraction coupling on the basis of calcium kinetics in multi-compartment model. *Journal of Molecular and Cellular Cardiology*, **6**, 543–59.

Morad, M. & Goldman, Y. (1973). Excitation–contraction coupling in heart muscle: membrane control of development of tension. *Progress in Biophysics and Molecular Biology*, **27**, 257–313.

Phillips, P. J., Gwathmey, J. K., Feldman, M. D., Schoen, F. J., Grossman, W. & Morgan, J. P. (1990). Post-extrasystolic potentiation and the force–frequency relationship: differential augmentation of myocardial contractility in working myocardium from patients with end-stage heart failure. *Journal of Molecular & Cellular Cardiology*, **22**, 99–110.

Seed, W. A., Noble, M. I. M., Walker, J. M., Miller, G. A. H., Pidgeon, J., Redwood, D., Wanless, R., Franz, M. R., Schoettler, M. & Schaefer, J. (1984). Relationships between beat-to-beat interval and the strength of contraction in the healthy and diseased human heart. *Circulation*, **70**, 799–805.

Suga, H. & Sagawa, K. (1974). Instantaneous pressure–volume relationships and their ratio in the excised, supported canine left ventricle. *Circulation Research*, **35**, 117–26.

Suga, H. & Sagawa, K. (1977). End-diastolic and end-systolic ventricular volume clamper for isolated canine heart. *American Journal of Physiology*, **233**, H718–22.

Wier, W. G. & Yue, D. T. (1986). Intracellular calcium transients underlying the short-term force–interval relationship in ferret ventricular myocardium. *Journal of Physiology*, **376**, 507–30.

Wohlfart, B. (1979). Relationships between peak force, action potential duration and stimulus interval in rabbit myocardium. *Acta Physiologica Scandinavica*, **106**, 395–409.

Wohlfart, B. (1982). Interval–strength relations of mammalian myocardium interpreted as altered kinetics of activator calcium during the cardiac cycle (PhD Thesis). Lund: University of Lund.

Wood, E. H., Heppner, R. L. & Weidmann, S. (1969). Inotropic effects of electric currents: 2. Hypotheses: calcium movements, excitation–contraction coupling and inotropic effects. *Circulation Research*, **24**, 409–45.

Yue, D. T., Burkhoff, D., Franz, M. R., Hunter, W. C. & Sagawa, K. (1985). Postextrasystolic potentiation of the isolated canine left ventricle: relationship to mechanical restitution. *Circulation Research*, **56**, 340–50.

Yue, D. T. & Sagawa, K. (1987). Insight into excitation–contraction coupling of heart derived from studies of the force–interval relationship. In *Activation, Metabolism and Perfusion of the Heart*, ed. S. Sideman & R. Beyar, pp. 261–277. Dordrecht: Martinus Nijhoff.

Interval–force effects in the pulse variation of atrial fibrillation: a statistical approach

K. P. PFEIFFER, T. KENNER and
S. M. HARDMAN

Introduction

Since the early work of Bowditch (1871), there has been consistent interest in the behaviour and mechanisms of the interval–force relationships of cardiac tissue. Much of the work has been performed in isolated tissue, but there is an important body of work from intact animal preparations and indeed from man showing that, where appropriate pacing or stimulation protocols have been employed, post-extrasystolic potentiation, mechanical restitution and frequency potentiation can be demonstrated with clarity (see chapter by Seed, pp. 317–54). However, the range of intervals studied in the intact heart is necessarily limited by the spontaneous rate and rhythm and another approach is to record from man during arrhythmias such as atrial fibrillation and then to try to extract information from these data about interval–force relationships (Meijler, 1986; Pfeiffer, Kenner & Schaefer, 1984). But there are difficulties inherent in this approach as well. For example, a short interval followed by a long one will cause potentiation of the beat following the long interval. If, however, the short interval is followed by another short interval, restitution will be incomplete and this will mask the potentiation. As the influence of more and more beats is considered, the analysis of interval–force relationships in atrial fibrillation becomes extremely difficult, and yet the attractions of deriving these relationships from patients with this arrhythmia are severalfold. Atrial fibrillation is a common arrhythmia and so such studies might be of interest to clinicians and physiologists alike. Specifically, because the arrhythmia occurs naturally and pacing is avoided, the spread of excitation follows the usual sequence rather than a pacing induced sequence. Finally, the actual range of intervals observed may exceed those which could be obtained in pacing experiments.

In this chapter a study in patients with atrial fibrillation is described and illustrates, with data from a typical patient, the methods by which interval– force relationships can be extracted from beat by beat recordings of ventricular function. In particular the use of statistical modelling to examine mechanical restitution and post-extrasystolic potentiation, and to assess the historical contribution of earlier beats, is discussed. It will be demonstrated that all such force–interval phenomena can be reproduced by this modelling without resort to conventional pacing protocols.

Patients and data

Patients with atrial fibrillation, but without mitral regurgitation, were studied during diagnostic cardiac catheterisation. A catheter was positioned to record high fidelity left ventricular pressure through a catheter tip manometer whilst an electromagnetic flowmeter set several centimetres proximally in the catheter (Mills & Shillingford, 1967) was used to record simultaneous aortic blood velocity. A surface electrocardiogram was recorded as a time base for the cardiac cycle, the interval between beats being measured as the RR interval for consecutive beats. Differentiation of the left ventricular pressure signal allowed the maximum rate of rise of left ventricular pressure (LV dP/dt_{max}) to be determined as a measure of contractility (Drake-Holland *et al.*, 1990). From the aortic velocity signal the systolic velocity integral was derived, which is proportional to stroke volume, but for the sake of simplicity most of the analyses are restricted to LV dP/dt_{max} rather than ejection indices. The data in all the subsequent examples are from a patient who had been in atrial fibrillation for several years and in whom attempted cardioversion was unsuccessful. The clinical diagnosis was of an alcoholic cardiomyopathy and the left heart catheter was performed to exclude coronary artery disease. His only medication at the time of investigation was digoxin.

Results

Descriptive analysis of relationships between successive beats

In each patient, one or more sequences of at least 100 consecutive beats free of ectopics were selected from the recorded data. The presence of ectopics dominates the mechanical response because of the abnormal spread of excitation that occurs and so obscures the interval–force relationships. These sequences were analysed in descriptive terms by plotting scattergrams. The first example shows a plot of preceding interval

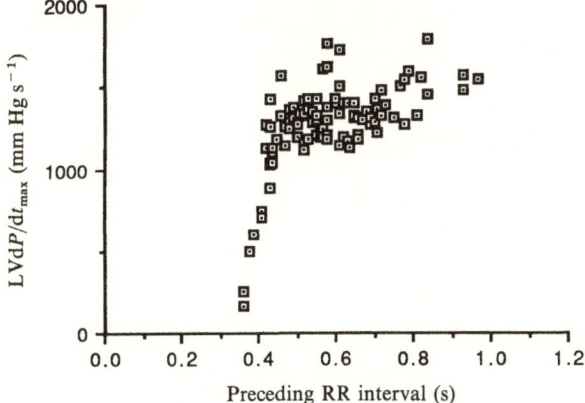

Fig. 1. Mechanical restitution during spontaneous atrial fibrillation. All data points for 105 consecutive beats are plotted.

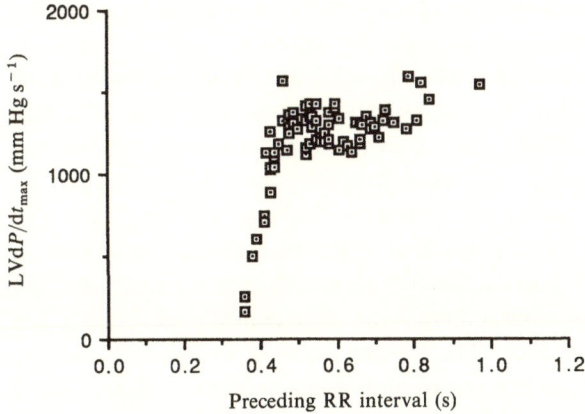

Fig. 2. Mechanical restitution during atrial fibrillation. Data gated to exclude points with pre-preceding intervals of less than 500 ms.

against LV dP/dt_{max} to examine for the presence or absence of mechanical restitution (see Fig. 1). Two observations are immediately evident; the first that mechanical restitution is present and the second that there is considerable 'scatter'. It was found that this 'scatter' could be reduced by imposing a form of gating, whereby limitations were set on pre-preceding intervals. Thus if preceding interval against LV dP/dt_{max} was plotted for those beats which had a pre-preceding interval of more than 500 milliseconds, as in Fig. 2, there was a reduction in the 'scatter'. These

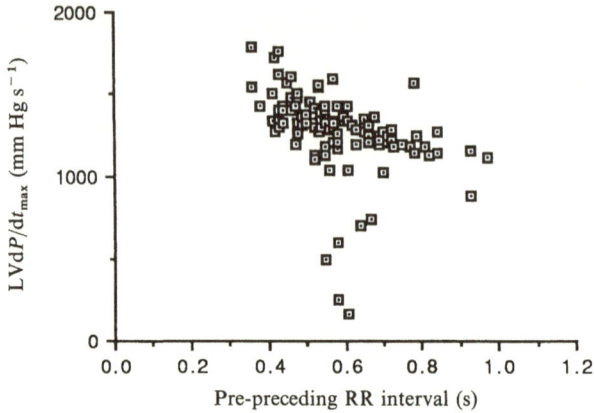

Fig. 3. Post-extrasystolic potentiation during spontaneous atrial fibrillation. All data points plotted.

results are consistent with an effect of post-extrasystolic potentiation being superimposed on the mechanical restitution curve.

The same approach was used when looking for a relationship between pre-preceding interval and the mechanical response. Fig. 3 shows a plot of all the data points. Whilst there is evidence of an inverse relationship between pre-preceding interval and contractility there is also 'scatter'. In this case those beats where the preceding interval was less than 500 milliseconds were gated out. The effect of this manoeuvre can be seen in Fig. 4 and suggests that in atrial fibrillation the effects of post-extrasystolic potentiation can be obscured if there is incomplete mechanical restitution of the beat being examined. The 'scatter' can be reduced further by excluding data for which the pre-pre-preceding interval is short. Fig. 5 shows the additional effect of gating out all points where the pre-pre-preceding interval is less than 500 milliseconds. This suggests that the effects of potentiation are still present two beats after a short beat during spontaneous atrial fibrillation. This is consistent with the observation that, during steady pacing in man, it may take up to six beats before the decay of potentiation resulting from a single short interval is complete (Seed *et al.*, 1984).

These results demonstrate the powerful relationships between preceding intervals and contractile force in atrial fibrillation and they suggest that factors influencing the beat to beat variation in contractility include mechanical restitution, and post-extrasystolic potentiation decaying over a number of beats.

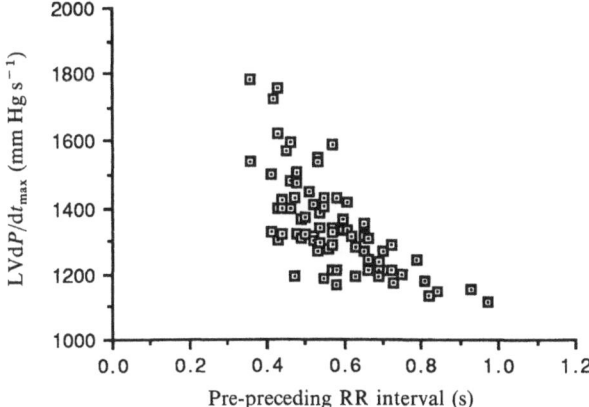

Fig. 4. Post-extrasystolic potentiation during atrial fibrillation. Data gated to exclude beats with preceding intervals of less than 500 ms. Note that the ordinate is scaled differently from Fig. 3.

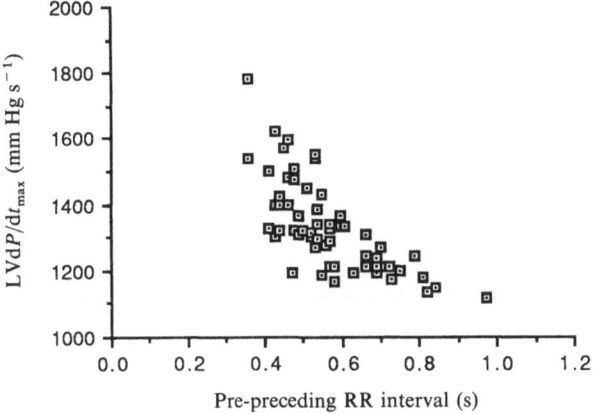

Fig. 5. Post-extrasystolic potentiation during atrial fibrillation. Data gated to exclude beats with preceding intervals and pre-pre-preceding intervals of less than 500 ms.

The same approach can be used to examine these influences on other variables, and to give one additional example, pre-preceding interval was plotted against systolic velocity integral as in Figs. 6 and 7. These results suggest that the pre-preceding interval not only has an inverse relationship with contractility but also with ejection indices and that this relationship is most clearly demonstrated on beats that are fully or near fully restituted.

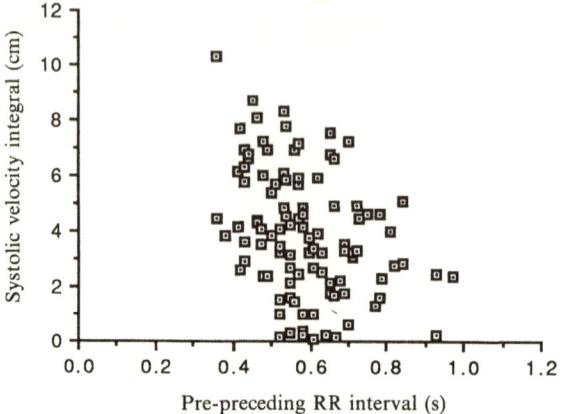

Fig. 6. The inverse relationship between pre-preceding interval and systolic velocity integral during spontaneous atrial fibrillation. All data points plotted.

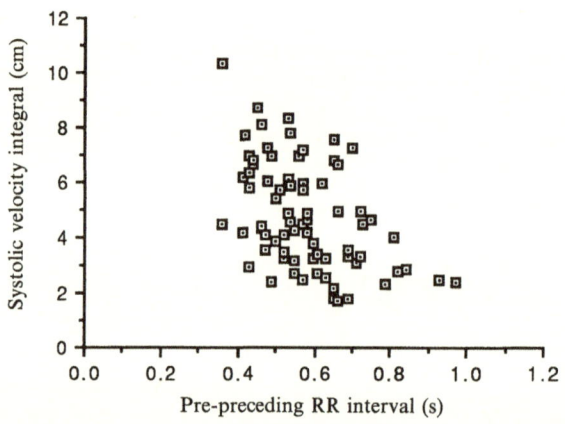

Fig. 7. The inverse relationship between pre-preceding interval and systolic velocity integral during atrial fibrillation. Data gated to exclude beats with a preceding interval of less than 500 ms.

Modelling and simulating the interval–force relationship

An analysis of sequences of RR intervals in patients with atrial fibrillation did not show any substantial dependence of RR interval on any properties of preceding beats. An example of the lack of correlation between RR interval and dP/dt_{max} of the preceding beat is shown in Fig. 8. This exclusivity of the RR interval is important for modelling and simulation,

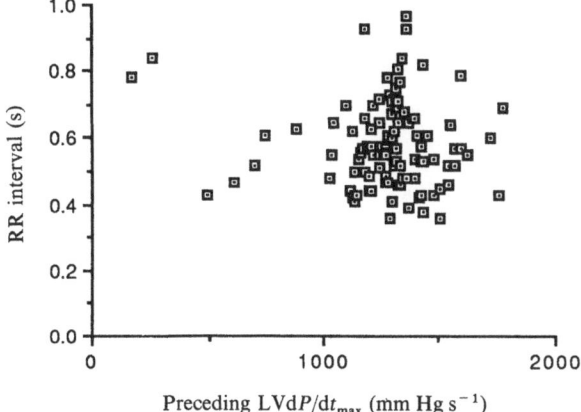

Fig. 8. The lack of dependence of RR interval on the preceding LV dP/dt_{max}.

because the demonstration that RR interval is a randomly determined, independent function allows its use as an input variable.

Modelling and simulation of the force–interval relationship can be approached by a mathematical technique called transfer function modelling (Box & Jenkins, 1970). Used in the study of atrial fibrillation, this effectively allows the mechanical characteristics of any beat in a consecutive series to be described by the added-together influence of the characteristics (for example, the RR interval, force, end-diastolic pressure) of any chosen number of preceding beats (plus a residual term for unexplained influences). The general form of the equation which does this is given below, but an explanation of how it works is useful first.

If we suspect that interval–force mechanisms are important determinants of mechanical function in atrial fibrillation, it would be reasonable to look for an influence of the preceding interval (mechanical restitution) and of the pre-preceding interval (post-extrasystolic potentiation) on the force of a beat. However, since post-extrasystolic potentiation decays over several beats in the normal human heart, it may be necessary to look for an influence of earlier beats as well. It is assumed that some measurement of the force of contraction of the ventricle such as dP/dt_{max} is being examined and that the influence of the preceding interval (mechanical restitution) is to be assessed. The influence might be expected to increase as the interval lengthens. So a term is entered in the equation which consists of the preceding interval multiplied by a scaling factor. However, such a term would assume that the influence of increasing interval was linear – increasing steadily as interval lengthened – whereas in reality it is non-linear, increasing rapidly at short intervals and then reaching a plateau. This can be allowed for in the equation by pairing the linear term with another, non-linear term. In its simplest form, this will include the square of the interval, again multiplied by a scaling constant. So for beat 100 in a sequence, an equation of the form:

$$dP/dt_{beat\,100} = k_0 + k_1 \times RR_{beat\,99} + k_2 \times RR^2_{beat\,99} + e$$

emerges, where k_0 is a constant term, k_1 and k_2 are the scaling constants, and e is the proportion of the beat force which is *not* explained by the two other terms – the residual.

For this modelling approach to have any practical value, values are needed for the constants. These are obtained by a statistical process which involves solving the equation of each of a successive sequence of beats, obtaining the summed value of the residual (squared to make all values positive) for all the beats, and then adjusting the value of the constants and repeating the process until the residual reaches a minimum value. This gives optimum values (partial regression coefficients) for the constants.

At this point, the power of the method becomes apparent, because terms can now be added into the equation for any other variable which it is suspected may have an influence on contractile force, to see if it reduces the size of the residual. If it does, it is having a real influence, at least in a statistical sense. Thus the determinants of contractile force can be explored. For example, an effect of post-extrasystolic potentiation can be tested for by adding to the equation linear and non-linear terms for the pre-preceding interval (and for any intervals further back which are expected to be relevant). Anything else which may have an influence can be tested for – the force of the preceding beat, for example, or the end-diastolic pressure. The equation may therefore become very complicated, but that is not a problem since it will be solved with the use of a computer. This process of stepwise selection of variables allows identification of the most important determinants and leads to the most economical model. As will be shown later, more than 80% of the variance of dP/dt_{max} in AF can often be described by considering the properties for the preceding 3–5 beats.

Once established, the model can also be used to *predict*, because it will predict the force on each beat of any sequence which is specified. So in the example of atrial fibrillation, the question of whether the beat-to-beat variations of force are, in part, determined by the Bowditch effect can be tested by asking the model to simulate the responses to a stepwise series of increases of rate. Examples of this sort of use will be given later.

This description has used familiar variables like preceding interval to show how the model works, but it is not necessary to have physiological insight to use the method; important determinants of a sequence of events can be identified by trial and error, as described. The essential requirements are that the events are a true sequence (no beats missed out) and that there are enough of them to give the statistical methods used to characterise the terms enough significance. A sequence of at least 100 consecutive beats is needed to study atrial fibrillation.

The general form of the equation which forms the transfer function model, describing the magnitude of a dependent variable y, on beat i of a sequence, in terms of the value on earlier beats of y (linear relation) and of another, independent variable x (non-linear relation), is:

$$y_i = a_0 + \sum_{k=1}^{p} a_k \times y_{i-k} + \sum_{k=1}^{q_1} b_k \times x_{i-k} + \sum_{k=1}^{q_2} c_k \times x_{i-k}^2 + e_i$$

where:

a_0	is a constant term,
i	is the beat number, in a sequence from $i = 1$ to n,
k	is a whole number from 1 upwards (determining which beat is considered; so $i - k$ identifies the preceding beat if k is set to 1),
p, q_1, q_2	are the maximum number of preceding beats which are included,
y_i	is the dependent variable (e.g. dP/dt_{max}),
x_i	is an independent variable (e.g. RR interval),
a_k, b_k, c_k	are the scaling constants (regression coefficients),
e_i	is the residual.

The optimum form of the model is identified by minimising the residual term; this is achieved when the sum of the squares of e_i $\left(\sum_{i=1}^{n} e_i^2 \right)$, for the n beats examined is a minimum. A further requirement is that there is no correlation between the residuals obtained from the examination of successive beats, since any such correlation would imply a relationship between the beats not accounted for by the model.

For comparison with experimental studies of interval force phenomena (e.g. Anderson et al., 1976; Edman & Jóhannsson, 1976; Pidgeon et al., 1980; Yue et al., 1985), two types of stimulation patterns are used as input sequences into the transfer function model:

1. stepwise changes from one regular stimulation frequency to another,
2. a single interval variation within a regular sequence of intervals.

After any change in the basic interval at least 10 to 20 pulses are computed to regain the steady state.

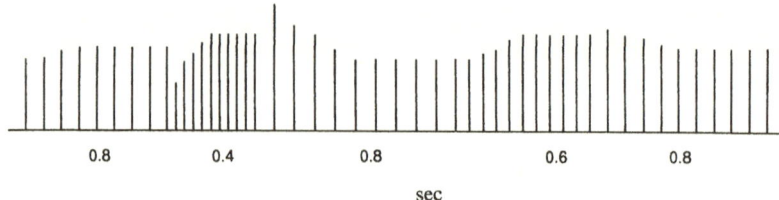

Fig. 9. Simulation of the effect of stepwise changes in steady-state stimulation frequency on dP/dt_{max}. dP/dt_{max} is expressed by the vertical height of each bar and interval by the separation between bars. Steady-state intervals of 0.8 s, 0.4 s, 0.8 s, 0.6 s and 0.8 s are shown. The simulation is derived from the transfer function model using data from a consecutive sequence of beats from the patient in atrial fibrillation.

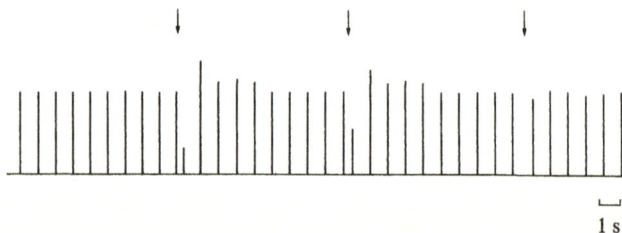

Fig. 10. Simulations of the effect of changing a single interval within a train of steady-state intervals on dP/dt_{max}. The effects of three intervals at 0.35, 0.4 and 0.9 s are shown. The steady-state interval (0.8 s) is long enough to allow full mechanical restitution between beats.

Such stimulation sequences have been used in many experimental protocols with isolated heart muscle preparations, and also in man. The behaviour in response to these protocols which examine beat to beat changes as well as steady state changes can be summarised, and indeed are well known, as:

1. staircase phenomenon (Bowditch, 1871; Kock-Weser & Blinks, 1963; Seed & Walker, 1988).
2. post-stimulation potentiation (Koch-Weser & Blinks, 1963; Yue *et al.*, 1985).
3. post-extrasystolic potentiation and decay (Langendorff, 1885; Woodworth, 1902; Hoffman, Bindler & Suckling, 1956; Siebens *et al.*, 1959; Seed *et al.*, 1984).
4. mechanical restitution (Braveny & Kruta, 1958; Meijler, 1962; Edman & Jóhannsson, 1976; Elzinga *et al.*, 1981; Fry *et al.*, 1983; Burkhoff *et al.*, 1984).

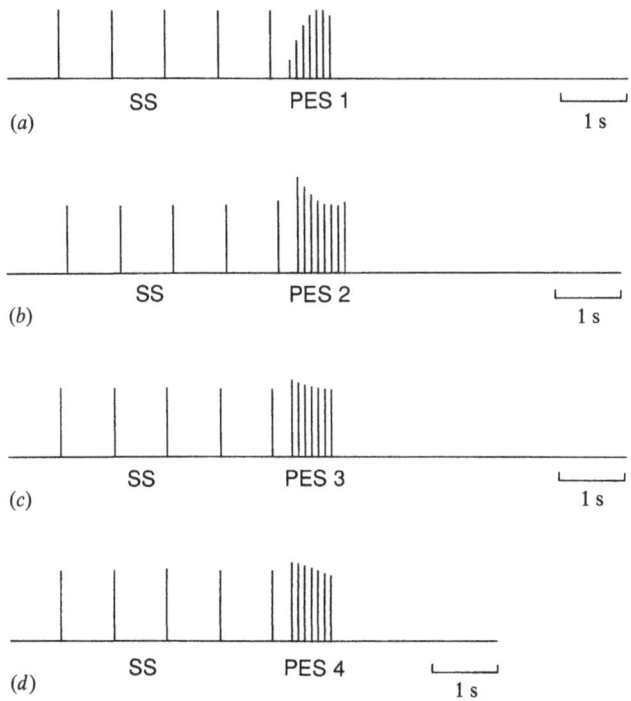

Fig. 11. Simulations of extrasystolic and post-extrasystolic behaviour. The steady state is 0.8 seconds throughout, and dP/dt_{max} is indicated by bars, as before. A series of interval changes, each within a train of steady-state beats as in Fig. 10, are shown. To emphasise the effect of the interval changes (0.3 s–0.9 s in steps of 0.1 s) on the contractile responses these responses have been grouped so that (a) shows the effect of this series of interval changes on the beat immediately following each interval change (PES1: mechanical restitution), and (b), (c) and (d) on each of the three successive beats (PES2,3,4) which are at the steady-state interval (these summarise post-extrasystolic potentiation and its decay).

Of special interest is the influence of a single interval variation within a regular sequence of intervals on the force indicators of the succeeding beats.

Figs. 9 to 11 show the simulated behaviour of dP/dt_{max}, in the patient already described, in response to particular stimulation sequences frequently used in experiments on the interval–force relationship.

Fig. 9 shows the behaviour of dP/dt_{max} in response to stepwise changes of stimulation frequency. Typical short-term and steady state changes in force due to stepwise frequency changes are visible. These phenomena are well known from experiments with isolated myocardial strips (Anderson *et al.*, 1976; Koch-Weser & Blinks, 1963), and here it is shown that they can also be inferred in the human heart during spontaneous arrhythmia. Simulations shown in Fig. 10 concentrate on the impact of a single interval change on a train of steady-state beats and the post-extrasystolic potentiation demonstrated here is similar to that described in isolated myocardial tissue. Fig. 11 explores the impact of such a single interval variation further, and summarises the effects of varying this interval on each of the four subsequent beats. Thus, by identifying a given variation in interval from the last steady-state beat, one can see the impact this interval has in terms of mechanical restitution, post-extrasystolic potentiation, and decay of post-extrasystolic potentiation simply by identifying the beat in Figs. 11(a) to 11(d).

In this patient, transfer function analysis of the data showed that LV dP/dt_{max} of a beat had some dependence on five preceding intervals, and on LV dP/dt_{max} of the two preceding beats. As might be expected from the curvilinear relationships between interval and force of both mechanical restitution and post-extrasystolic potentiation, the influence of the two immediately preceding intervals was non-linear.

Discussion

Simple analysis by scattergrams and sequential gating, as described, demonstrates convincingly that left ventricular dP/dt_{max} in atrial fibrillation is influenced by preceding interval (mechanical restitution as in Figs. 1 and 2), and inversely by the pre-preceding interval (post-extrasystolic potentiation as in Figs. 3–7). Whilst there may be other influences such as variations in pre-load and afterload, it is clear that interval–force mechanisms contribute to the variation in pulse properties seen in atrial fibrillation.

A transfer function model, whose parameters have been estimated from an arrhythmic sequence of pulses, can be used to predict the behaviour of the heart in response to certain stimulation sequences such as single or sustained interval changes. This procedure takes advantage of the natural irregularity of beat to beat intervals in atrial fibrillation to study the interval–force relationship in man without artificial stimulation. Since interval–force processes may provide information about the state of the heart from a clinical viewpoint it may also prove to have some diagnostic or prognostic application (Anderson, Manring & Johnson, 1977; Seed et al., 1984). The quality of the model was evaluated in a previous study by analysis of the isometric force development of isolated heart muscle stimulated with a random sequence of intervals (Pfeiffer & Kenner, 1983;

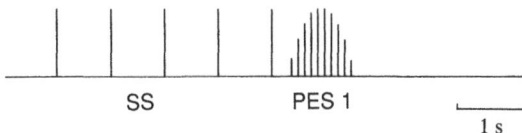

Fig. 12. The simulation shows dP/dt_{max} on a series of steady-state beats (SS), and on a range of extrasystoles, as in Fig. 11(*a*). However, in this simulation the predictions include extrasystolic intervals outside the range of those occurring in the patient.

Pfeiffer *et al.*, 1984). Comparison between predictions about contractile behaviour from the model and response to actual stimulation sequences in the muscle showed good agreement.

It should be stressed that simulations produced using the transfer function model will only be accurate for data within the range of data entered from the patient. Fig. 12 shows a simulation for mechanical restitution, as in Fig. 11(*a*), but the predictions have extended outside the range of data measured, and the predicted behaviour does not reflect the sort of mechanical response one would expect in man at these intervals (Seed *et al.*, 1984).

Of course, this transfer function model is just a phenomenological model and cannot be interpreted from a physiological point of view, but the power of the model is such that it allows the investigator to test for the relevance of any variable that has been measured. If such a variable reduces the size of the residual, it is clear that the variable is relevant. The model has clearly identified that properties of more than one preceding interval are important. Such long-term effects can be interpreted in terms of recirculation mechanisms (Burkhoff *et al.*, 1984).

Acknowledgements

We would like to thank W. A. Seed and M. I. M. Noble for their help in data collection and for many stimulating discussions.

This work was supported by the Garfield Weston and Wellcome Trusts.

References

Anderson, P. A. W., Manring, A. & Johnson, E. A. (1977). The force of contraction of isolated papillary muscle; a study of the interaction of its determining factors. *Journal of Molecular and Cellular Cardiology*, **9**, 131–50.
Anderson, P. A. W., Rankin, J. S., Arentzen, C. E., Anderson, R. W. & Johnson,

E. A. (1976). Evaluation of the force–frequency relationship as a descriptor of the inotropic state of canine left ventricular myocardium. *Circulation Research*, **39**, 832–9.

Bowditch, H. P. (1871). Über die Eigenthümlichkeiten der Reizbarkeit, welche die Muskelfasern des Herzens zeigen. *Berichte der Königlich-Sächsischen Gesellschaft der Wissenschaften*, **23**, 652–89.

Box, G. E. P. & Jenkins, G. M. (1970). *Time Series Analysis, Forecasting and Control*. San Francisco: Holden Day.

Braveny, P. & Kruta, V. (1958). Dissociation de deux facteurs: restitution et potentiation dans l'action de l'intervalle sur l'amplitude de la contraction du myocarde. *Achives Internationales de Physiologie et de Biochimie*, **66**, 633–52.

Burkhoff, D., Yue, D. T., Franz, M. R., Hunter, W. C. & Sagawa, K. (1984). Mechanical restitution of isolated perfused canine left ventricles. *American Journal of Physiology*, **246**, H8–16.

Drake-Holland, A. J., Mills, C. J., Noble, M. I. M. & Pugh, S. E. (1990). Response to changes in filling and contractility of indices of human left ventricular mechanical performance. *Journal of Physiology*, **422**, 29–39.

Edman, K. A. P. & Jóhannsson, M. (1976). The contractile state of rabbit papillary muscle in relation to stimulation frequency. *Journal of Physiology*, **254**, 565–81.

Elzinga, G., Lab, M. J., Noble, M. I. M., Papadoyannis, D., Pidgeon, J., Seed, W. A. & Wohlfart, B. (1981). The action potential duration and contractile response of the intact heart related to the preceding interval and the preceding beat in the dog and cat. *Journal of Physiology*, **314**, 481–500.

Fry, C. H., Walker, J. M., Webb-Peploe, M. M. & Williams, B. T. (1983). Restitution of contractility *in vitro* of human and guinea-pig ventricular myocardium. *Journal of Physiology*, **339**, 26–27P.

Hoffman, B. F., Bindler, E. & Suckling, E. E. (1956). Postextrasystolic potentiation of contraction in cardiac muscle. *American Journal of Physiology*, **185**, 95–102.

Koch-Weser, J. & Blinks, J. R. (1963). The influence of the interval between beats on myocardial contractility. *Pharmacological Reviews*, **15**, 601–52.

Langendorff, O. (1885). Über die elektrische Reizung des Herzens. *Archiv für Physiologie*, **8**, 284–7.

Meijler, F. L. (1962). Staircase, rest contractions, and potentiation in the isolated rat heart. *American Journal of Physiology*, **202**, 636–40.

Meijler, F. L. (1986). The pulse in atrial fibrillation. *British Heart Journal*, **56**, 1–3.

Mills, C. J. & Shillingford, J. P. (1967). A catheter tip electromagnetic velocity probe and its evaluation. *Cardiovascular Research*, **1**, 263–73.

Pfeiffer, K. P. & Kenner, T. (1983). A statistical approach to the analysis of phenomena of frequency potentiation of isolated myocardial strips. *Basic Research in Cardiology*, **78**, 239–55.

Pfeiffer, K. P., Kenner, T. & Schaefer, J. (1984). Application of statistical methods for the analysis of interval related cardiac performance variations during cardiac arrhythmia in man. *Cardiovascular Research*, **18**, 80–98.

Pidgeon, J., Lab, M., Seed, A., Elzinga, G., Papadoyannis, D. & Noble, M. I. M. (1980). The contractile state of cat and dog heart in relation to the interval between beats. *Circulation Research*, **47**, 559–67.

Siebens, A. A., Hoffman, B. F., Cranefield, P. F. & Brooks, C. McC. (1959). Regulation of contractile force during ventricular arrhythmias. *American Journal of Physiology*, **197**, 971–7.

Seed, W. A., Noble, M. I. M., Walker, J. M., Miller, G. A. H., Pidgeon, J., Redwood, D., Wanless, R., Franz, M. R., Schoettler, M. & Schaefer, J. (1984). Relationships between beat to beat interval and the strength of contraction in the healthy and diseased human heart. *Circulation*, **70**, 799–805.

Seed, W. A. & Walker, J. M. (1988). Review: Relation between beat interval and force of the heartbeat and its clinical implications. *Cardiovascular Research*, **22**, 303–14.

Woodworth, R. S. (1902). Maximal contraction, 'staircase' contraction, refractory period, and compensatory pause of the heart. *American Journal of Physiology*, **8**, 213–49.

Yue, D. T., Burkhoff, D., Franz, M. R., Hunter, W. C. & Sagawa, K. (1985). Postextrasystolic potentiation of the isolated canine left ventricle: relationship to mechanical restitution. *Circulation Research*, **56**, 340–50.

Interval–force processes in the intact animal and human heart

W. A. SEED

Introduction

The study of interval–force mechanisms in the intact heart is a relatively recent phenomenon. Most descriptions of cardiac function have concentrated on the roles of the diastolic muscle fibre length (the Frank–Starling mechanism), the load that the ventricle must overcome in ejecting blood (aortic pressure), and neural and other influences that affect force independently of muscle length (inotropic mechanisms). These three factors have long provided a framework for understanding cardiac function (Elzinga & Westerhof, 1976, 1978; Sagawa, 1981) and the Frank–Starling mechanism in particular has had a dominant role.

The neglect of interval–force mechanisms is interesting, since the original observations of Bowditch (Bowditch, 1871) predate those of Frank (Frank, 1895) and Starling (Patterson, Piper & Starling, 1914), and, as will be seen, there was abundant evidence in early human and animal studies of a possible role for interval–force mechanisms in normal cardiac function. Some of the reasons for the neglect are discussed elsewhere in this book (see the historical note with the Bowditch translation); and, in addition, the early literature was probably a deterrent, particularly to clinical scientists, since it was largely concerned with isolated cardiac muscle and contained many inconsistencies attributable to differences in experimental conditions, species, and frequency of stimulation. Another reason may have been the facility with which possible interval–force effects can be explained away as manifestations of the effects of ventricular filling or load. Thus a change of interval may alter both filling (Fig. 1) and loading conditions of the subsequent beat (Fig. 2), masking any direct inotropic effect of the interval change itself. Instances where this may have biased the interpretation of experiments away from interval–force mechanisms abound in the literature. Thus

317

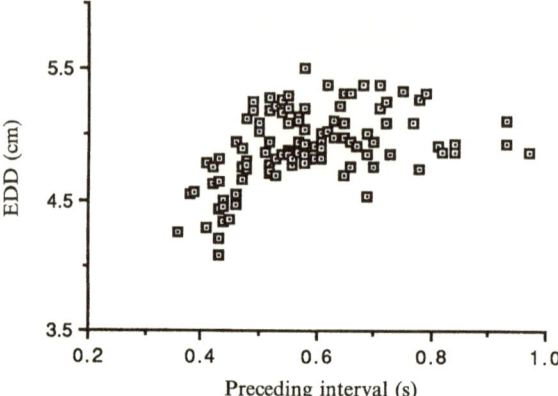

Fig. 1. Time course of filling in the human left ventricle. End-diastolic diameter (EDD) of a large number of beats with continuously varying intervals (due to atrial fibrillation) measured by echocardiography. Filling follows a time course not dissimilar to that of mechanical restitution (see Fig. 4).

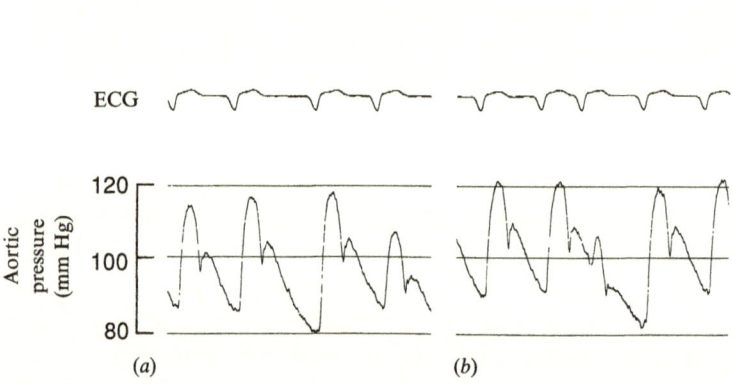

Fig. 2. Effect of variation in beat to beat interval on left ventricular load. Pressure was measured in the ascending aorta with an end-catheter manometer while the patient was paced at a steady state interval of 600 msec. Aortic end-diastolic pressure was markedly lower after a pause (panel (a), interval 800 ms) than after steady-state beats, and higher at the onset of a premature beat (panel (b), interval 400 ms).

descriptions of the recovery of function after a beat, and the pulse fluctuations seen in atrial fibrillation, pulsus alternans and postextra-systolic potentiation were, until the late 1950s, almost without exception couched in terms of the Frank–Starling mechanism or the effect of aortic pressure. Since these views were put by figures like Lewis, Wenckebach, Wiggers, Katz, and Braunwald they created a strong legacy.

More recently, however, awareness of the potential contribution of interval–force processes to cardiac function, and of the need to disentangle haemodynamic and interval-related influences has increased, and this chapter presents the evidence for an influence of interval–force processes on events in the intact heart. Its purpose is to identify where, and how, these processes may be determining or modifying both normal and abnormal cardiac function. The experimental problem has been tackled on several levels. At one extreme, an isolated preparation (usually the canine left ventricle) has been studied, either *in situ* or after excision, with coronary perfusion maintained and ventricular filling and load regulated or measured. Such a preparation gives great control and allows sophisticated measurements of contractile function. Alternatively, acute studies in animals have been employed. These are not so demanding, but offer less control and still involve anaesthesia and surgery with invasive methods of measurement. Studies in conscious animals have usually involved previous implantation of transducers for the measurement of pressure, flow, or chamber dimensions, and allow little or no control of ventricular filling or aortic pressure. The same is true of studies in man, where measurements have been made during cardiac surgery or diagnostic catheterisation. In many studies, therefore, particularly in man, the conditions have not allowed clear separation of interval–force from length- and load-dependent events.

Another approach to the problem of separating these influences in the intact heart has been to look for an index of cardiac contractile function which is sensitive to inotropic influences, but not to length or load changes. Then, as long as reflex or hormonal inotropic effects can be avoided, interval–force effects can be identified. Since the use of such indices of contractility is central to the interpretation of many of the studies mentioned in this chapter, their problems and limitations need to be reviewed.

Measurement of force in the intact heart

Since the force with which a muscle fibre contracts depends on the velocity of concomitant shortening, studies of contractile behaviour in isolated cardiac muscle are usually conducted with the muscle held at constant length (isometric contraction). Force is measured by attaching one end of the muscle strip to a transducer which does not significantly change length, and which can be calibrated against known small weights. Such a calibration is in units of force (mass × acceleration, the acceleration being that due to the earth's gravitational field), expressed in grams or in newtons, and often referred to in the literature as tension. It is firmly established that changes in peak tension or its maximum rate of rise, in a muscle contracting at constant length, are sensitive indicators of the contractile state (contractility) of the muscle.

Unfortunately, tension is not measurable in the intact heart wall except in very special circumstances, and for most studies, particularly in man, a compromise must be adopted; an index of contractile state must be chosen which is both accessible to measurement and related to muscle tension development. Since left ventricular pressure and wall tension are directly related (the law of Laplace, see below) such indices frequently are derived from pressure measurements, obtained during the period before the aortic valve opens in order to avoid muscle shortening. Actually, there are changes of ventricular shape even during this isovolumic period, so that the proportionality between pressure and tension may not be constant, but the effect is probably small.

Isovolumic indices of contractile force

A number of possible indices have been explored, both theoretically and experimentally (Braunwald & Ross, 1979). Of these, the maximum rate of rise of intraventricular pressure during systole (dP/dt_{max}) has particular relevance, because it is easily measured with high fidelity catheter-tip micromanometers and is in widespread use in both animals and man. Many of the observations on interval–force effects in the intact heart have been based on measurements of dP/dt_{max}, and its validity and limitations need consideration. There is no doubt that interventions which increase the contractile force of the left ventricle produce substantial increases in dP/dt_{max} in both experimental animals (Reeves *et al.*, 1960; Schaper, Lewi & Jageneau, 1965; Fisher *et al.*, 1967; Furnival, Linden & Snow, 1970; Patterson, Kent & Peirce, 1972; Mahler *et al.*, 1975; Schmidt & Hoppe, 1978; Kass *et al.*, 1987) and in man (Mason, 1969; Gleason & Braunwald, 1962*a*; Drake-Holland *et al.*, 1990). Thus it is certainly capable of registering changes in inotropic state. However, as Figs. 1 and 2 show, changes of interval may influence both left ventricular filling and the end-diastolic pressure in the aorta, so that the sensitivity of dP/dt_{max} to these influences is important.

The evidence with respect to aortic pressure is fairly consistent, with a consensus (though not unanimity (Wallace, Skinner & Mitchell, 1963; Wildenthal, Mierzwiak & Mitchell, 1969)) from animal experiments that, as long as dP/dt_{max} is reached during the isovolumic period, it is largely unaffected by changes in aortic diastolic pressure (Schaper *et al.*, 1965; Furnival *et al.*, 1970; van den Bos *et al.*, 1973; Little, 1985; Kass *et al.*, 1987). This condition is likely to be met as long as the heart is healthy (Furnival *et al.*, 1970) and the aortic diastolic pressure above 50 mm Hg (Schaper *et al.*, 1965) at least up to intervals of one second (Fisher *et al.*, 1967) and probably applies in man (Quinones, Gaasch & Alexander, 1976) even at intervals in excess of a second (Pidgeon *et al.*, 1982). At very long intervals or low aortic pressures, dP/dt_{max} will be limited by aortic valve opening, with an underestimation of contractile force.

The effect of changes in left ventricular filling on dP/dt_{max} is more difficult to establish. Most studies on the isolated heart, or the heart *in situ* in anaesthetised animals, show a positive dependence of dP/dt_{max} on indices of diastolic filling such as left ventricular end-diastolic pressure, volume, or diameter (Reeves *et al.*, 1960; Wallace *et al.*, 1963; Schaper *et al.*, 1965; Patterson *et al.*, 1972; Grossman *et al.*, 1972; van den Bos *et al.*, 1973; Schmidt & Hoppe, 1978; Kass *et al.*, 1987). However, it has not been seen in all studies (Furnival *et al.*, 1970) and it has often been modest or absent in the conscious animal at normal filling pressures (Fisher *et al.*, 1967; Noble *et al.*, 1969; van den Bos *et al.*, 1973; Davidson *et al.*, 1974; Anderson *et al.*, 1976) being clearly seen only when venous return to the heart was reduced (Little, 1985). In patients studied during cardiac catheterisation, the dependence of dP/dt_{max} on ventricular volume has generally been slight (see Fig. 3, and Grossman *et al.*, 1972; Sanghvi *et al.*, 1972; Pidgeon *et al.*, 1982; Drake-Holland *et al.*, 1990) irrespective of whether ventricular function was normal or impaired. Thus the evidence is conflicting.

One explanation suggested for these inconsistencies (Burkhoff *et al.*, 1984) was that sensitivity to ventricular filling in patient studies was masked by baroreceptor reflexes. This seems unlikely; in one of the studies heart rate and mean aortic pressure were reported unchanged (Grossman *et al.*, 1972) and in others some (Pidgeon *et al.*, 1982) or all (Drake-Holland *et al.*, 1990) of the patients were on beta-adrenergic blocking therapy.

It seems more likely that the explanation is at least partly methodological. The range of ventricular fibre lengths corresponding to particular end-diastolic pressures is likely to vary in different preparations, depending for example on the heart rate and whether the thorax and pericardium

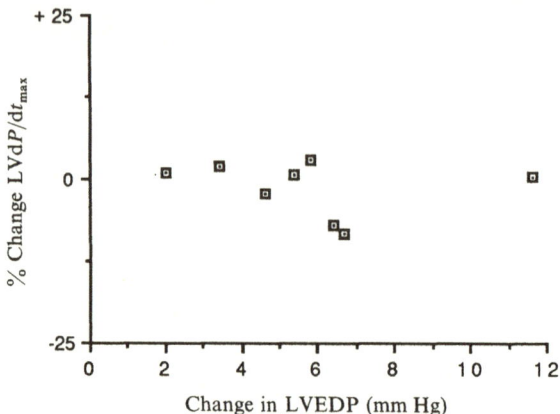

Fig. 3. Lack of influence of left ventricular filling on dP/dt_{max} in man. A consecutive series of eight patients with normal left ventricular function were paced at a constant heart rate whilst left ventricular filling was transiently increased by passive leg raising or head down tilt during cardiac catheterisation. Increased filling (rise in left ventricular end-diastolic pressure, abscissa) had no significant effect on left ventricular dP/dt_{max}.

are open. This makes comparison between studies uncertain, as does the recently reported time dependence of the effect of a given degree of filling on dP/dt_{max} (Lew, 1988). Another possible explanation lies in the physical nature of the measurement. The rate of rise of pressure is linked to the rate of rise of wall tension in the left ventricle (the direct measure of contractile force) by the geometry of the ventricle (Reeves *et al.*, 1960; van den Bos *et al.*, 1973). In the very simplest analysis, treating the ventricle as a sphere, the relevant geometric terms in the Law of Laplace are the radius and the wall thickness. The mathematics for a more realistic ventricular shape becomes complicated but the basic relationship between pressure, tension, and ventricular dimensions still holds. Therefore, dP/dt during the isovolumic phase of systole would be expected to depend directly on the rate of rise of tension in the wall and inversely on the starting dimensions of the ventricle – end-diastolic diameter or volume. As the size of the ventricle increases, the rate of rise of wall tension will inevitably increase, simply because of the length–tension relationship. This will oppose the inverse effect of increasing size, so that dP/dt_{max} will be unaffected only if the two balance. This may hold over a particular range, but is unlikely to be generally true, since chamber geometry may vary with heart size and between species. Uncertainties about the reliability of the relationship between heart size and end-diastolic pressure in assessing end-diastolic volume add to the problem. Thus the discordances in the literature are unsurprising and the conclusion must be that the volume independence of dP/dt_{max} can only be accepted where it has been experimentally established, ideally in each experiment. On the available evidence, it seems probable that dP/dt_{max} is sensitive to left ventricular filling in many experimental situations, but the effect has been shown to be small when volume changes are both modest, and within the physiological range, in the conscious dog and man.

Non-isovolumic indices – stroke volume and related measurements

Many haemodynamic studies which have relevance to interval–force processes, particularly in man, have relied on indices of left ventricular function during ejection. Older studies used measurements of arterial pulse pressure or peak systolic pressure. Within an individual, pulse pressure correlates well with stroke volume (Hamilton & Remington, 1947; Starr *et al.*, 1954) but peak systolic pressure is an unreliable guide; for example, it is normally lower on the potentiated beat following an extrasystole than on the one preceding it (Beck, Chesler & Schrire, 1971; Kvasnicka *et al.*, 1975; and see Fig. 8), whilst both stroke volume and pre-ejection indices of contractility are higher. More modern studies have examined ventricular dimensions obtained during angiography, which can provide information about end-diastolic and end-systolic volumes and wall movement, or by ultrasound methods, which allow non-invasive measurements of left ventricular dimensions and ejection fraction, or (by Doppler techniques) stroke volume or stroke distance.

Measurements of stroke volume and ejection fraction have limitations in the study of interval–force processes. An alteration in ventricular inotropic state may affect them only modestly (Noble, Trenchard & Guz, 1969; Drake-Holland *et al.*, 1990). Thus all such measurements are likely to be much more sensitive to alterations of ventricular filling than of contractility, and provide reliable evidence of interval–force effects only if ventricular filling is controlled or shown to have no influence. Equally, such measurements are sensitive to load – the extreme example being the isovolumic beat. This has been examined by Kass *et al.* (1987). The only volume-related index which is largely insensitive to load is the slope of the end-systolic pressure–volume relationship (Sagawa *et al.*, 1977) which is technically demanding and has been applied on a very limited scale in clinical work, though it has proved a powerful tool in animal studies.

Recovery of mechanical function after a beat – mechanical restitution

The time course of recovery of contractile function after each beat in the intact heart is similar to that in isolated ventricular muscle from many mammalian species at 37 °C. There is a mechanical restitution curve (see chapter by Jóhannsson in this book) which rises to a plateau at about 800 ms. This has been demonstrated in the isolated, perfused ventricle of the cat (Pidgeon *et al.*, 1980) and dog (Burkhoff *et al.*, 1984) and in the intact dog heart (Mahler & Rogel, 1970; Pidgeon *et al.*, 1980). It has also been shown in man, where typical curves have been recorded for tension in isolated human cardiac muscle (Fry *et al.*, 1983) and for dP/dt_{max} during pacing studies in the intact circulation (Fig. 4, and Anderson *et al.*, 1979; Pidgeon *et al.*, 1982). Numerous studies which employed ejection indices have demonstrated similar curves, whether intervals were controlled by pacing (Schaefer *et al.*, 1971) or varied spontaneously because of atrial fibrillation (see later).

As in isolated muscle, the position of the restitution curve relative to the time axis in the intact heart may show small shifts following interventions which alter the duration of the myocardial action potential (Burkhoff *et al.*, 1984). The speed of restitution may also be affected by disease, being slowed in cardiac muscle obtained from patients with impairment of ventricular function (Fry *et al.*, 1983). The position of the curve relative to the force axis is also influenced by various factors that affect the inotropic state of the muscle. Thus the whole curve is moved

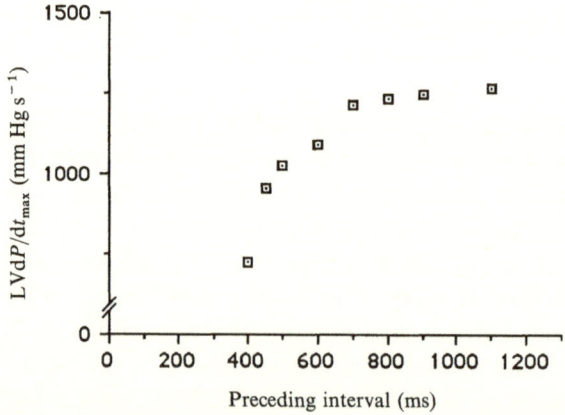

Fig. 4. Mechanical restitution in man. Left ventricular contractile force (LV dP/dt_{max}) measured on test beats introduced at the intervals shown during steady pacing.

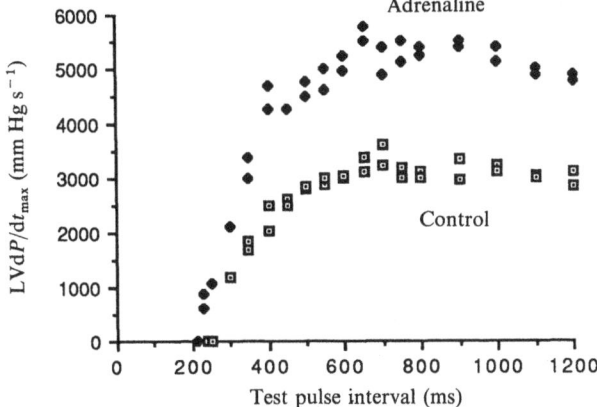

Fig. 5. Effect of adrenaline (12 μg/min) on mechanical restitution of canine left ventricle. Heart rate was maintained constant throughout by pacing.

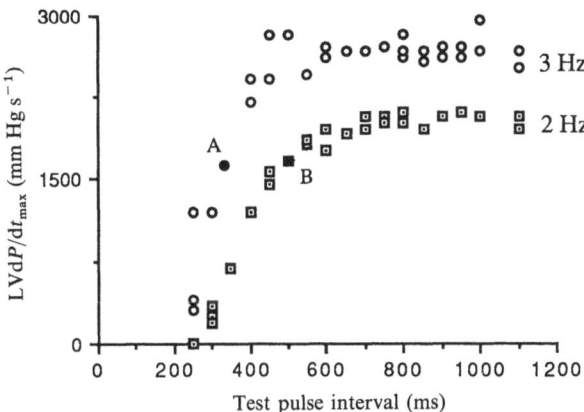

Fig. 6. Effect of increased heart rate on mechanical restitution of canine left ventricle. The steady-state pacing frequencies are indicated, and the force of the steady-state beats at each of these frequencies given by the filled symbols A and B.

upwards by adrenaline (Fig. 5, and Pidgeon *et al.*, 1980) and isoprenaline (Goodyer & Wong, 1977), or by an increase in the preceding heart rate (Fig. 6, and Goodyer & Wong, 1977; Pidgeon *et al.*, 1980, 1982; Burkhoff *et al.*, 1984) and downwards by beta-adrenergic blockade (Goodyer & Wong, 1977). All these properties mirror those seen in isolated muscle.

Effects of sustained changes of beat to beat interval: the steady-state interval–force response

An increase of stimulation frequency in isolated cardiac muscle from many mammals causes a progressive increase in tension on the first few beats up to a plateau (Bowditch's staircase; see Bowditch translation in this book). The tension reached by the beats on the plateau often increases progressively as the stimulation frequency increases (Woodworth, 1902; Koch-Weser & Blinks, 1963). This steady-state interval–force behaviour (sometimes referred to as the steady-state staircase) has been studied in both isolated human cardiac muscle and the intact heart.

Steady-state staircase in isolated human cardiac muscle

Early studies with isolated human ventricular muscle obtained at cardiac surgery did not demonstrate a positive steady-state force staircase (Sonnenblick, Braunwald & Morrow, 1965). Indeed, a negative response, with diminishing force production at increasing rates, has also been described in human muscle (Buckley, Penefsky & Litwak, 1972; Penefsky & Butler, 1974) but this was at unphysiologically low frequencies of stimulation (<1 Hz) in tissue from severely hypertrophied hearts. More recent work at both low and physiological stimulation rates has demonstrated that a positive steady-state staircase response can be found in human ventricular myocardium (Gennser, Jóhannsson & Nilsson, 1972; Walker, 1984; Gwathmey *et al.*, 1990), although it may be diminished or reversed in muscle from severely ill patients (Walker, 1984; Gwathmey *et al.*, 1990). This latter observation may explain the earlier results, which were obtained in muscle specimens from patients operated on late in their disease when cardiac function was severely compromised. A negative steady-state staircase has also been described in the canine ventricle during global ischaemia (Weber & Janicki, 1978).

Steady-state staircase in the intact heart

There is no clear consensus about the steady-state staircase in the intact heart. The confusion probably stems from methodological differences; results have been shown to be influenced by temperature (Kahn, Kavaler & Fisher, 1976), anaesthesia (Higgins *et al.*, 1973), the particular variable measured (Sonnenblick, Morrow & Williams, 1966; Kahn *et al.*, 1976) and the absolute range of heart rate examined (Maughan *et al.*, 1985). In

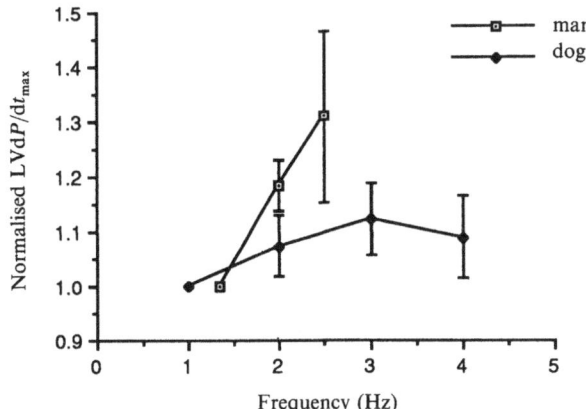

Fig. 7. Steady-state staircase in canine ($n = 12$) and normal human ($n = 6$) left ventricle. Contractile force (as dP/dt_{max}, normalised to the lowest pacing frequency) plotted (± 1 SD) against the obtainable range of steady pacing frequencies.

addition, many studies have examined ejection indices, and changes in rate in the intact heart may affect ventricular volume (Ingels *et al.*, 1977) and aortic pressure (Powers, Foster & Powell, 1976) both of which may influence such measurements. In those animal studies where ventricular filling and aortic pressure were known or controlled, or the index of contractility was independent of them, a modest positive steady-state staircase was observed (Lendrum *et al.*, 1960; Monroe & French, 1961; Mitchell, Wallace & Skinner, 1963; Covell *et al.*, 1967; Boerth *et al.*, 1969; Furnival *et al.*, 1970; Higgins *et al.*, 1973; Pidgeon *et al.*, 1980). Typical results from the anaesthetised dog are illustrated in Fig. 7. In experiments with conscious animals, measurements of dP/dt_{max} have usually shown a flat (Arentzen *et al.*, 1978; Pouleur *et al.*, 1983) or only modestly rising (Higgins *et al.*, 1973; Mahler, Yoran & Ross, 1974; Freeman, Little & O'Rourke, 1987) response to increased heart rate. In several of these studies, reflex effects were minimised with beta-adrenergic and/or vagal blockade without significantly affecting the outcome. In man, no positive steady-state staircase was seen in either working or bypassed hearts at the time of cardiac surgery (Sonnenblick *et al.*, 1966) and it was absent or modest in patients with normal haemodynamic function (Fig. 7, and Schwarz, Thormann & Winkler, 1975; Pidgeon *et al.*, 1982) and in patients with ischaemic heart disease unless the disease was severe, when a negative steady-state staircase might be seen (O'Brien *et al.*, 1969, Schwarz *et al.*, 1975).

The steady-state staircase would therefore appear to be a more prominent phenomenon in the isolated myocardium than in the intact heart. Direct support for this comes from experiments which demonstrated a much weaker positive steady-state staircase in the intact dog heart than in isolated canine cardiac muscle, in some cases taken from the same hearts (Kavaler *et al.*, 1971; Kahn *et al.*, 1976). Thus it plays an uncertain, but probably small, role in muscle function in the normal heart, as opposed to the heart exposed to anaesthetic agents or isolated in an organ bath, and the reason for the difference is unclear.

Relevance of the steady-state staircase to human cardiac performance

The staircase phenomenon is of clinical interest because it bears on the question of whether there is an optimum heart rate. If the interval–force behaviour of the heart was described by a single mechanical restitution curve (i.e. was influenced by only the preceding interval), one would expect a negative steady-state staircase, since force decreases with shorter interval (Fig. 4). This is masked by the fact that rate changes themselves have an inotropic effect, moving the entire restitution curve relative to the force axis, as shown in Fig. 6. Thus there is a family of restitution curves, and a rate change both shifts contractile force along the curve and changes the position of the whole curve relative to the force axis. For example, in Fig. 6 the contractile response of the steady-state beats changed little following an increase of heart rate from 2 Hz (point B) to 3 Hz (point A). Since other inotropic influences can also shift the restitution curve in human cardiac muscle (Walker, 1984; Gwathmey *et al.*, 1990) as in other species, it follows that, even if haemodynamic and reflex effects are eliminated, the force developed by a beat may depend on the interplay of several influences (here the preceding heart rate as well as the preceding interval). Therefore not only may there be no optimum heart rate, but the form of the steady-state staircase may depend heavily on prevailing circumstances. This may well explain many of the differences between experimental studies described above.

Effects of transient changes of beat to beat interval

Post-extrasystolic potentiation

Effects on contractility in the intact heart

The first detailed studies were those of Hoffman and his colleagues in the isovolumically contracting right ventricle of the dog heart (Siebens *et al.*, 1959). They showed that the weakness of the extrasystole is not attributable to insufficient ventricular filling, asynchrony of contraction due to aberrant conduction, or subnormal excitability of the muscle. Instead, it is a manifestation of the recovery process described earlier, i.e. mechanical restitution. The potentiation of the subsequent beat, the magnitude of which was inversely related to the prematurity of the extrasystole, was a direct consequence of the presence of the premature beat preceding it, and could not be explained purely on the basis of a longer than normal interval preceding it (mechanical restitution) or an increased filling time (Frank–Starling mechanism), though it was emphasised that these mechanisms might augment the extent of potentiation in the intact circulation. This early proof was later supported by a wide spectrum of other evidence that post-extrasystolic potentiation is an intrinsic contractile property of the intact heart, not dependent on ventricular filling or load. In the canine heart post-extrasystolic potentiation is still observed when diastolic volume is kept constant and contractile state is assessed using indices that are independent of aortic pressure (Lendrum *et al.*, 1960; Hoffman *et al.*, 1965; Yue *et al.*, 1985). Also, potentiation of dP/dt_{max} has been seen consistently in studies where dP/dt_{max} was confirmed to be unaffected by changes in ventricular filling (Elzinga *et al.*, 1981) or was held constant on the pre- and post-extrasystolic beats by control of their intervals (Kuijer *et al.*, 1978). In the intact human circulation, dP/dt_{max} has also consistently shown potentiation following spontaneous or induced extrasystoles (Fig. 8, and Schwarz, Thormann & Winkler, 1975; Kvasnicka *et al.*, 1975; van der Werf *et al.*, 1976; Katus *et al.*, 1980; Seed *et al.*, 1984), with a degree of potentiation directly related to the prematurity of the extrasystole (Fig. 9) and the completeness of restitution of the post-extrasystolic beat, and which decays gradually over the following beats.

Effects of post-extrasystolic potentiation on ejection indices in the intact heart

There is also a wealth of evidence that post-extrasystolic potentiation can affect the pumping function of the ventricle. Thus ejection indices also

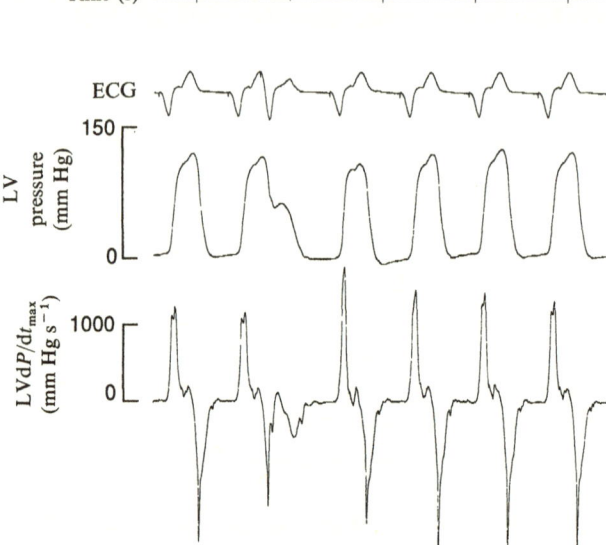

Fig. 8. Post-extrasystolic potentiation in the normal human left ventricle. Effect of a single premature beat at 350 ms on left ventricular pressure and dP/dt. All other intervals 750 ms, i.e. fully restituted beats.

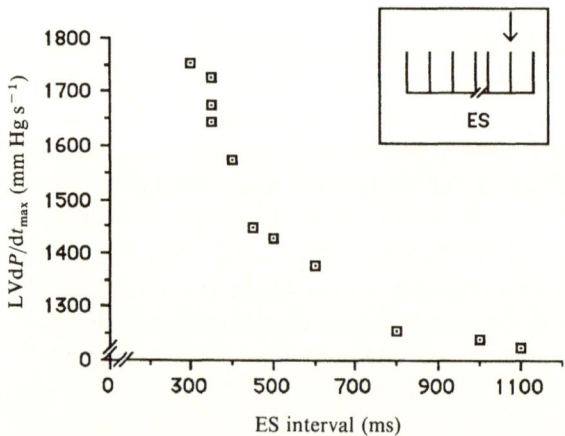

Fig. 9. Relationship between prematurity of an extrasystole and the extent of post-extrasystolic potentiation in man. Pacing protocol inset; all intervals except that of the extrasystole (ES, abscissa) were 800 ms; thus the post-extrasystolic beat was fully restituted.

show potentiation in both animals and man. In the intact canine circulation, major changes in the stroke volume of post-extrasystolic beats may occur with only marginal changes in the preceding diastolic volume (Yellin *et al.*, 1979) and echocardiographic and isovolumic indices of left ventricular function still show augmentation where the timing of the post-extrasystolic beat is adjusted to match its filling to that of the pre-extrasystolic beat (Kuijer *et al.*, 1978; Lust *et al.*, 1982; Cooper, Lutherer & Lust, 1982).

The latter technique has also been used during angiography in man, and has shown potentiation of ejection indices (Cooper *et al.*, 1986; Kuijer, van der Werf & Meijler, 1990); and other angiographic studies have shown post-extrasystolic increases in ejection fraction and other ejection indices without significant changes in end-diastolic volume of the post-extra-systolic beat (Sung C.-S. *et al.*, 1980; Hamby *et al.*, 1975). In these latter studies, and in the dog studies of Yellin *et al.* (1979), the end-diastolic volume was not augmented despite the fact that the interval before the post-extrasystolic beat was always longer than that before the control beats. The implication of all these studies is that post-extrasystolic potentiation augments left ventricular emptying, so that end-systolic volume falls in comparison with the pre-extrasystolic beat.

Clinical aspects of post-extrasystolic potentiation

Detection of ischaemia Clinical interest in post-extrasystolic potentiation initially followed a report that during acute ischaemia in the canine heart, post-extrasystolic potentiation could be used to differentiate between muscle that would recover its function on reperfusion and that which was irrevocably damaged by ischaemia (Dyke *et al.*, 1975). The same group also found that in patients with coronary artery disease the degree of potentiation observed during pre-operative angiography correlated with prognosis from coronary artery bypass surgery (Cohn *et al.*, 1975). A number of clinical studies followed in which ventricular function was assessed by measurements of wall motion from angiograms; such studies allowed regional as well as global measurements, so that the value of post-extrasystolic potentiation in identifying local areas of abnormal wall movement which could be improved by surgical revascularisation could be assessed (Hamby *et al.*, 1975; Popio *et al.*, 1977). However, there were inconsistencies. Crozatier and colleagues (Crozatier *et al.*, 1977) could not confirm the original results in animals of Dyke and colleagues (1975). In retrospect, this may have been because they did not control the interval between beats, since later studies (Boden, Liang & Hood, 1980) with intervals controlled by pacing supported the original results. An alternative was put forward later by Crozatier (Crozatier, 1982) when he found that local systolic length changes following an extrasystole differed depending upon the degree of ischaemia. He suggested that the differences between previous studies could be reconciled when similar degrees of ischaemia were compared. A further problem with such studies is that results from measurements related to stroke volume (such as ejection fraction) have not always been consistent with those using isovolumic events. For example, the augmentation of the ejection fraction has not always been clearly related to the prematurity of the preceding extrasystole (Markis *et al.*, 1976; Katus *et al.*, 1980) nor has ejection fraction always shown mechanical restitution (Klausner *et al.*, 1976). These results may reflect the effect on ejection fraction of ventricular filling and aortic diastolic pressure, which will inevitably vary in such experiments. However, there have been other criticisms of the reliability of the method (Cornish *et al.*, 1981; Gibson, Fleck & Rudolph, 1983), and it has not remained in general use.

Force–interval ratio The actual magnitude of the potentiation evoked by an extrasystole has also received clinical attention. Anderson and colleagues described a force–interval ratio – the ratio between the force of the post-extrasystolic beat and that of the steady state beats preceding the extrasystole (Anderson, Manring & Johnson, 1977). This was suggested as an indicator of the inotropic state of the heart, since in isolated muscle it was independent of muscle length and responded appropriately to positive and negative inotropic interventions. The ratio has been examined, or can be calculated from the data, in a number of human studies in which the intervals before and after the extrasystole have been controlled, so that comparison between subjects with normal and abnormal cardiac function is possible (Kvasnicka *et al.*, 1975; Anderson *et al.*, 1979; Seed *et al.*, 1984). Some of these data are presented in Fig. 10, and show that the ratio tends to be increased in the presence of impaired left ventricular function. In other words, potentiation of the first beat after an extrasystole is exaggerated in the abnormal left ventricle. The mechanism is obscure, and it remains to be seen whether the ratio is sensitive enough to be useful; but the force–interval ratio merits further study, particularly since the same trend can be detected in a recent study employing ejection indices of ventricular function obtained angiographically (Kuijer *et al.*, 1990). A further indication that the ratio reflects the

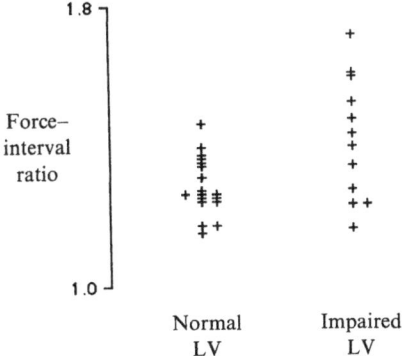

Fig. 10. Force–interval ratio (see text) in patients with normal ($n = 18$) and impaired ($n = 12$) left ventricular function. Data calculated from Seed *et al.* (1984) and Kvasnicka *et al.* (1975) for fully restituted beats and an extrasystolic interval of 400 ms. Difference between means significant at 5% level.

integrity of cardiac muscle function can be found in a study which examined interval–force properties of both the intact heart and isolated ventricular muscle strips in the rabbit (Wohlfart & Elzinga, 1982). The degree of potentiation evoked by an optimally timed extrasystole was considerably greater in the isolated muscle.

Recirculation fraction The effect of an extrasystole is to inject an extra bolus of activator calcium into the contractile system of cardiac muscle (Wier & Yue, 1986), and there is a fixed relation between the extent of potentiation of the first and second post-extrasystolic beats (as long as the intervals before both allow full restitution). This has been found in isolated cardiac muscle and the intact heart in both animals and man (Wohlfart, 1979; Wohlfart & Elzinga, 1982; Drake-Holland *et al.*, 1983; Seed *et al.*, 1984). In terms of calcium handling, it suggests that a fixed proportion of the extra bolus is recirculated from the first to the second beat – the recirculation fraction (Seed *et al.*, 1984) – and that this is independent of the degree of potentiation (see chapter by ter Keurs in this book). This has pathophysiological relevance. It has been shown that the recirculation fraction is lower in biopsy specimens from patients in cardiac failure than in samples from a more normal group (Walker *et al.*, 1984). This observation in isolated muscle has been confirmed in a catheter-based study of normal subjects and patients with cardiomyopathic or ischaemic heart failure (Seed *et al.*, 1984), in which the recirculation

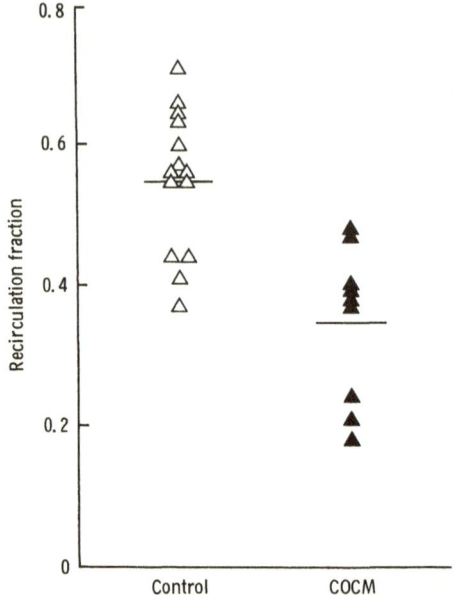

Fig. 11. Recirculation fraction (see text) in patients with normal left ventricular function (control) and left ventricular function impaired by dilated cardio-myopathy (COCM). Difference significant at 1% level. (Data from Seed *et al.*, 1984.)

fraction was found to be significantly lower in the abnormal than the normal hearts (Fig. 11). Thus the abnormal heart not only potentiates more strongly than the normal after an extrasystole, but that potentiation decays more rapidly. These properties might form the basis of clinically useful functional tests.

Paired pacing

If the coupling interval of an extrasystole is progressively shortened, a point is reached where the second depolarisation still occurs, but too early for mechanical restitution to have begun. Thus there is a single contraction. The subsequent contraction is still potentiated, and this process can be maintained by trains of such paired stimuli. In isolated cardiac muscle, such paired pacing causes sustained increases in contractile force; and the same was found in isolated human muscle obtained during cardiac surgery.

Paired pacing has been explored intensively as an alternative to pharmacological interventions in increasing the inotropic state of the heart. Studies addressed whether haemodynamic benefit (increased cardiac output, lowered left ventricular diastolic pressure, or both) ensued, whether any beneficial effects were seen in the abnormal heart, and at what cost in terms of oxygen demand by the myocardium. The subject was extensively documented in two reviews (Braunwald *et al.*, 1965; Symposium, 1965), and will only be summarised here.

The inotropic effect of paired pacing in the intact heart has been unequivocally shown in animal studies where haemodynamic variables were controlled by cardiopulmonary bypass (Ross *et al.*, 1965) or by isolation from the circulation (Serur & Urschel, 1973). Studies of the intact circulation in animals are numerous but are less easy to interpret because of possible reflex and load changes. Initially, a clear increase in inotropic state is seen, together with a fall in ventricular end-diastolic pressure. However, there was no consistent augmentation of cardiac output in the normal heart. Myocardial oxygen consumption and coronary blood flow increased appreciably even if stroke volume, effective heart rate, and mean aortic pressure were held constant (Ross *et al.*, 1965). In other words, the increased inotropic state has an oxygen cost comparable to that seen with catecholamines, even if external work does not increase.

The benefit obtainable from paired pacing in the failing heart appears to depend on the adequacy of myocardial blood flow. Early animal studies showed an increase in cardiac output, with a fall in end-diastolic pressure and heart size (Cranefield, 1965). However, coronary blood flow increased, implying an increase in myocardial oxygen demand. These improvements in ventricular function in the failing dog heart were modest and shortlived, with a transient fall below control values when paired pacing ceased (King & Taylor, 1968). In the ischaemic, isolated canine heart initial inotropic effects were rapidly attenuated and contractility became subnormal on reverson to single pacing (Serur & Urschel, 1973). Thus ischaemic myocardium could not sustain its response.

Early studies of paired pacing in man were disappointing and do not appear to have been pursued (Braunwald *et al.*, 1964, 1965). A sustained positive inotropic effect was certainly obtained, as judged by indices such as dP/dt_{max}, and left ventricular end-diastolic pressure fell, particularly if it had been high. However, there was no consistent increase in cardiac output. The reasons for this were not clear but may have included haemodynamic and reflex circulatory effects. Also, ventricular pacing was used, which may itself cause a fall in cardiac output because of the loss of atrial function and asynchrony of ventricular activation. There is a good case for a further study of the method, at least in circumstances such as non-ischaemic cardiomyopathy and postoperative intropic support. Safety does not appear to have been a problem, despite the fact that the extrasystolic stimuli were being applied close to or during the vulnerable period of the previous beat. This has been attributed to limitation of the duration and amplitude of the stimuli (Braunwald *et al.*, 1967).

Clinical interval–force phenomena

Pulses alternans

Precipitating factors

The phenomenon of alternating weak and strong beats in a heart contracting with a regular rhythm was first described clinically by Traube (Traube, 1872) and observed experimentally by Gaskell (Gaskell, 1882). In animal experiments on the intact heart, mechanical alternans may occur spontaneously (usually during long experiments where heart muscle contractility is flagging) but much more commonly it is provoked by a rhythm disturbance such as a pause, an extrasystole, or an abrupt increase in heart rate (Mitchell, Sarnoff & Sonnenblick, 1963; Guntheroth *et al.*, 1969; Noble & Nutter, 1970; Mahler & Rogel, 1970), and in such circumstances is frequently transient, dying out over a few beats (Fig. 12(*a*)). It is more likely to occur, and to be sustained, at high heart rates (Fig. 12(*b*) and Gilbert *et al.*, 1965; Guntheroth *et al.*, 1969) and can often be initiated by negative inotropic interventions such as beta-adrenergic blockade (Miller, Liedtke & Nellis, 1986), vagal stimulation (Guntheroth *et al.*, 1969) or carotid sinus stimulation (Mitchell, Sarnoff & Sonnenblick, 1963) and abolished by positive inotropic interventions such as catechol-amines, calcium infusion, or cardiac glycosides (Friedman, Daily & Sheffield, 1953; Ferrer *et al.*, 1956; Mitchell, Sarnoff & Sonnenblick, 1963; Badeer *et al.*, 1967). It has also been provoked experimentally by ischaemia (Green, 1935–6; Parmley *et al.*, 1972; Weber & Janicki, 1978; Crozatier *et al.*, 1979). In isolated cardiac muscle preparations it is also promoted by cooling (Nayler & Robertson, 1965; Lu, Lange & Brooks, 1968; Spear & Moore, 1971) and by reduction of calcium concentration in the bathing medium (Lu *et al.*, 1968; Wohlfart, 1982).

Clinical occurrence of pulsus alternans

As a clinical observation in man, pulses alternans is nowadays uncommon, and it is unclear whether its prevalence has diminished or whether it no

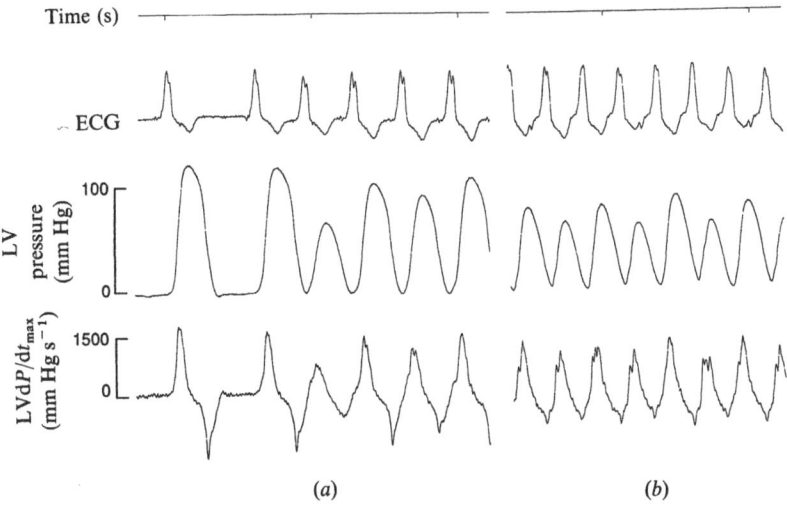

Fig. 12. Pulses alternans of pressure and dP/dt_{max} in the canine left ventricle: (a) transient, provoked by a step increase in pacing frequency from 1.67 to 3 Hz; (b) sustained, at very high pacing rate (4 Hz).

longer arouses interest and is not sought. Early reports emphasised its frequency; for example White (White, 1915), who made careful recordings of brachial pulse pressure, detected ten cases a month in the wards of Massachusetts General Hospital, a frequency equal to that of atrial fibrillation. Certainly, there are strong grounds for suspecting that alternans can often not be detected by simple observation of the pulse. During catheterisation it has been reported in an appreciable proportion (15–55%) of cases, but has often been transient and of small amplitude (Cooper, Braunwald & Morrow, 1958; Cohn, Sandler & Hancock, 1967; Hada, Wolfe & Craige, 1982). Also, in aortic stenosis, which is one of the commonest conditions to provoke it, alternans of left ventricular pressure may be greatly attenuated during passage of the pressure wave across the aortic valve (Cooper *et al.*, 1958; Swanton *et al.*, 1976) and may be undetectable peripherally. Alternans is only palpable in the peripheral arterial pulse if there is a difference of 20 mm Hg or more between beats (Harris *et al.*, 1966). This is uncommon, although in extreme cases the pulse difference may be up to 60 mm Hg, so that alternate beats may not eject, and a false impression of bradycardia may be created (Liu & Luisada, 1955; Harris *et al.*, 1966).

Underlying causes of the left ventricular damage which may provoke

alternans include hypertension (Spodick, Khan & Quarry, 1974), ischaemia (Spodick *et al.*, 1974; Hada *et al.*, 1982), cardiomyopathy (Cooper *et
al.*, 1958; Harris *et al.*, 1966; Cohn *et al.*, 1967; Spodick *et al.*, 1974; Lewis,
Lewis & Gotsman, 1975, Hada *et al.*, 1982) and valve disease, particularly
aortic (Cooper *et al.*, 1958; Swanton *et al.*, 1976; Hess *et al.*, 1984).
Mechanical alternans can also occur in the pulmonary artery, usually in
the presence of pulmonary hypertension secondary to left-sided heart
disease or lung disease (Ferrer *et al.*, 1956, Harris *et al.*, 1966, Hada *et
al.*, 1982).

Severe alternans (sustained, with a magnitude great enough to be
detectable by palpation of the pulse, and at normal heart rates) indicates
severe ventricular disease or failure and has a sinister outlook (White
recorded over 50% mortality in less than a year in this group). Less severe
cases do better, and there is some correlation with the degree of ventricular
dysfunction (Cooper *et al.*, 1958; Ryan *et al.*, 1956). As in animals, it is
more likely to occur at high heart rates (Ryan *et al.*, 1956), and may be
initiated by a transient rhythm disturbance such as an extrasystole. It
may also be provoked (perhaps related to cardioacceleration) by deep
inspiration (Liu & Luisada, 1955) and by sitting or standing upright
(Friedman *et al.*, 1953; Liu & Luisada, 1955; Ryan *et al.*, 1956; Lewis *et
al.*, 1975). Finally, alternans is not always an indicator of disease; it may
occur transiently at the onset of severe tachycardia in subjects with normal
myocardial function (Saunders & Ord, 1962).

Possible mechanisms of pulsus alternans

There has been a long debate about whether alternans is due to length
and load dependent, or to inotropic, effects. The view that alternans was
caused by alternation of ventricular filling was promoted by Wenckebach
(1902) and Wiggers (1927). They held that the strong beat would have a
larger stroke volume than the weak beat, so that its systole would last
slightly longer and its end-systolic volume be lower. Therefore the
ventricle would start to fill later and from a lower volume after the strong
beat, so that systole on the weak beat would begin from a slightly lower
end-diastolic volume. Confirmation that end-systolic and end-diastolic
volumes alternated in an appropriate way was provided by Gleason and
Braunwald (1962b), who measured left ventricular volume on four beats
of alternans following an extrasystole during angiography. Further support came from both isolated muscle and intact heart experiments
(Mitchell *et al.*, 1963).

The other argument postulated an intrinsic defect in contractility of at least some myocardial fibres on alternate beats, and originated with Gaskell (1882). Further support for an inotropic mechanism (which could not be excluded in the studies cited above) steadily accumulated. Alternans was reported in isovolumic canine heart preparations (Lendrum *et al.*, 1960; Weber & Janicki, 1978), and in isolated muscle at constant length and resting tension (Nayler & Robertson, 1965). It was also seen in the intact dog heart without any correlation between end-diastolic diameter and stroke volume (Guntheroth *et al.*, 1969). It was seen as a local phenomenon in ischaemic segments of the ventricular wall of the dog when the rest of the wall was contracting regularly (Parmley *et al.*, 1972; Crozatier *et al.*, 1979). Finally, increased ventricular size at the onset of the stronger beat was variably reported in angiographic studies in man to be seen consistently (Harris *et al.*, 1966), inconsistently (Cohn *et al.*, 1967; Swanton *et al.*, 1976) or not at all (Hess *et al.*, 1984).

The direct evidence of a contractile disturbance as the cause of alternans, and a discussion about its mechanisms are presented in detail elsewhere in this book (see chapter by Lab & Spencer, pp. 277–82).

Atrial fibrillation

Mechanism of the pulse variation in atrial fibrillation: haemodynamic versus interval–force effects

The marked variations in the pulse pressure in atrial fibrillation (Fig. 13) have been a source of clinical interest for years. The haemodynamics of atrial fibrillation were first studied by Lewis, who noted a general relationship between cycle length and arterial pressure (Lewis, 1912). Perhaps not surprisingly, since he was working across the road from Starling and using his cardiometer to measure heart volume, he attributed this to filling effects, but he did not examine it in detail. The first detailed study of beat by beat relationships was that of Einthoven & Korteweg (1915). They correlated ECG intervals with externally recorded carotid pulse pressure and showed two important features. First, long pauses were followed by larger pulse pressures, and short pauses by smaller pulses; this relationship, which showed a lot of scatter, was attributed to the degree of filling of the ventricle at the start of each contraction (the Frank–Starling mechanism). Secondly, the scatter was in considerable part due to variation of the pulse pressure of the previous beat. The relationship was inverse, so that a strong previous beat tended to be

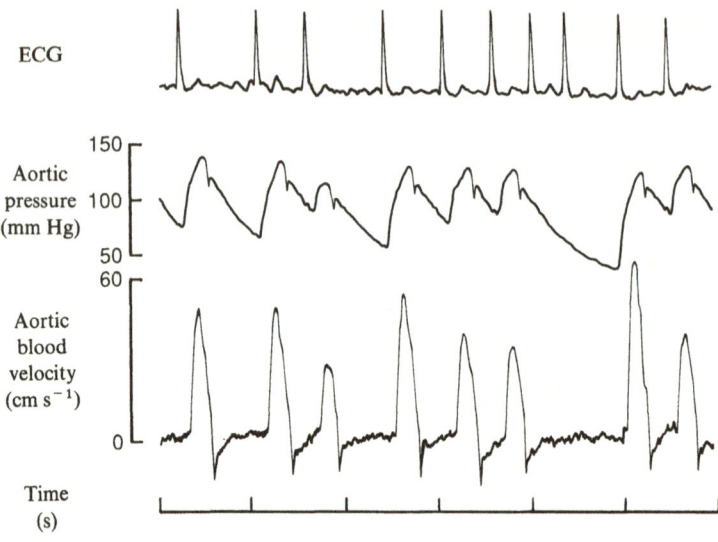

Fig. 13. Atrial fibrillation. Recordings during cardiac catheterisation, showing variations in beat to beat interval and ascending aortic pressure and flow.

followed by a smaller beat than would be expected from the interval alone. This was explained on the basis of fluctuations of aortic pressure.

This paper, which attributed almost all the irregularity of the pulse in atrial fibrillation to haemodynamic causes, was enormously influential. The relationship between amplitude of the ventricular pressure pulse and preceding interval was confirmed in both animals (Wiggers, 1915) and man (Katz & Feil, 1923; Buchbinder & Sugarman, 1940). Later, indirect measurements of human left ventricular volume (Dodge, Kirkham & King, 1957) and direct measurements of left ventricular wall segment length (Braunwald *et al.*, 1960) both showed a relationship between end-diastolic dimension and the pulse pressure of the ensuing beat. Concluding (as had every other study quoted) that this was evidence of the operation of Starling's law, Braunwald and colleagues commented:

The possibility that some other parameter which is the true determinant of ventricular contraction always correlates closely with left ventricular end-diastolic segment length or left ventricular end-diastolic pressure cannot be excluded from these studies. . . .

In defence of this view, it should be pointed out that all these studies were examining ejection function of the ventricle, so that it was natural to seek a length-dependent explanation rather than exploring interval–force possibilities. In addition, the concept of mechanical restitution was a brand new idea at that time, very recently described in animals (Siebens *et al.*, 1959; Lendrum *et al.*, 1960) and never in man. On the other hand, it had been quite explicitly shown that preceding interval *did* correlate closely with end-diastolic volume (Dodge *et al.*, 1957), so that it is difficult to escape the suspicion of a bias in favour of the Frank–Starling mechanism.

It is perfectly possible to argue for either interval–force or length and load related mechanisms in explaining most of these findings. On the one hand, a strong beat might follow a long interval because end-diastolic volume was augmented, or aortic end-diastolic pressure was reduced, or both. Also, the negative effect of the strength of one beat on the next might be due to the levels of ventricular filling and load passed on from the previous weak or strong beat. On the other hand, the beat that follows a long pause might be strong because of mechanical restitution, whereas the tendency for a strong beat to be followed by a weaker one would be consistent with the recirculation process (see section on post-extrasystolic potentiation).

The negative correlation between successive beat strengths merits special mention because it has provoked some misunderstanding. Einthoven & Korteweg (1915), when they described the effect for the first time, thought that weakened ventricular muscle would be particularly sensitive to aortic pressure. Since this would be high after a strong beat, and low after a weak one, a mechanism for alternating beat strength could be established (though it would frequently be masked by the primary influence of beat irregularity on ventricular filling). They suggested that the same mechanism might explain true pulsus alternans.

Lewis (1925) accepted this view, particularly because he had often seen alternans in the closely allied (though regular) rhythm disturbance of rapid atrial flutter. However he followed Gaskell's view (see section on alternans) that the ventricular weakness was an alternating failure of contraction of some fibres. This materially altered the argument, since it implied that contractile alternation was a primary mechanism contributing to the pulse variation of atrial fibrillation.

Subsequent to this, the relationship began to be referred to as alternans, which is unfortunate because the definition of alternans is based on a regular rhythm. However, the possibility that the same underlying mechanism is at work in atrial fibrillation bears inspection. Several authors have shown records of atrial fibrillation with short sequences of alternating pulse pressure (Dodge *et al.*, 1957; Edmands, Greenspan & Fisch, 1970) or, like Einthoven & Korteweg, demonstrated a negative correlation between the force of successive beats statistically (Pfeiffer, Kenner & Schaefer, 1984; Rawles & Rowland, 1986; Rawles, 1988). Often, this pattern of alternation has been attributed to the haemodynamic or inotropic mechanisms postulated to underlie true alternans, but an alternative suggestion (Rawles & Rowland, 1986; Meijler, 1986) is that it follows inevitably from the interaction of two opposing time-dependent processes (mechanical restitution and post-extrasystolic potentiation). Thus each interval has an opposing effect on the first and second subsequent beats, and it is unnecessary to invoke any interaction between the amplitude of the beats themselves. This is, in effect, to say that alternation in atrial fibrillation has nothing to do with the mechanism which underlies true pulsus alternans. Support for this comes from the repeated observation of the phenomenon in patients without any evidence of left ventricular abnormality (Lewis, 1925; Dodge *et al.*, 1957; Rawles & Rowland, 1986). However, since the mechanism of alternans is unclear, it still remains possible that it could make an independent contribution to pulse variation in the abnormal ventricle.

One further characteristic of the pulse variation in atrial fibrillation is difficult to explain in terms of length and load. Most of the studies mentioned above identified a negative correlation between pulse pressure and pre-preceding interval, and described this as an expression of post-extrasystolic potentiation; and the evidence is compelling (see section on post-extrasystolic potentiation) that this is an inotropic process. Thus none of these studies excluded an interval–force contribution (or *proved* the influence of the Frank–Starling effect), and several of them (Einthoven & Korteweg, 1915; Buchbinder & Sugarman, 1940; Dodge *et al.*, 1957) and others subsequently (Greenfield *et al.*, 1968; Päuser, Kenner & Bachmann, 1968; Pfeiffer *et al.*, 1984; Iwase *et al.*, 1989), include plots which show pulse pressure or stroke volume rising with increase of preceding interval in a way which, though usually attributed to the Frank–Starling effect, is consistent with mechanical restitution.

However, evidence in favour of mechanical restitution rather than the Frank–Starling mechanism is limited, particularly in man. Gibson and colleagues (Gibson, Broder & Sowton, 1971) provided some evidence to exclude an important influence of end-diastolic volume in a study of patients after cardiac valve replacement, but an effect of aortic diastolic pressure could not be excluded. In addition, they and Karliner and colleagues (Karliner *et al.*, 1974) observed an inverse relation between ventricular ejection performance of a beat and the duration of the pre-preceding interval – a situation analogous to post-extrasystolic potentiation – which both groups concluded had an inotropic rather than a haemodynamic origin. Greenfield and colleagues (Greenfield *et al.*, 1968) made a similar observation.

There is some evidence from isolated tissue experiments that wholly excludes haemodynamic influences, but it is indirect. In guinea-pig papillary muscle maintained at constant length (Pfeiffer & Kenner, 1983) and in the isolated perfused rat heart maintained at constant load and end-diastolic dimensions (Meijler *et al.*, 1968), sequences of random stimulation with a spectrum of intervals matching those of human atrial fibrillation gave patterns of contractile variation that were very reminiscent of the pulse variation seen in clinical atrial fibrillation whilst being explicable in terms of known interval–force processes. Thus the strength of individual contractions was strongly positively correlated with preceding interval (mechanical restitution) and negatively correlated with pre-preceding intervals (postextrasystolic potentiation).

Two studies in the dog, using measurements independent of ventricular filling, have provided more direct evidence (Rogel & Mahler, 1969; Edmands *et al.*, 1970). In both, wall tension was measured with strain-gauge arches sewn to the ventricular wall and adjusted to slightly stretch the muscle so that diastolic tension remained constant regardless of filling volume. Episodes of atrial fibrillation were then induced by electrical or chemical stimulation of the atria.

In the first study (Rogel & Mahler, 1969) peak isometric tension was plotted against preceding and pre-preceding interval, and provided clear evidence of mechanical restitution and post-extrasystolic potentiation. In the second (Edmands *et al.*, 1970) the rate of rise of tension, which is also a valid contractile index, was examined and compared with beat to beat intervals and aortic and left ventricular pressures. Again, there was evidence for restitution and post-extrasystolic potentiation. In addition, pulse pressure (which is a valid index of stroke volume) was better correlated with maximum rate of rise of tension than with left ventricular end-diastolic pressure or aortic end-diastolic pressure at the start of the beat. This important result indicates that the inotropic state of the muscle attached to the strain gauge (at a length unaffected by ventricular filling and measured at a time before aortic valve opening) was a better predictor of ventricular performance than were the end-diastolic ventricular or aortic pressures.

These experiments demonstrate that interval-dependent inotropic mechanisms can no longer be dismissed as causes of the pulse variation of atrial fibrillation. The topic needs further investigation, particularly in man; atrial fibrillation may yet prove to be a natural demonstration of interval–force mechanisms. Some recent evidence in support of this view can be found in the chapter by Kenner *et al.* in this book.

Summary

The study of interval–force effects in the intact heart poses a difficult experimental problem because of the confounding effects of length and load-dependent mechanisms – particularly the Frank–Starling mechanism. The two main approaches have been either to control ventricular filling and load whilst an interval intervention is applied, or to observe cardiac responses to an interval intervention using an index of contractile behaviour which is to a greater or lesser degree insensitive to ventricular filling and load.

Many human studies have transgressed both these principles, and have yielded ambiguous results consistent with both interval–force and load-dependent interpretations. For historical reasons, the latter have almost always been favoured.

In both animals and man, studies which do allow separation of different effects have systematically confirmed that interval–force properties of isolated muscle are mirrored in the intact heart. Thus:

1. Mechanical restitution of force after a beat occurs, with a contractile response to a second stimulus becoming detectable shortly after the end of the preceding action potential and showing an exponential or near-exponential increase of force to a plateau 0.8–1 second after the previous beat. Behaviour at longer intervals is disputed.
2. The absolute level of force of a beat is determined by the previous contractile history. The influence of interval extends back several beats, the most powerful influence being the pre-preceding interval. If this is short, the beat is potentiated (post-extrasystolic potentiation). Potentiation is more marked after a series of short intervals than after just one (post-stimulation potentiation). The true magnitude of such potentiation is only revealed if it is measured on a fully restituted beat. Frequency potentiation as assessed by the magnitude of the steady state beats (the steady-state staircase) appears to be more modest in the intact heart than it is in isolated muscle. The same is true of post-extrasystolic potentiation.
3. Post-extrasystolic potentiation can be sustained if successive beats are separated by short and long intervals (paired pacing). In the healthy

heart this leads to maintained increases in contractile force, but the effect on cardiac output may be modest, and clinical usefulness is usually limited by increased myocardial oxygen demand.

In the abnormal heart, both restitution and post-extrasystolic potentiation may be modified, although the mechanisms and possible diagnostic usefulness remain largely unexplored. There is also strong evidence that interval–force effects have relevance to pulsus alternans and atrial fibrillation. Pulsus alternans appears to be due to a disturbance of normal cellular contractile control mechanisms, provoked by tachycardia or transient rhythm disturbances. In atrial fibrillation, the variations of interval constantly modulate mechanical restitution and post-extrasystolic potentiation, contributing to the variation in pulse amplitude.

There is a fascinating parallelism in the mammalian heart between basic interval–force effects on cardiac function and Frank–Starling effects. For example, mechanical restitution has a time course similar to diastolic filling of the ventricle; thus in normal regular rhythm, both may contribute to contractile function. Similarly, a premature beat, weak because of limited filling and incomplete restitution, is followed by a beat which is augmented by post-extrasystolic potentiation as well as the carryover of volume from the weak beat. The relative role of the two mechanisms in such situations has rarely been objectively explored; historically, precedence has usually been given to the Frank–Starling mechanism.

Acknowledgements

I am grateful for the help of Professor M. Noble and Dr S. Hardman with the figures in this chapter, which are taken from our own animal and human studies.

References

Anderson, P. A. W., Manring, A. & Johnson, E. A. (1977). The force of contraction of isolated papillary muscle: a study of the interaction of its determining factors. *Journal of Molecular and Cellular Cardiology*, **9**, 131–50.

Anderson, P. A. W., Manring, A., Serwer, G. A., Benson, D. W., Edwards, S. B., Armstrong, B. E., Sterba, R. J. & Floyd, R. D. (1979). The force–interval relationship of the left ventricle. *Circulation*, **60**, 334–48.

Anderson, P. A. W., Rankin, J. S., Arentzen, C. E., Anderson, R. W. & Johnson, E. A. (1976). Evaluation of the force–frequency relationship as a descriptor of the inotropic state of canine left ventricular myocardium. *Circulation Research*, **39**, 832–9.

Arentzen, C. E., Rankin, J. S., Anderson, P. A. W., Feezor, M. D. & Anderson, R. W. (1978). Force–frequency characteristics of the left ventricle in the conscious dog. *Circulation Research*, **42**, 64–71.

Badeer, H. S., Ryo, U. H., Gassner, W. F. *et al.* (1967). Factors affecting pulsus alternans in the rapidly driven heart and papillary muscle. *American Journal of Physiology*, **213**, 1095–101.

Beck, W., Chesler, E. & Schrire, V. (1971). Postextrasystolic ventricular pressure responses. *Circulation*, **44**, 523–33.

Boden, W. E., Liang, C. & Hood, W. B. (1980). Postextrasystolic potentiation of regional mechanical performance during prolonged myocardial ischemia in the dog. *Circulation*, **61**, 1063–70.

Boerth, R. C., Covell, J. W., Pool, P. E. & Ross, J., Jr. (1969). Increased myocardial oxygen consumption and contractile state associated with increased heart rate in dogs. *Circulation Research*, **24**, 725–34.

Bowditch, H. P. (1871). Über die Eigenthümlichkeiten der Reizbarkeit, welche die Muskelfasern des Herzens zeigen. *Berichte der Königlich-Sächsische Gesellschaft der Wissenschaften*, **23**, 652–89.

Braunwald, E., Frye, R. L., Aygen, M. M. & Gilbert, J. W. Jr. (1960). Studies on Starling's law of the heart. III. Observations in patients with mitral stenosis and atrial fibrillation on the relationships between end-diastolic segment length, filling pressure, and the characteristics of ventricular contraction. *Journal of Clinical Investigation*, **39**, 1874–84.

Braunwald, E. & Ross, J., Jr. (1979). Control of cardiac performance. In *Handbook of Physiology*, Section 2, vol. I. Chap. 15, pp. 533–580, ed. R. Berne & N. Sperelakis. Bethesda: American Physiological Society.

Braunwald, E., Ross, J. Jr., Frommer, P. L., Williams, J. F., Sonnenblick, E. H. & Gault, J. H. (1964). Clinical observations on paired electrical stimulation of the heart. *American Journal of Medicine*, **37**, 700–11.

Braunwald, E., Ross, J. Jr., Sonnenblick, E. H., Frommer, P. L., Braunwald, N. S. & Morrow, A. G. (1965). Slowing of heart rate, electroaugmentation of ventricular performance, and increase of myocardial oxygen consumption produced by paired electrical stimulation. *Bulletin of the New York Academy of Medicine*, **41**, 481–97.

Braunwald, E., Sonnenblick, E. H., Frommer, P. L. & Ross, J. Jr. (1967). Paired electrical stimulation of the heart: physiologic observations and clinical implications. *Advances in Internal Medicine*, **13**, 61–96.

Buchbinder, W. C. & Sugarman, H. (1940). Arterial blood pressure in cases of atrial fibrillation, measured directly. *Archives of Internal Medicine*, **66**, 625–42.

Buckley, N. M., Penefsky, Z. J. & Litwak, R. S. (1972). Comparative force–frequency relationships in human and other mammalian ventricular myocardium. *Pfügers Archiv*, **332**, 259–70.

Burkhoff, D., Yue, D. T., Franz, M. R., Hunter, W. C. & Sagawa, K. (1984). Mechanical restitution of isolated perfused canine left ventricles. *American Journal of Physiology*, **246**, H8–16.

Cohn, K. E., Sandler, H. & Hancock, E. W. (1967). Mechanisms of pulsus alternans. *Circulation*, **36**, 372–80.

Cohn, P. F., Gorlin, R., Herman, M. W. *et al.* (1975). Relation between contractile reserve and prognosis in patients with coronary artery disease and a depressed ejection fraction. *Circulation*, **51**, 414–20.

Cooper, M. W., Lutherer, L. O. & Lust, R. M. (1982). Postextrasystolic potentiation and echocardiography. *Circulation*, **66**, 771–6.

Cooper, M. W., Lutherer, L. O., Stanton, M. W. & Lust, R. M. Jr. (1986).

Postextrasystolic potentiation: analysis of methods of induction. *American Heart Journal*, **111**, 330–3.

Cooper, T., Braunwald, E. & Morrow, A. G. (1958). Pulsus alternans in aortic stenosis. *Circulation*, **18**, 64–70.

Cornish, A. L., Hanley, H. G., Patrick, T. A., Cole, J. S. & O'Connor, W. (1981). Failure of postextrasystolic potentiation to identify viable, but ischaemic myocardium. *American Journal of Physiology*, **241**, H654–61.

Covell, J. W., Ross, J. Jr., Taylor, R., Sonnenblick, E. H. & Braunwald, E. (1967). Effects of increasing frequency of contraction on the force velocity relation of left ventricle. *Cardiovascular Research*, **1**, 2–8.

Cranefield, P. F. (1965). Paired pulse stimulation and postextrasystolic potentiation in the heart. *Progress in Cardiovascular Diseases*, **8**, 446–60.

Crozatier, B. (1982). Relations between myocardial blood flow and postextrasystolic potentiation in epicardial and endocardial left ventricular regions early after coronary occlusion in dogs. *Circulation*, **66**, 938–44.

Crozatier, B., Caillet, D., Jouannot, P. & Hatt, P. Y. (1979). Pulsus alternans in regionally hypoxic ventricles of open chest dogs: regional mechanical alternation of potentiation and attenuation of the inotropic state. *Basic Research in Cardiology*, **74**, 639–48.

Crozatier, B., Franklin, D., Theroux, P., Tomoike, H., Sasayama, S. & Ross, J., Jr. (1977). Loss of regional ventricular postextrasystolic potentiation after coronary occlusion in dogs. *American Journal of Physiology*, **233**, H392–8.

Davidson, D. M., Covell, J. W., Malloch, C. I. & Ross, J., Jr. (1974). Factors influencing indices of left ventricle contractility in the conscious dog. *Cardiovascular Research*, **8**, 299–312.

Dodge, H. T., Kirkham, F. T. Jr. & King, C. V. (1957). Ventricular dynamics in atrial fibrillation. *Circulation*, **15**, 335–47.

Drake-Holland, A. J., Mills, C. J., Noble, M. I. M. & Pugh, S. (1990). Responses to changes in filling and contractility of indices of human left ventricular mechanical performance. *Journal of Physiology*, **422**, 29–39.

Drake-Holland, A. J., Noble, M. I. M., Pieterse, M. *et al.* (1983). Cardiac action potential duration and contractility in the intact dog heart. *Journal of Physiology*, **345**, 75–85.

Dyke, S. H., Urschel, C. W., Sonnenblick, E. H., Gorlin, R. & Cohn, P. F. (1975). Detection of latent function in acutely ischemic myocardium in the dog. *Circulation Research*, **36**, 490–7.

Edmands, R. E., Greenspan, K. & Fisch, C. (1970). The role of inotropic variation in ventricular function during atrial fibrillation. *Journal of Clinical Investigation*, **49**, 738–46.

Einthoven, W. & Korteweg, A. J. (1915). On the variability of the size of the pulse in cases of auricular fibrillation. *Heart*, **6**, 107–20.

Elzinga, G., Lab, M. J., Noble, M. I. M., Papadoyannis, D. E., Pidgeon, J., Seed, W. A. & Wohlfart, B. (1981). The action-potential duration and contractile response of the intact heart related to the preceding interval and the preceding beat in the dog and cat. *Journal of Physiology*, **314**, 481–500.

Elzinga, G. & Westerhof, N. (1976). The pumping ability of the left heart and the effect of coronary occlusion. *Circulation Research*, **38**, 297–302.

Elzinga, G. & Westerhof, N. (1978). The effect of an increase in inotropic state and end-diastolic volume on the pumping ability of the feline left heart. *Circulation Research*, **42**, 620–8.

Ferrer, M. I., Harvey, R. M., Cournard, A. & Richards, D. W. (1956). Cardiocirculatory studies in pulsus alternans of the systemic and pulmonary circulations. *Circulation*, **14**, 163–74.

Fisher, V. J., Lee, R. J., Marlon, A. M. & Kavaler, F. (1967). Paired electrical stimulation and the maximum contractile response of the ventricle. *Circulation Research*, **20**, 520–33.

Frank, O. (1895). Zur Dynamik des Herzmuskels. Zeitschrift für Biologie, **32**, 370–447. Translated by: Chapman C. B., Wasserman E. On the dynamics of heart muscle. *American Heart Journal*, 1959; **58**, 282–317, 467–78.

Freeman, G. L., Little, W. C. & O'Rourke, R. A. (1987). Influence of heart rate on left ventricular performance in conscious dogs. *Circulation Research*, **61**, 455–64.

Friedman, B., Daily, W. M. & Sheffield, R. S. (1953). Orthostatic factors in pulsus alternans. *Circulation*, **8**, 864–73.

Fry, C. H., Walker, J. M., Webb-Peploe, M. M. & Williams, B. T. (1983). Restitution of contractility *in vitro* of human and guinea-pig ventricular myocardium. *Journal of Physiology*, **339**, 26–27P.

Furnival, C. M., Linden, R. J. & Snow, H. M. (1970). Inotropic changes in the left ventricle: the effect of changes in heart rate, aortic pressure, and end-diastolic pressure. *Journal of Physiology*, **211**, 359–87.

Gaskell, W. (1882). On the rhythm of the heart of the frog, and on the nature of the action of the vagus nerve. *Philosophical Transactions of the Royal Society, London, series B*, **173**, 993–1034.

Gennser, G., Jóhannsson, M. & Nilsson, E. (1972). The influence of contraction frequency and of a local anaesthetic (mepivacaine) on human fetal myocardium. *Acta Physiologica Scandinavica*, **85**, 559–68.

Gibson, D. G., Broder, G. & Sowton, E. (1971). Effect of varying pulse interval in atrial fibrillation on left ventricular function in man. *British Heart Journal*, **33**, 388–93.

Gibson, D. G., Fleck, E. & Rudolph, W. (1983). Effect of postextrasystolic potentiation on amplitude and timing of regional left ventricular wall motion in ischaemic heart disease. *British Heart Journal*, **49**, 466–76.

Gilbert, J. L., Janse, M. J., Lu, H. H., Pinkston, J. O. & Brooks, C. McC. (1965). Production and abolition of alternation in mechanical action of the ventricle. *American Journal of Physiology*, **209**, 945–50.

Gleason, W. L. & Braunwald, E. (1962a). Studies on the first derivative of the ventricular pressure pulse in man. *Journal of Clinical Investigation*, **41**, 80–91.

Gleason, W. L. & Braunwald, E. (1962b). Studies on Starling's law of the heart: IV Relation between left ventricular end-diastolic volume and stroke volume in man, with observation on the mechanism of pulsus alternans. *Circulation*, **25**, 841–8.

Goodyer, A. V. N. & Wong, B. Y. S. (1977). Physiologic determinants of left ventricular strength–interval curve of the dog. *American Journal of Physiology*, **233**, H555–61.

Green, H. D. (1935–36). The nature of ventricular alternation resulting from reduced coronary blood flow. *American Journal of Physiology*, **114**, 407–13.

Greenfield, J. C. Jr., Harley, A., Thompson, H. K. & Wallace, A. G. (1968). Pressure-flow studies in man during atrial fibrillation. *Journal of Clinical Investigation*, **47**, 2411–21.

Grossman, W., Haynes, F., Paraskos, J. A., Saltz, S., Dalen, J. E. & Dexter, L. (1972). Alterations in preload and myocardial mechanics in the dog and in man. *Circulation Research*, **31**, 83–94.

Guntheroth, W. G., Morgan, B. C., McGough, G. A. & Scher, A. M. (1969). Alternate deletion and potentiation as the causes of pulsus alternans. *American Heart Journal*, **78**, 669–81.

Gwathmey, J. K., Slawsky, M. T., Hajjar, R. J., Briggs, G. M. & Morgan, J. P. (1990). Role of intracellular calcium handling in force–interval relationships of human ventricular myocardium. *Journal of Clinical Investigation*, **85**, 1599–613.

Hada, Y., Wolfe, C. & Craige, E. (1982). Pulsus alternans determined by biventricular simultaneous systolic time intervals. *Circulation*, **65**, 617–26.

Hamby, R. I., Aintablian, A., Wisoff, G. & Hartstein, M. L. (1975). Response of the left ventricle in coronary artery disease to postextrasystolic potentiation. *Circulation*, **51**, 428–35.

Hamilton, W. F. & Remington, J. W. (1947). The measurement of the stroke volume from the pressure pulse. *American Journal of Physiology*, **148**, 14–24.

Harris, L. C., Nghiem, Q. X., Schreiber, M. H. & Wallace, J. M. (1966). Severe pulsus alternans associated with primary myocardial disease in children. *Circulation*, **34**, 948–61.

Hess, O. M., Surber, E. P., Ritter, M. & Krayenbuehl, H. P. (1984). Pulsus alternans: its influence on systolic and diastolic function in aortic valve disease. *Journal of the American College of Cardiology*, **4**, 1–7.

Higgins, C. B., Vatner, S. F., Franklin, D. & Braunwald, E. (1973). Extent of regulation of the heart's contractile state in the conscious dog by alteration in the frequency of contraction. *Journal of Clinical Investigation*, **52**, 1187–94.

Hoffman, B. F., Bartelston, H. J., Scherlag, B. J. & Cranefield, P. F. (1965). Effects of postextrasystolic potentiation in normal and failing hearts. *Bulletin of the New York Academy of Medicine*, **41**, 498–534.

Ingels, N. B. Jr., Ricci, D. R., Daughters, G. T., Alderman, E. L. & Stinson, E. B. (1977). Effects of heart rate augmentation on left ventricular volumes and cardiac output of the transplanted human heart. *Circulation*, **56** (suppl 2), 1132–7.

Iwase, M., Aoki, T., Maeda, M., Yokota, M. & Hayashi, H. (1989). Relationship between beat to beat interval and left ventricular function in patients with atrial fibrillaton. *International Journal of Cardiac Imaging*, **3**, 217–26.

Kahn, M. L., Kavaler, F. & Fisher, V. J. (1976). Frequency–force relationships of mammalian ventricular muscle *in vivo* and *in vitro*. *American Journal of Physiology*, **230**, 631–6.

Karliner, J. S., Gault, J. H., Bouchard, R. & Holzer, J. (1974). Factors influencing the ejection fraction and the mean rate of circumferential fibre shortening during atrial fibrillation in man. *Cardiovascular Research*, **8**, 18–25.

Kass, D. A., Maughan, W. L., Guo, M., Kono, A., Sunagawa, A. & Sagawa, K. (1987). Comparative influence of load versus inotropic state on indices of ventricular contractility: experimental and theoretical analysis based on pressure–volume relationships. *Circulation*, **76**, 1422–36.

Katus, H., Mehmel, H. C., von Olshausen, K., Stockins, B. & Kübler W. (1980). Influence of timing of the extrasystolic beat on the extent of postextrasystolic potentiation in the intact human left ventricle. *Basic Research in Cardiology*, **75**, 657–67.

Katz, L. N. & Feil, H. S. (1923). Clinical observations on the dynamics of ventricular systole. I. Auricular fibrillation. *Archives of Internal Medicine*, **32**, 672–80.

Kavaler, F., Harris, R. S., Lee, R. J. & Fisher, V. J. (1971). Frequency–force behavior of *in situ* ventricular myocardium in the dog. *Circulation Research*, **28**, 533–44.

King, A. J. & Taylor, D. E. M. (1968). The inotropic action of paired pulse stimulation in the normal and failing heart. An experimental study. *Cardiovascular Research*, **2**, 122–9.

Klausner, S. C., Ratshin, R. A., Tyberg, J. V., Lappin, H. A., Chatterjee, K. & Parmley, W. W. (1976). The similarity of changes in segmental contraction patterns induced by postextrasystolic potentiation and nitroglycerin. *Circulation*, **54**, 615–23.

Koch-Weser, J. & Blinks, J. R. (1963). The influence of the interval between beats on myocardial contractility. *Pharmacological Reviews*, **15**, 601–52.

Kuijer, P. J. P., Heethaar, R. M., Herbschleb, J. N., Zimmerman, A. N. E. & Meijler, F. L. (1978). Postextrasystolic potentiation in the dog heart. *European Journal of Cardiology*, **7** (suppl.), 133–45.

Kuijer, P. J. P., van der Werf, T. & Meijler, F. L. (1990). Post-extrasystolic potentiation without a compensatory pause in normal and diseased hearts. *British Heart Journal*, **63**, 284–6.

Kvasnicka, J., Liander, B., Broman, H. & Varnauskas, E. (1975). Quantitative evaluation of postectopic beats in the normal and failing human heart using indices derived from catheter-tip manometer readings. *Cardiovascular Research*, **9**, 336–41.

Lendrum, B., Feinberg, H., Boyd, E. & Katz, L. N. (1960). Rhythm effects on contractility of the beating isovolumic left ventricle. *American Journal of Physiology*, **199**, 1115–20.

Lew, W. Y. W. (1988). Time-dependent increase in left ventricular contractility following acute volume loading in the dog. *Circulation Research*, **63**, 635–47.

Lewis, T. (1912). Fibrillation of the auricles: its effect upon the circulation. *Journal of Experimental Medicine*, **16**, 395–420.

Lewis, T. (1925). *The Mechanism and Graphic Registration of the Heart Beat.* Chicago: Chicago Medical Book Co.

Lewis, B. S., Lewis, N. & Gotsman, M. S. (1975). Effect of postural changes on pulsus alternans. *Chest*, **75**, 634–6.

Little, W. C. (1985). The left ventricular dP/dt_{max}-end-diastolic volume relation in closed-chest dogs. *Circulation Research*, **56**, 808–15.

Liu, C. K. & Luisada, A. A. (1955). Halving of the pulse due to severe alternans (pulsus bisectus). *American Heart Journal*, **50**, 927–33.

Lu, H.-H., Lange, G. & Brooks, C. McC. (1968). Comparative studies of electrical and mechanical alternans in heart cells. *Journal of Electrocardiology*, **1**, 7–17.

Lust, R. M. Jr., Lutherer, L. O., Gardner, M. & Cooper, M. W. (1982). Postextrasystolic potentiation and contractile reserve: requirements and restrictions. *American Journal of Physiology*, **243**, H990–7.

Mahler, F., Ross, J. Jr., O'Rourke, R. J. & Covell, J. W. (1975). Effects of changes in preload, afterload, and inotropic state on ejection and isovolumic phase measures of contractility in the conscious dog. *American Journal of Cardiology*, **35**, 626–34.

Mahler, F., Yoran, C. & Ross, J. (1974). Inotropic effect of tachycardia and post-stimulation potentiation in the conscious dog. *American Journal of Physiology*, **227**, 569–75.

Mahler, Y. & Rogel, S. (1970). Interrelation between restitution time-constant and alternating myocardial contractility in dogs. *Clinical Science*, **39**, 625–39.

Markis, J. E., Cohn, P. F., Roberts, B. H., Skelton, C. L. & Sonnenblick, E. H. (1976). Effect of varying the coupling interval on post extrasystolic potentiation. [Abstract]. *Clinical Research*, **24**, 229A.

Mason, D. T. (1969). Usefulness and limitations of the rate of rise of intraventricular pressure (dP/dt_{max}) for the evaluation of myocardial contractility. *American Journal of Cardiology*, **23**, 516–27.

Maughan, W. L., Sunagawa, K., Burkhoff, D., Graves, W. L., Hunter, W. C. & Sagawa, K. (1985). Effect of heart rate on the canine end-systolic pressure-volume relationship. *Circulation*, **72**, 654–9.

Meijler, F. L. (1986). The pulse in atrial fibrillation. *British Heart Journal*, **56**, 1–3.

Meijler, F. L., Strackee, J., van Capelle, F. J. L. & du Perron, J. C. (1968). Computer analysis of the RR interval–contractility relationship during random stimulation of the isolated heart. *Circulation Research*, **22**, 695–702.

Miller, W. P., Liedtke, A. J. & Nellis, S. H. (1986). End-systolic pressure–diameter relationships during pulsus alternans in intact pig hearts. *American Journal of Physiology*, **250**, H606–11.

Mitchell, J. H., Sarnoff, S. J. & Sonnenblick, E. H. (1963). The dynamics of pulsus alternans: alternating end-diastolic fibre length as a causative factor. *Journal of Clinical Investigation*, **42**, 55–63.

Mitchell, J. H., Wallace, A. G. & Skinner, N. S. (1963). Intrinsic effects of heart rate on left ventricular performance. *American Journal of Physiology*, **205**, 41–8.

Monroe, R. G. & French, G. N. (1961). Left ventricular pressure–volume relationships and myocardial oxygen consumption in the isolated heart. *Circulation Research*, **9**, 362–74.

Nayler, W. G. & Robertson, P. G. C. (1965). Mechanical alternans and the staircase phenomenon in dog papillary muscle. *American Heart Journal*, **70**, 494–8.

Noble, M. I. M., Trenchard, D. & Guz, A. (1966). Left ventricular ejection in conscious dogs: II. Determinants of stroke volume. *Circulation Research*, **19**, 148–52.

Noble, M. I. M., Wyler, J., Milne, E. N. C., Trenchard, D. & Guz, A. (1969). Effect of changes in heart rate on left ventricular performance in conscious dogs. *Circulation Research*, **24**, 285–95.

Noble, R. J. & Nutter, D. O. (1970). The demonstration of alternating contractile state in pulsus alternans. *Journal of Clinical Investigation*, **49**, 1166–77.

O'Brien, K. P., Higgs, L. M., Glancy, D. L. & Epstein, S. E. (1969). Hemodynamic accompaniments of angina. *Circulation*, **39**, 735–43.

Parmley, W. W., Tomoda, H., Fujimura, S. & Matloff, J. M. (1972). Relation between pulsus alternans and transient occlusion of the left anterior descending coronary artery. *Cardiovascular Research*, **6**, 709–15.

Patterson, R. E., Kent, B. B. & Peirce, E. C. II. (1972). A comparison of empiric contractile indices in intact dogs. *Cardiology*, **57**, 277–94.

Patterson, S. W., Piper, H. & Starling, E. H. (1914). The regulation of the heart beat. *Journal of Physiology*, **48**, 465–513.

Päuser, P., Kenner, T. & Bachmann, K. (1968). Beurteilung des Verhaltens der Gleichgewichtskurven des menschlichen Herzens auf Grund arterieller Druckpulse. *Zeitschrift für Kreislaufforschung*, **57**, 1049–60.

Penefsky, Z. J. & Buckley, N. M. (1974). Effects of low sodium on myocardium of human and other species. In: *Myocardial Biology: Recent Advances in*

Studies on Cardiac Structure and Metabolism, vol. 4, ed. N. Dhalla, pp. 31–39. Baltimore MD: University Park Press.

Pfeiffer, K. P. & Kenner, T. (1983). A statistical approach to the analysis of phenomena of frequency potentiation of isolated myocardial strips. *Basic Research in Cardiology*, **78**, 239–55.

Pfeiffer, K. P., Kenner, T. & Schaefer, J. (1984). Application of statistical methods for the analysis of interval related cardiac performance variations during cardiac arrhythmia in man. *Cardiovascular Research*, **18**, 80–98.

Pidgeon, J., Lab, M., Seed, W. A., Elzinga, G., Papadoyannis, D. & Noble, M. I. M. (1980). The contractile state of cat and dog heart in relation to the interval between beats. *Circulation Research*, **47**, 559–67.

Pidgeon, J., Miller, G. A. H., Noble, M. I. M., Papadoyannis, D. & Seed, W. A. (1982). The relationship between the strength of the human heart beat and the interval between beats. *Circulation*, **65**, 1404–10.

Popio, K. A., Gorlin, R., Bechtel, D. & Levine, J. A. (1977). Postextrasystolic potentiation as a predictor of potential myocardial viability: preoperative analyses compared with studies after coronary bypass surgery. *American Journal of Cardiology*, **39**, 944–53.

Pouleur, H., Rousseau, M. F., Petein, M., Van Mechelen, H. & Charlier, A. A. (1983). Effects of chronic volume overload on left ventricular response to tachycardia. *American Journal of Physiology*, **245**, H218–28.

Powers, E. R., Foster, J. R. & Powell, W. J. Jr. (1976). Interaction of interval–force relationship with aortic pressure and stroke volume. *American Journal of Physiology*, **230**, 893–900.

Quinones, M. A., Gaasch, W. H. & Alexander, J. K. (1976). Influence of acute changes in preload, afterload, contractile state and heart rate on ejection and isovolumic indices of myocardial contractility in man. *Circulation*, **53**, 293–302.

Rawles, J. M. (1988). A mathematical model of left ventricular function in atrial fibrillation. *International Journal of Biomedical Computing*, **23**, 56–68.

Rawles, J. M. & Rowland, E. (1986). Is the pulse in atrial fibrillation irregularly irregular? *British Heart Journal*, **56**, 4–11.

Reeves, T. J., Hefner, L. L., Jones, W. B., Coghlan, C., Prieto, G. & Carroll, J. (1960). The hemodynamic determinants of the rate of change of pressure in the left ventricle during isometric contraction. *American Heart Journal*, **60**, 745–61.

Rogel, S. & Mahler, Y. (1969). Myocardial tension in atrial fibrillation. *Journal of Applied Physiology*, **27**, 822–5.

Ross, J. Jr., Sonnenblick, E. H., Kaiser, G. A., Frommer, P. L. & Braunwald, E. (1965). Electroaugmentation of ventricular performance and oxygen consumption by repetitive application of paired electrical stimuli. *Circulation Research*, **16**, 332–42.

Ryan, J. M., Schieve, J. F., Hull, H. B. & Oser, B. M. (1956). Experiences with pulsus alternans. Ventricular alternation and the stage of heart failure. *Circulation*, **14**, 1099–103.

Sagawa, K. (1981). The end-systolic pressure–volume relation of the ventricle: definition, modifications and clinical use. *Circulation*, **63**, 1223–7.

Sagawa, K., Suga, H., Shoukas, A. A. & Bakalar, K. M. (1977). End-systolic pressure/volume ratio: a new index of ventricular contractility. *American Journal of Cardiology*, **40**, 748–53.

Sanghvi, V. R., Khaja, F., Mark, A. L. & Parker, J. O. (1972). Effects of blood volume expansion on left ventricular hemodynamics in man. *Circulation*, **46**, 780–7.

Saunders, D. E. & Ord, J. W. (1962). The hemodynamic effects of paroxysmal supraventricular tachycardia in patients with the Wolff–Parkinson–White syndrome. *American Journal of Cardiology*, **9**, 223–36.

Schaefer, J., Reichel, H., Schwarzkopf, H. J., Rumberger, E., Nordmann, K. J., Sedlmeyer, I. & Bleichert, A. (1971). Untersuchungen zur Kraft-Frequenz-Beziehung des menschlichen Herzens. *Verhandlung Deutschen Gesellschaft Kreislaufforschung*, **37**, 356–9.

Schaper, W. K. A., Lewi, P. & Jageneau, A. H. M. (1965). The determinants of the rate of change of the left ventricular pressure (dp/dt). *Archiv für Kreislaufforschung*, **46**, 27–41.

Schmidt, H. D. & Hoppe, H. (1978). Preload dependence of dP/dt_{max}, $V_{CE_{max}}$ and calculated V_{max} compared to the inotropic sensitivity of these indices of cardiac contractility. *Basic Research in Cardiology*, **73**, 380–93.

Schwarz, F., Thormann, J. & Winkler, B. (1975). Frequency potentiation and postextrasystolic potentiation in patients with and without coronary arterial disease. *British Heart Journal*, **37**, 514–19.

Seed, W. A., Noble, M. I. M., Walker, J. M., Miller, G. A. H., Pidgeon, J., Redwood, D., Wanless, R., Franz, M. R., Schoettler, M. & Schaefer, J. (1984). Relationships between beat-to-beat interval and the strength of contraction in the healthy and diseased human heart. *Circulation*, **70**, 799–805.

Serur, J. R. & Urschel, C. W. (1973). Attenuation of inotropic interventions by myocardial ischaemia. *Cardiovascular Research*, **7**, 458–63.

Siebens, A. A., Hoffman, B. F., Cranefield, P. F. & Brooks, C. McC. (1959). Regulation of contractile force during ventricular arrhythmias. *American Journal of Physiology*, **197**, 971–7.

Sonnenblick, E. H., Braunwald, E. & Morrow, A. G. (1965). Contractile properties of human heart muscle: studies on myocardial mechanics of surgically excised papillary muscles. *Journal of Clinical Investigation*, **44**, 966–77.

Sonnenblick, E. H., Morrow, A. G. & Williams, J. F. (1966). Effects of heart rate on the dynamics of force development in the intact human ventricle. *Circulation*, **33**, 945–51.

Spear, J. F. & Moore, E. N. (1971). A comparison of alternation in myocardial action potentials and contractility. *American Journal of Physiology*, **220**, 1708–16.

Spodick, D. H., Khan, A. H. & Quarry, V. M. (1974). Systolic and diastolic time intervals in pulsus alternans. *American Heart Journal*, **87**, 5–10.

Starr, I., Schnabel, T. G. Jr., Askovitz, S. I. & Schild, A. (1954). On the relation between pulse pressure and cardiac stroke volume, leading to a clinical method of estimating cardiac output from blood pressure and age. *Circulation*, **9**, 648–63.

Sung, C.-S., Mathur, V. S., Garcia, E., de Castro, C. M. & Hall, R. J. (1980). Is postextrasystolic potentiation dependent on Starling's law? *Circulation*, **62**, 1032–5.

Swanton, R. H., Jenkins, B. S., Brooksby, I. A. B. & Webb-Peploe, M. M. (1976). An analysis of pulsus alternans in aortic stenosis. *European Journal of Cardiology*, **4**, 39–47.

Symposium on paired pulse stimulation and postextrasystolic potentiation in the heart. (1965). *Bulletin of the New York Academy of Medicine*, **41**, 417–47.

Traube, L. (1872). Ein Fall von Pulsus Bigeminus nebst Bemerkungen über die Leberschwellungen bei Klappenfehlern und über acute Leberatrophie. *Berliner Klinische Wochenschrift*, **9**, 185–8.

van den Bos, G. C., Elzinga, G., Westerhof, N. & Noble, M. I. M. (1973). Problems in the use of indices of myocardial contractility. *Cardiovascular Research*, **7**, 834–48.

van der Werf, T., van Poelgeest, R., Herbschleb, H. H. & Meijler, F. L. (1976). Postextrasystolic potentiation in man. *European Journal of Cardiology*, **4** (suppl.), 131–41.

Walker, J. M. (1984). The contractility of human and guinea-pig ventricular myocardium *in vitro*. MD thesis, University of Birmingham, UK.

Walker, J. M., Seed, W. A., Noble, M. I. M., Lincoln, J. R. C., Williams, B. T. & Oldershaw, P. J. (1984). Force interval relationships in the human heart studied *in vivo* and *in vitro* [Abstract]. *Clinical Science*, **67**, 30P.

Wallace, A. G., Skinner, N. S. & Mitchell, J. H. (1963). Hemodynamic determinants of the maximal rate of rise of left ventricular pressure. *American Journal of Physiology*, **205**, 30–6.

Weber, K. T. & Janicki, J. S. (1978). Interdependence of cardiac function, coronary flow, and oxygen extraction. *American Journal of Physiology*, **235**, H784–93.

Wenckebach, K. F. (1902). Zur Analyse des unregelmassingen Pulses: IV. Über den Pulsus Alternans. *Zeitschrift für Klinische Medizin*, **44**, 218–25.

White, P. D. (1915). Alternation of the pulse: a common clinical condition. *American Journal of Medical Science*, **150**, 82–97.

Wier, W. G. & Yue, D. (1986). Intracellular calcium transients underlying the short-term force–interval relationship in ferret ventricular myocardium. *Journal of Physiology*, **376**, 507–30.

Wiggers, C. J. (1915). Studies on the pathological physiology of the heart. I. The intra-auricular, intra-ventricular, and aortic pressure curves in auricular fibrillations. *Archives of Internal Medicine*, **15**, 77–91.

Wiggers, C. J. (1927). The dynamics of ventricular alternation. *Annals of Clinical Medicine*, **5**, 1022–7.

Wildenthal, K., Mierzwiak, D. S. & Mitchell, J. H. (1969). Effect of sudden changes in aortic pressure on left ventricular dp/dt. *American Journal of Physiology*, **216**, 185–90.

Wohlfart, B. (1979). Relationships between peak force, action potential duration and stimulus interval in rabbit myocardium. *Acta Physiologica Scandinavica*, **106**, 395–409.

Wohlfart, B. (1982). Analysis of mechanical alternans in rabbit papillary muscle. *Acta Physiologica Scandinavica*, **115**, 405–14.

Wohlfart, B. & Elzinga, G. (1982). Electrical and mechanical responses of the intact rabbit heart in relation to the excitation interval. *Acta Physiologica Scandinavica*, **115**, 331–40.

Woodworth, R. S. (1902). Maximal contraction, 'staircase' contraction, refractory period, and compensatory pause of the heart. *American Journal of Physiology*, **8**, 213–49.

Yellin, E. L., Kennish, A., Yoran, C., Laniado, S., Buckley, N. M. & Frater, R. W. M. (1979). The influence of left ventricular filling on postextrasystolic potentiation in the dog heart. *Circulation Research*, **44**, 712–22.

Yue, D. T., Burkhoff, D., Franz, M. R., Hunter, W. C. & Sagawa, K. (1985). Postextrasystolic potentiation of the isolated canine left ventricle: relationship to mechanical restitution. *Circulation Research*, **56**, 340–50.

Author index

Subject index

For EU product safety concerns, contact us at Calle de José Abascal, 56–1°,
28003 Madrid, Spain or eugpsr@cambridge.org.

www.ingramcontent.com/pod-product-compliance
Ingram Content Group UK Ltd.
Pitfield, Milton Keynes, MK11 3LW, UK
UKHW010853090126
466816UK00011B/209